BEYOND LABELS

A Doctor and a Farmer Conquer Food Confusion One Bite at a Time

By

Sina McCullough, PhD

and

Joel Salatin, Farmer

ISBN: 978-1-7336866-0-0
Library of Congress Control Number: 2020902787

Edited by Janet Smith, Owen Finnegan and Donald McCullough III
Cover Design © Bonnie Watson. All rights reserved.
Author photo (Sina McCullough) by Julie Massie © www.juliemassie.com All rights reserved.
Author photo (Joel Salatin) by Rachel Salatin. All rights reserved.
Desktop Publishing by Jennifer Dehoff Design.

This book is dedicated to anyone who wants to eat better
and doesn't know how.
You are not alone and there is a solution.

Praise for Beyond Labels

Most folks know there's something wrong with our food. And this book proves it unequivocally. But it doesn't stop there. It offers dozens of proven, practical ways to beat a system that seems rigged against us. The ideas, evidence and takeaways from this book have the power to reshape America's declining health. This is the most-fascinating, scariest and flat out most-useful book I've ever read. Joel and Sina have done what no other authors have managed to do. They've created a survival guide for the war on our gut microbiome.

-Andy Snyder, Founder of Manward Press

In their groundbreaking book, *Beyond Labels*, Dr. Sina McCullough and Joel Salatin offer a thought-provoking network of strategies to take charge of our health and well-being through food choices adapted to individuals. You get to build your own pathway. You won't find the magic bullet or any prescribed, mindless fad diets here, rather a complete atlas-makers toolkit for drawing custom pathways to the modern Mecca of good health through a diversity of whole foods. This book should be on the shelves of all eaters.

-Hank Will, Editor At Large, Mother Earth News & Food Farmer at Prairie Turnip Farm

Beyond Labels is the best possible investment you can make to guide you on your way toward optimal health. Don't expect a book that will lecture you or make you feel badly about your current eating habits. Joel and Sina offer budget-friendly tips and break down the choices into easily manageable changes that anyone can make. You won't be overwhelmed by confusing technical jargon or grim warnings that you're going to die if you don't throw away everything in your kitchen right this very moment. Instead, you'll be warmly encouraged to nurture and heal yourself with high-quality food.

-Daisy Luther, Founder of Luther Inc. & TheOrganicPrepper.com

The labels we put on ourselves as eaters are as mired in dogma and misinformation as the labels on our packaged food: paleo, vegan, keto, pescatarian and beyond. *Beyond Labels* makes the complex simple, but more importantly, it is an opportunity for our unity and reconnection to the land, our communities, and our humanity through real food. Let the feast begin...

-Zach Bush MD, Triple Board-Certified Physician & Founder of Seraphic Group, Inc.

Beyond Labels unpacks one of the most undervalued powers humans possess: the ability to choose what we eat. With practical advice and no judgment, the authors provide clear entry points to an authentic organic food system, bringing our plates closer to our ideals.

- Michele Marchetti, Co-director of Communications, The Cornucopia Institute

Do you count yourself among the bewildered? Think you should eat better but don't know where to start? Then *Beyond Labels* is the book for you! Sina McCullough, PhD and Joel Salatin, Celebrity Farmer, lead the way with fascinating discussion coupled with Practical Bites to help you start over with a more nutritious diet and better health.

-Sally Fallon Morell, President of The Weston A. Price Foundation

A successful, all-natural farmer and a savvy PhD nutritionist/scientist get together to write a book about food. What a concept! Finally, a story about eating that invites you, the reader, to co-create your own personalized roadmap to finding the best food options for you and your loved ones.

-Will Winter, DVM, Holistic Veterinarian

This book has the power to change the way the food industry operates and thus, MOST IMPORTANTLY, the health of Americans! We have been gifted, by Joel and Sina, a transparent look into the way food is grown and handled, and the information is packaged in bright, amusing, swirls of color, that left me feeling that this gift could keep on giving. I finished this book feeling empowered to make simple, step by step changes in my personal life and in my business. This book should be included in every high school and university health and wellness class.

-Michelle Walrath, Producer of FedUp & Co-Founder of Organic Krush

Liberating! Fascinating! Transformational! The farmer, world-renowned Joel Salatin of Polyface Farm, and nutritionist Sina McCollough, PhD, are exactly what the world needs right now. Their conversational story-telling style in this delightful book is not only informational, pertinent, crucial and fascinating....it is transformational.

- Zen Honeycutt, Moms Across America

Dr. Sina McCullough and Joel Salatin bridge the gap between producer, consumer and healthcare practitioner in their amazing book *Beyond Labels*. Whether you are just embarking on your health or you are a nutrition ninja, this book is for you.

-Robb Wolf, New York Times Best-Selling Author of The Paleo Solution and Wired To Eat

This is a remarkably well-structured book, which unusually educates consumers on the simple steps they need to take to improve their diets rather than just outlining the problems surrounding the products on grocery store shelves. A must read for everyone who cares about food!

-Henry Rowlands, Director of The Detox Project

More Praise for Beyond Labels

Hands down, the best book I've read in years. As a mother, wife, meal planner, and budget calculator, I have found myself overwhelmed standing in the grocery checkout line with the multitude of fad diets or quick mental health fixes available. The colorful pictures with seemingly happy healthy people conflict with what the grocery store offers in their coupons or incentives for me as the grocery shopper. *Beyond Labels* has given me a simple guided approach for success not only nutritionally, but mentally and emotionally.

-Christine Fauver, Mother of Two

Only solutions at the intersection of the food system and community health have the potential to deliver the lasting, sustainable cure we are desperately searching for. This book is a roadmap to that future.

-James Maskell, Founder of Evolution of Medicine

Beyond Labels tackles the very root of the cause of most modern diseases: diet! In this time of "food-like substances" as Joel likes to say, we need a return to home-cooked meals. Reading this book will help you better understand how real food can truly heal. We need more collaboration like this between food producers and healthcare providers.

-Diana Rodgers, RD, Director of the film and Co-Author of the book Sacred Cow: The Case for Better Meat

The beauty of this book is that it addresses both ends of the value-chain and builds stronger connections between the plight of both growers and eaters. We share that goal on the Land to Market team at the Savory Institute - cultivating new market opportunities for farmers while empowering consumers with real-world data about environmental impact and soil health that allows them to vote with their dollar, in a transparent food democracy, like never before.

-Chris Kerston, Chief Commercial Officer of Land to Market - Savory Institute

Other Books & Resources By Sina McCullough, PhD

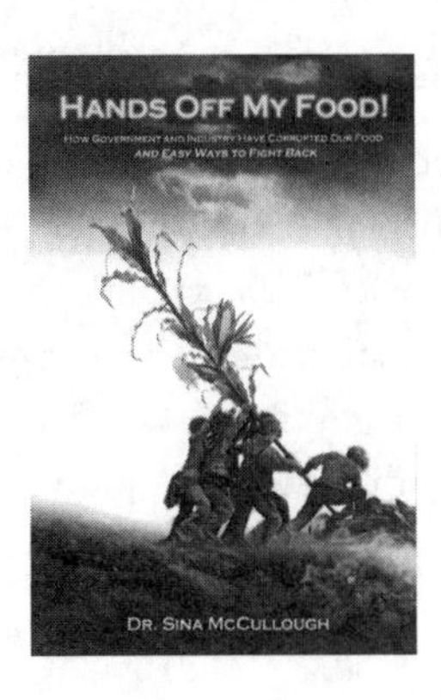

Hands Off My Food: How Government and Industry Have Corrupted Our Food and Easy Ways to Fight Back

Americans have stopped being watchdogs over their own food supply. Roughly 100 years ago, with the birth of the FDA, we handed that responsibility over to the government and the food industry. They, in turn, have fundamentally transformed our food supply and it's making us sick, including our children. Not only are we losing our health to food related illnesses like cancer and heart disease, we are losing our freedom. Did you know that government and the food industry have already chosen your dinner for you? In fact, the government nudges you to pick the foods they want you to eat. They've been doing it your whole life.

In *Hands Off My Food!* Dr. McCullough, a Ph.D. in Nutrition from the University of California at Davis, walks you through the truth behind what's currently in our food and how it got there. You may be surprised to learn that our food system is not designed to protect our long-term health. Both the food industry and the government have played a major role in the demise of our food supply, but they are not the root of the problem. Dr. McCullough reveals who is ultimately responsible for the adulteration of our food and how each of us has the power to restore the integrity of the food we eat by taking back our consent. Together we can reclaim our voice by becoming the watchdogs we were meant to be. It's easier than you might think!

How to Prevent & Reverse Disease

Through a series of online videos, Dr. McCullough walks you through the steps involved in preventing and reversing disease. Physical, emotional, and spiritual aspects are addressed to help you identify the root cause of your symptoms. Practical tools are also provided to help you implement the necessary changes, including: cooking videos, sample menus, a list of Dr. McCullough's go-to prepared foods, suggestions on how to make healthy food more affordable, and solutions for handling social situations and eating outside of your home. This program will inspire you to take charge of your health so you can finally be healthy, happy, and free!
Available at www.HandsOffMyFood.com

Rattlesnake Treats: Take the Bite Out of Sweets

This electronic cookbook features 14 grain-free dessert recipes, including two recipes that won first place at the Virginia State Fair! In addition, each recipe contains a product comparison designed to help empower children to make healthier food choices by teaching them what's in their food. Ingredient sources are also provided.
Available at www.HandsOffMyFood.com

Other Books By Joel Salatin

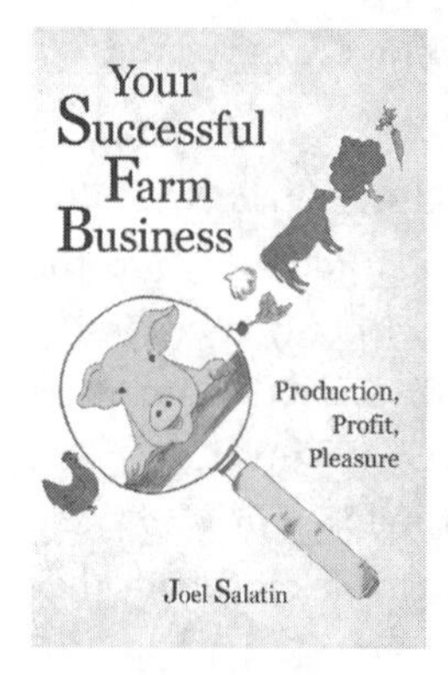

Your Successful Farm Business: Production, Profit, Pleasure

Twenty years ago Joel wrote You Can Farm, which has launched thousands of farm entrepreneurs around the world. With another 20 years of experience under his belt, he decided to build on that foundation with a sequel, a graduate level curriculum. In those 20 years, Polyface Farm progressed from a small family operation to a 20-person, 6,000-customer, 50-restaurant business, all without sales targets, government grants, or an off-farm nest egg. Salatin offers a pathway to success, with production, profit, and pleasure thrown in for good measure.

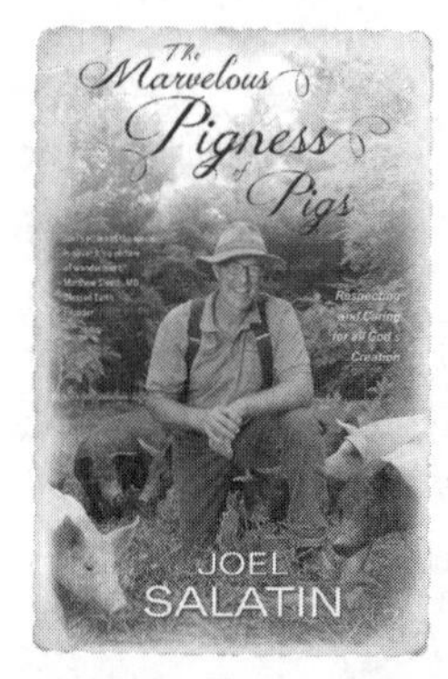

The Marvelous Pigness of Pigs: Nurturing and Caring for All God's Creation

Growing up straddling the tension between the environmental and faith-based community, several years ago Joel poked good-naturedly at the stereotypes with his self-acclaimed moniker: Christian libertarian environmentalist capitalist lunatic farmer. Friends in both camps have marveled at how he could be so ecological but yet read the Bible. Aren't the two mutually exclusive? The thesis of the book is simple: All physical creation is an object lesson of spiritual truth. The question is simple: Do the beliefs in the pew align with what's on the menu?

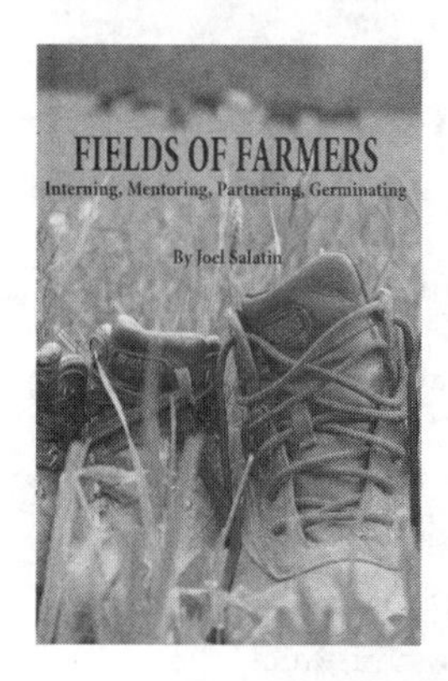

Fields of Farmers: Interning, Mentoring, Partnering, Germinating

America's average farmer is sixty years old. When young people can't get in, old people can't get out. Approaching a watershed moment, our culture desperately needs a generational transfer of millions of farm acres facing abandonment, development, or amalgamation into ever-larger holdings. Based on his decades of experience with interns and multigenerational partnerships at Polyface Farm, farmer and author Joel Salatin digs deep into the problems and solutions surrounding this land and knowledge-transfer crisis. This book empowers aspiring young farmers, midlife farmers, and nonfarming landlords to build regenerative, profitable agricultural enterprises.

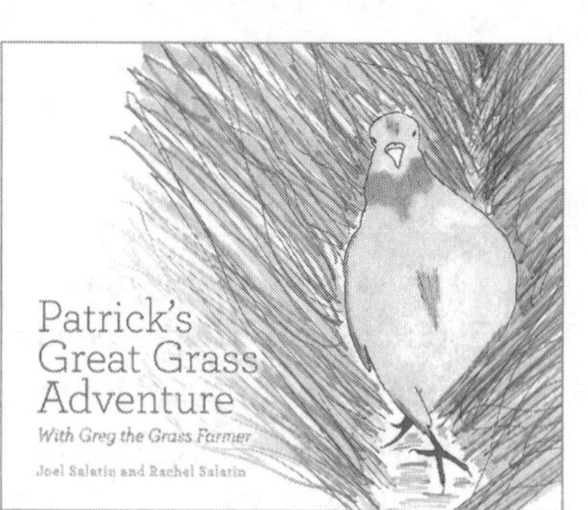

Patrick's Great Grass Adventure: With Greg the Grass Farmer

In his first children's book, Joel Salatin and his daughter Rachel team up on a whimsical tale about a pigeon, a farmer, and grass. This beautifully illustrated edu-tainment book introduces 4-7 year-olds to Greg the grass farmer through the eyes of Patrick Pigeon. What better way to discover ecology-enhancing grass farming than from an aerial view? Grass as crop, insect haven, and diversity blanket comes to life as Patrick Pigeon watches and reports on Greg the grass farmer's activities. Discover a real farm from a real farmer through captivating explanation and illustration.

Other Books By Joel Salatin

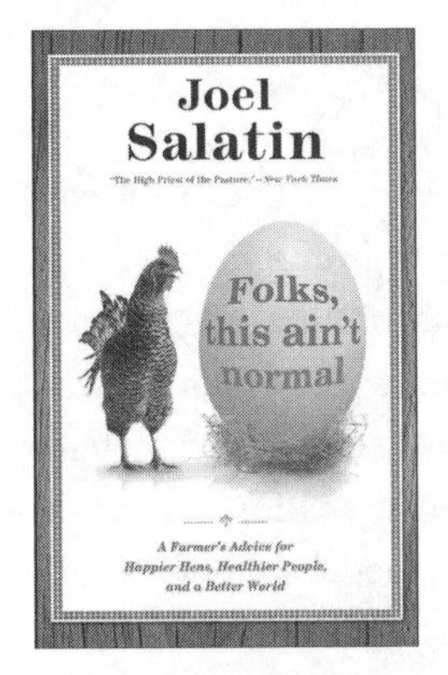

Folks, This Ain't Normal: A Farmer's Advice for Happier Hens, Healthier People, and a Better World

From Joel Salatin's point of view, life in the 21st century just ain't normal. He discusses how far removed we are from the simple, sustainable joy that comes from living close to the land and the people we love. Salatin has many thoughts on what normal is and shares practical and philosophical ideas for changing our lives in small ways that have big impact. Salatin understands what food should be: Wholesome, seasonal, raised naturally, procured locally, prepared lovingly, and eaten with a profound reverence for the circle of life.

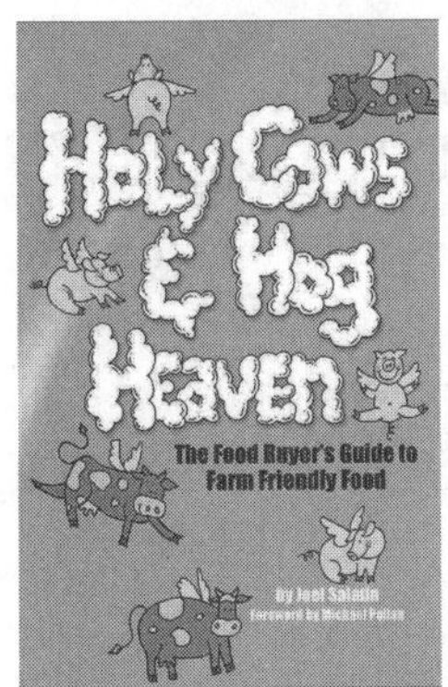

Holy Cows and Hog Heaven: The Food Buyer's Guide to Farm Friendly Food

Written for food buyers to empower them in their dedication to food with integrity, this book changes people's lives. Farmers who give it to their customers say that folks who have read it have a new level of understanding and a delightful attitude about the farmer-consumer relationship. A short, easy read, this book will make you laugh and cry, all in a matter of minutes. Any consumer wanting to peek in to the life behind the local food farmer will be delighted at the insights and real-life stories Joel shares from his own marketing experience.

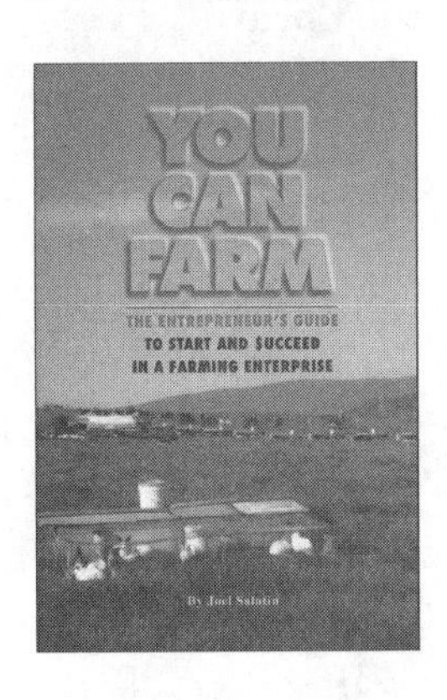

You Can Farm: The Entrepreneur's Guide to Start and $ucceed in a Farming Enterprise

For all the wannabes and newbies. A veritable compendium of information, Joel pulls from his eclectic sphere of knowledge, combines it with a half century of farming experience, and covers as many topics as he can think of that will affect the success of a farming venture. He offers his 10 best picks for profitable ventures, and the 10 worst. He covers insurance, record keeping, land acquisition, and equipment. A hard hitting, practical view from a successful farmer, if this book scares you off, it will be the best reality check you ever spent.

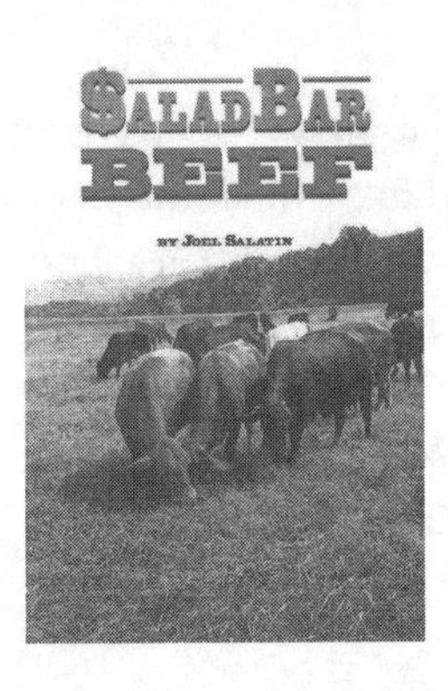

$alad Bar Beef

Fishing for a phrase to describe this ultimately land-healing and nutrition-escalating production model, Joel realized that he was offering the cows a salad bar. He coined the phrase to describe the farm's beef, and thereby stimulate questions from potential customers. This book describes herd effect, mobbing, moving, field design, water systems, manure monitoring, soil fertility, and even pigaerating. A fundamentally fresh way to look at the symbiosis between farmer, field, and cow, this book is now a classic in the pasture-based livestock movement.

Other Books By Joel Salatin

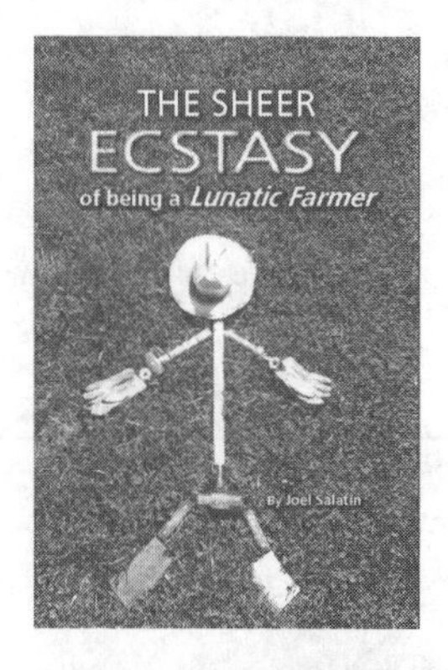

The Sheer Ecstasy of Being a Lunatic Farmer

Have you ever wondered: So what really is the difference, anyway? Can there really be that much difference between the way two farmers operate? After all, a cow is a cow and the land is the land, isn't it? Gleaning stories from his fifty years as localized, compost-fertilized, pasture-based, beyond organic farmer, Salatin explores the differences. From how farmers view soil and water, to how they build fences, market their products or involve their families, this book shows a depth of thought that expresses itself through his family's Polyface Farm. In the international spotlight for this different kind of farm, Salatin explains a different food model and shows with good humor and stories how this alleged lunacy actually offers a life of sheer ecstasy.

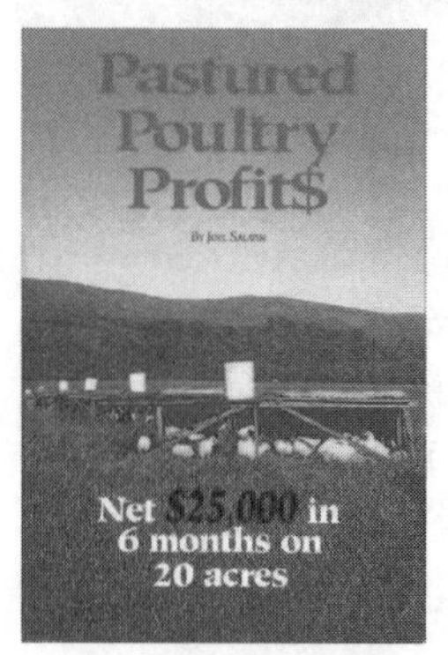

Pastured Poultry Profit$: Net $25,000 on 20 Acres in 6 Months

Joel began raising chickens when he was 10 years old and serendipitously fell into the pastured poultry concept a couple of years later. Still the centerpiece of the farm, and the engine that drives sales, notoriety, and profit, pastured poultry has revolutionized countless farming endeavors around the world. A how-to book, this includes all the stories and tips, from brooding to marketing. Centered around meat chickens, it includes a section on layers and turkeys. Many would say this book started the American pastured poultry movement.

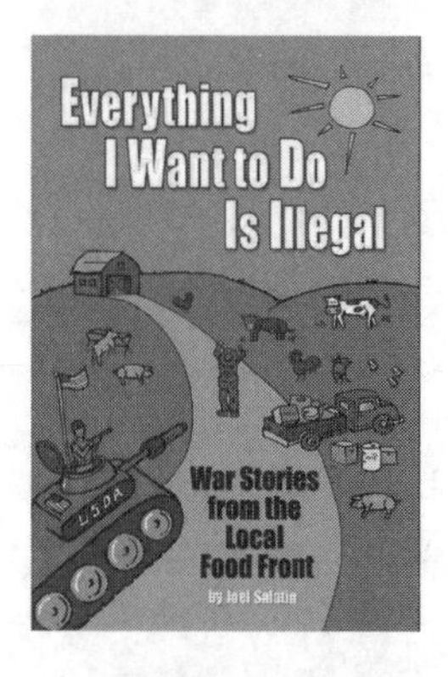

Everything I Want to Do Is Illegal: War Stories from the Local Food Front

Although Polyface Farm has been glowingly featured in countless national print and video media, it would not exist if the USDA and the Virginia Department of Agriculture and Consumer Services had their way. From a lifetime of noncompliance, frustration, humor, and passion come the behind-the-scenes real stories that have brought this little family farm into the forefront of the non-industrial food system. You may not agree with all of his conclusions, but this book will force you to think about things that most people didn't even know existed.

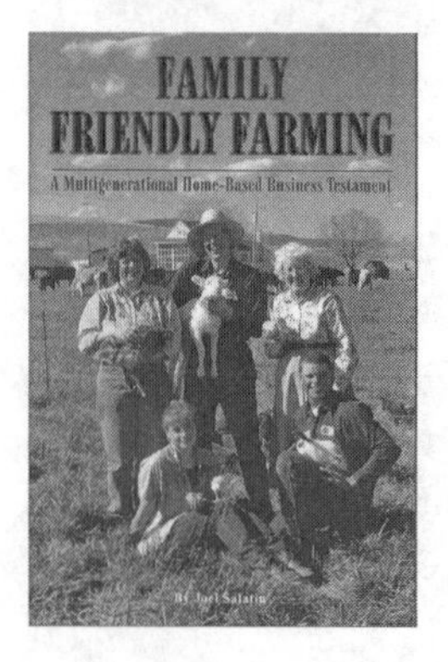

Family Friendly Farming: A Multi-Generational Home-Based Business Testament

Few life circumstances are as hard to navigate as family business. Today, four generations of Salatins work and live on Polyface Farm. It's not easy, but this book describes the rules and relational principles to harmonize in what is too often a tense environment. The chapters on how to get your children to enjoy working with you are worth the price of the book. But beyond that, it delves into the quagmire of inheritance, family meetings, and personal responsibility. These are thorny situations, but a pathway exists to leverage the strengths of family business. The goal of this book is to hold families, and especially family farms, together.

Other Resources By Joel Salatin

Primer Series: Pigs 'n Glens DVD

Pigs are omnivores, like humans. We don't use the word glens much anymore, but you'll find it in old fairy tales and fold lore with names like Rip Van Winkle and Ichabod Crane. It describes a forested setting in which the story will take place. This video combines the most ancient hog production techniques with the best of modern technology, using pigs to massage the ecological landscape in exercise. So hold onto your hats, here we go... Released June 2013 (40 minutes).

Primer Series: Techno Stealth: Metropolitan Buying Clubs DVD

Over the years, we have developed a local food distribution system that we call the Metropolitan Buying Club. We think it combines the real-time interfaces of online marketing with community-based interaction. These kinds of interfaces, without bricks and mortar, using the internet, create efficiencies and economies of scale in local food distribution that we think you will find very exciting. Released July 2014 (45 minutes).

Polyfaces: A World of Many Choices DVD

One Australian family spent 4 years documenting a style of farming that will help change the fate of humanity! Produced over 4 years it follows the Salatin's, a 4th generation farming family who do 'everything different' as they produce food in a way that works with nature, not against it. Using the symbiotic relationships of animals and their natural functions, they produce high quality, nutrient-dense products. Set amidst the stunning Shenandoah Valley in northern Virginia, 'Polyface Farm' is led by "the world's most innovative farmer" (TIME) and uses no chemicals and feeds over 6,000 families and many restaurants and food outlets within a 3 hour 'food-shed' of their farm. This model is being replicated throughout our global village, proving that we can provide quality produce without depleting our planet. Released 2015 (1 hour 32 minutes).

Other Resources By Joel Salatin

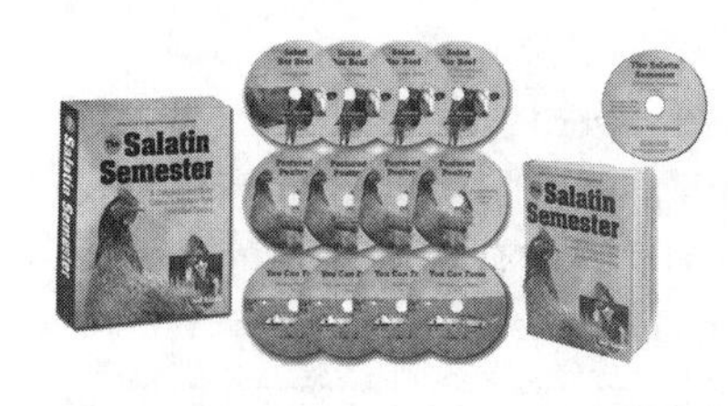

The Salatin Semester: A Complete Homestudy Course in Polyface-Style Diversified Farming

This amazing multimedia production conveys the Salatin family's methods of profitable diversified farming like no other. Joel Salatin presents his farming system in professional edited, live-cut video, engaging audio, and in a detail-rich reference guide. This package is a veritable fount of pertinent and crucial knowledge, a unique compilation of synergistic wisdom to help you earn a living as a farmer. The live presentations are presented in DVD video; the audio interviews with Q&A are in digital audio; and the myriad questions and answers from the resulting discussion are transcribed and edited in a detailed reference guide. The end result is an amazingly extensive – and affordable – training guide to help you reinvent your farm. This beautifully produced comprehensive tutorial contains:
18 hours of video on 12 DVDs
6 hours of audio Q&A
Digital slideshow farm tour
256-page guidebook

Joel Salatin's Books Available From

Polyface Farm Gift Shop	1-540-885-3590	www.polyfacefarms.com
Chelsea Green Publishing	1-800-639-4099	www.chelseagreen.com
Acres USA Magazine	1-800-355-5313	www.acresusa.com
Amazon.com		www.amazon.com
Your local bookstore		

Warning:

This is not a diet book.

The information contained within this book is not meant to be medical or diet advice, nor is it designed to replace advice, information, or prescriptions you receive from your health care provider. This book provides solutions that are used by the authors. It is not advice.

The information provided in this book is for informational purposes only. You should not use the information in this book for diagnosis or treatment of any health problem. Consult with a healthcare professional before starting any diet, exercise, or supplementation program.

Proceed at your own risk.

CONTENTS

Foreword xix
Introduction xxii

Section 1: Your Roadmap to Health, Happiness & Freedom

Chapter 1: Meet Your Roadmap 2
Chapter 2: Personalize Your Roadmap 6
Chapter 3: Set Yourself Up For Success 23

Section 2: Step Up Your Game with Convenience

Chapter 4: Shift from Low to High Quality Processed Food 34
Practical Bites
#1: Harness Your Power 36
#2: Find A Buddy 46
#3: Say No To Antibiotics When Eating Out 49
#4: Look For The 100% USDA Organic Label 55
#5: Mirror, Mirror 61
#6: Switch to Organic Eggs 66
#7: Say No To Chlorinated Eggs 71
#8: Choose Organic Chicken 75
#9: Choose Your Disinfectant On Your Chicken 80
#10: Don't Waste Your Money on "Free Range" Or "Pasture Raised" 90
#11: Eat 100% Grass-Finished, Organic Beef 93
#12: Eat What You Can Pronounce 98
#13: Avoid Artificial & "Natural" Flavor 103
#14: Choose Preservative Free 107
#15: Don't Fear The Fat Label 112
#16: Throw Out Artificial Sweeteners 123
#17: Get To Know Fake Meat 127
#18: Drink Soda With Intention 131
#19: Hydrate Your Cells 134
#20: Say Yes to rBGH-free Milk Products.... 145
#21: Be Informed At Restaurants 151
#22: Look For The Duo 155
#23: Look For The Trio 163
#24: Look For The Quartet 176
#25: Eat Real Salt 181
#26: Say Yes To Wild-Caught Fish 184
#27: Bring Your Lunch 190
#28: Be Prepared With Snacks 193

#29: Bring Your Own Solutions 194
#30: Step Outside The Grocery Store Box 200
#31: Stock Up On Sale Items 204
#32: Give Your Family The Freedom To Opt-In 207
#33: Create Convenience 212
#34: Sprout & Grind Your Grains 216

Section 3: Meet Real Food

Chapter 5: Shift From High Quality Processed Food To Whole Food 224
Practical Bites
#35: Count Quality, Not Calories 227
#36: Avoid The Dirty Dozen®; Choose The Clean Fifteen® 236
#37: Buy A Slow Cooker Or Pressure Cooker 240
#38: Use Your Slow Cooker Or Pressure Cooker 242
#39: Don't Trust The "Gluten-Free" Label 244
#40: Peel Your Apples 250
#41: Cook A Whole Chicken 253
#42: Cook One Meal Using Whole Foods 256
#43: Save Time & Money By Batching & Storing 262
#44: Eat A Daily Helping Of Microbes From Ferments 267
#45: Add One Prebiotic Each Week 273
#46: Spice It Up! 276
#47: Breathe In Microbial Diversity 281
#48: Say No To Arsenic In Rice 284
#49: Listen To Your Body 288
#50: Cycle Your Foods 298

Section 4: Meet Your Neighbor

Chapter 6: Shift From Whole Food To Locally Grown Whole Food 308
Practical Bites
#51: Choose Local In The Grocery Store 312
#52: Eat Ecologically Grown Produce From Your Local Farmer 314
#53: Eat Ecologically Raised, Pastured Chickens From Your Local Farmer 317
#54: Eat Ecologically Raised, Pastured Eggs From Your Local Farmer 319
#55: Eat Ecologically Raised, Grass-Finished Beef From Your Local Farmer 321
#56: Eat Ecologically Raised, Pastured Pork From Your Local Farmer 324
#57: Meet Your Local Farmers 327
#58: Thank Your Farmers 330
#59: Say No To Subsidies 332
#60: Eat Mindfully 335
#61: Meditate Daily 339

Section 5: Get Your Hands Dirty
Chapter 7: Shift From Locally Grown to Home-Grown Whole Food 344
Practical Bites
#62: Grow One Herb In Your Kitchen 346
#63: Grow One Edible Plant Indoors 349
#64: Grow Your Sprouts 354
#65: Start A Small Garden 356
#66: Cover Your Soil 360
#67: Create Your Own Compost 363
#68: Add A Solarium On Your Home 369
#69: Catch The Rain 370
#70: Save Money By Preserving One Fruit Or Vegetable 372
#71: Adopt Chickens & Feed Them Kitchen Scraps 374
#72: Relocate To A Homestead 376

Section 6: Spread Your Wings
Chapter 8: Become Your Own Headliner 378

Appendix
Joel's Story 384
Sina's Story 389
A Farmer and a PhD Unite! 392

Trademark Acknowledgment 395
References & Permissions 398
Index 419

Foreword

It helps to bring reading glasses when you go food-shopping. You'll need to read some very small print. The government-mandated labels on bottles, bags, boxes and jars are there to tell you what a product contains, and it's a good thing they do. The ingredients are listed in order of percentage of the whole, so if a can of soda puts sugar first, it means there is more sugar than anything else in the can. Take a squint at the Froot Loops® box. It does not list actual fruit because there isn't any.

I'm thankful for such admissions. But what can you make of the string of polysyllabic items that often follow them? They might as well be written in conversational Sanskrit.

Most labels tell only a partial story. A product's USDA Certified Organic label, for example, is pretty good proof that the ingredients are not genetically modified, or toxic. It does not assure that a vegetable or fruit was, as you might have supposed, grown in living soil rather than a hydroponic operation, or that an animal was honestly given "free range" of a pasture. And few labels will guarantee that your food has never, on its way to your table, been embalmed, disinfected, irradiated or spiked with any of the 10,000 chemical additives that can be legally added. And some labels are simply ridiculous, like the little "Gluten Free" stickers I once saw on broccoli heads in a supermarket bin.

Anyone eager to find a path through the label jungle in search of safe, honest, and highly nutritious food would do well to have Joel Salatin and Dr. Sina McCullough's book in their knapsack. You might already know some of the signposts, but these two have given us an encyclopedic guide to the good and the bad parts of our nation's food system. Joel, as a farmer, and Sina, as an expert in Nutrition, save you a lot of time trying to sort out what would otherwise be a vast, confusing, deliberately obfuscated mess.

This could be a depressing book, but it's not. Its positive, optimistic take on things stems from both authors' belief in the glory of real, living, unprocessed food. They explain how the nutritive and healing properties of food can only be derived from nature's own systems, whether you're looking at the biological diversity of a well-managed farm, or the self-balancing microbial populations of a well-fed human gut.

Many books have been written about America's food system: an industrial food Goliath that values the shelf life of groceries more than the life span of its customers -- a Goliath with a stranglehold on government regulation. Yes, the problem is political. But you could die waiting for a political solution. This book places the power directly in the hands of us, its readers, who are more powerful than we think. We have the power to question our food purveyors, ask that they give us better choices, and vote with our dollars. And we can improve the way we eat. The key lies in a continuum the authors have created that show the stages of food independence, from total helplessness to total command of our own food supply. It starts with shopping organic, moves through stages of a basic, whole, unprocessed and local diet and ends with growing some of your own. With each stage, they give you little steps – "small bites" – that can move you in the right direction, right now. Sometimes finding a local farmer you trust, or a farmers' market, is all you need to do.

As someone who grows food and also writes about it, I'm all too aware of how hard it is to change food-buying habits. The current system addicts us to inferior food by means of sophisticated flavor chemistry and lures us with convenience. Worst of all it exploits the susceptibility of children and the harried parents whose job it is to feed them. I've found that if you focus on the wholesome items that kids are willing to eat, however few, and keep adding others as their willingness to try new things grows, you can gradually succeed.

"But I don't have time to cook!" my readers have sometimes wailed. Like Joel and Sina, I've found that making a big quantity of something and freezing it in smaller batches can save hours of time with almost-instant meals.

"But organic food is too expensive", the wail continues. "And it's elitist! Only rich people can afford it" That's the one that really galls me. Industrial, processed food is kept artificially cheap by means of government subsidies for the crops that go into it. And when you add up all the sticky snacks and frozen pizzas we buy, we probably spend more than we would stocking up on unpackaged basics such as rice, dried beans, potatoes, onions, carrots, cabbages and winter squash. Add a little meat and you have the makings of stews, hearty soups and other time-honored peasant dishes. These are the foundation on which all the world's great cuisines stand.

Whether we are rich, poor, or just average folks, we all have some choice in how we spend what we earn, and if we want to be in good health, we have to eat good food. A friend once shared with me an old Sicilian proverb: "Che non si paglia alla tavola, si paglia al dottore." What you don't pay for at the table, you pay for at the doctor. I couldn't have said it better.

Barbara Damrosch,

Co-owner of Four Seasons Farm and author of *The Garden Primer*

Introduction

Do you want to be healthy, happy and free? But find yourself stuck in your healing journey and want some guidance and encouragement? Perhaps you are overwhelmed by all of the conflicting diet advice. Maybe you don't know where to start or who to trust. Or, maybe you just need a little motivation.

You're not alone. We're constantly bombarded with ever-changing diet recommendations and the latest diet crazes - Paleo, Keto, Whole 30, Specific Carbohydrate Diet, and the list goes on. Eggs are bad one day and good the next. Kale is good for you today. Tomorrow it contains high levels of thallium and is toxic to your thyroid gland. How do you know what to put on your plate that will bring you toward greater health and wellness?

In this information age, it should be easier than ever to figure out which foods your individual body needs in order to achieve optimal health and experience abundant energy throughout the day. But, it's not. While we're connected electronically and processing incoming information all day, we're disconnected from our food and our bodies. We can't discern the massive onslaught of information because we don't know what's in our food or how it was grown. And, we've outsourced our power to "experts" for so long that we have forgotten how to listen to our own bodies to know what they need to thrive. Consequently, we are becoming fatigued, sick, and enslaved.

So, where do you start? How do you wade through the massive database of conflicting research and opinions to find the truth? How do you finally figure out the diet your body needs to be healthy, happy and free?

Joel Salatin, a farmer who is blazing the trail in regenerative farming, and Sina McCullough, a PhD in Nutrition who reversed a chronic disease by changing her diet and lifestyle, have joined forces to take you on a healing journey. Through friendly banter and common-sense conclusions, Joel and Sina offer a well-rounded perspective on what's in your food, from farm to fork, while providing solutions that have been the most practical and impactful in their own lives.

Most importantly, they meet you where you are, and encourage you to move forward in your journey, one small step at a time. They call these small steps "Practical Bites," because they contain actionable items that are *actually* useful in your daily life, such as:

- What to eat
- How to procure it
- How to prepare it
- How to eat it
- How to save time in the kitchen
- How to save money on your grocery bill
- How to stay true to your principles in our modern culture (i.e. during family gatherings and lunch meetings, while traveling, or when surrounded by fast food).

Many of the Practical Bites take 5 minutes or less to implement. And, there are no deadlines! You choose your pace. You can pick one Practical Bite a day, one a week, or one a year. The timing doesn't matter. Move forward at a pace that works for you.

You also choose the length of your healing journey. Each Practical Bite begins with a short "How" followed by a longer "Why." If you're seeking a short journey, only read the "How." If you'd like to join Joel and Sina as they walk through the ins and outs of your food supply and wade through the conflicting dietary advice then also read the "Why." The choice is yours.

To provide you with a richer experience and better understanding of how Joel and Sina think about the food supply and how they make decisions about which foods to eat, *Beyond Labels* is written in a conversational format. Think of this book as your front-row ticket to a dinner theater featuring the rare pairing of a farmer and a PhD who exchange friendly banter while delving into difficult nutrition and health topics. Without further ado, here are your headliners, Joel and Sina.

Joel: Sina, you and I have been at this a long time and feel comfortable toward what I call "Food Paradise:" know what's in your food, know your farmer, know your body. But you didn't start out that way, did you?

Sina: Absolutely not! I started at the bottom of the barrel. For most of my life, I ate the way I was raised, which was based on the Standard American Diet. I ate mostly processed foods. And, I chose meat based on fat content and price, which means I only ate conventional. I didn't even know the difference between organic and conventional, which is crazy when I think about it because my PhD is in Nutrition! But we weren't taught that type of practical information. So, I completed graduate school not knowing how to navigate a grocery store.

When I started to get sick with an autoimmune disease, I realized I needed to make changes. So, I began to teach myself. I spent hours and hours reading articles, scientific studies, government documents, company statements, and textbooks. I quickly realized that the ins and outs of our food supply are complicated, especially when it comes to labels.

There are a lot of loopholes, exceptions, and confusing statements regarding labels. In fact, the more I learned about our food, the more I didn't know who to trust or what was true. It was overwhelming and frankly, upsetting. So, I didn't change everything all at once; I took it one step at a time.

Joel: Yes, moving toward Paradise takes experience and skill, both as a consumer and as a farmer. I know I've become much better at handling livestock over the course of my life. There's no question that my animals are happier, more in tune genetically with our environment, and healthier than they were a half century ago when we were feeling our way. Discernment is like a muscle, isn't it? It needs exercise.

Sina: Exactly. Now I'm healthy and completely disease-free, but it took a lot of decision-making to get to this point. If I could go back and do it all over again, there are choices that I would change. And, that's okay. Some people might say I made a lot of mistakes, but I think that's part of the journey. You make the best decisions you can in each moment, given the information you have. Then, you have the opportunity to re-assess when you have more information. It's all about baby steps.

I started my healing journey by learning how to read labels, which was more challenging than I could have imagined. I quickly realized that you can't take the label at face value. You have to learn to read beyond the label in order to truly understand what's in that box of cereal or package of cookies.

Joel: Labels are misleading and they don't tell you the truth about what's in your food and how it got there. I'd love to help people get out of the grocery stores and onto their local farms, where they can see the food for themselves. Now that's food freedom! But that's a process that requires coaching and many small steps. And, that's where we come in.

Sina: We'd like to invite you to join us on a healing journey where we teach you how to navigate the grocery store labyrinth and then show you how to move beyond those labels - to a place where you will find foods that truly heal.

Joel: We're going to show you how we think about the food supply because knowing how to think, how to decide, is more important than the ultimate decision. That's the real treasure of our journey together – the unique pairing of a farmer and a PhD.

We've all heard "experts" talk about silos. It's a hot word these days to describe tunnel vision and narrow expertise. I've always called it "knowing more and more about less and less." The agronomist doesn't know anything about grasshoppers and the entomologist doesn't know anything about organic matter. This is not only true in academics disciplines, it's also true in practical life.

We tend to gravitate toward people who know what we know, where we can converse with common lingo and understanding. The more different the disciplines or vocations, the less likely their practitioners are to get together. With that in mind, a farmer and a scientist teaming up together creates an eclectic conversation that would never happen with two farmers talking or two scientists talking. That broad conversation is critical to tease out the nuances and ramifications of an issue.

Complementary discussion broadens awareness and understanding. Too often in significant issue discussions, farmers get left off the table because after all, we're just a bunch of hillbilly bumpkins who don't really have anything worth saying. For an academically-accomplished scientist to engage a farmer as an equal is both unusual and special. I'm deeply grateful that Sina is a credentialed scientist who never condescends to me; who actually listens as if I have important things to contribute to the conversation.

By the same token, too often farmers like me dismiss scientists as impractical eggheads who don't know how to tie their shoes and walk around with their heads in the clouds. That's equally incorrect. We both need each other. In fact, we're both stronger listening to each other. But silos divide us more often than not. *This partnership*, then, creates a platform for a conversation unusual enough to interest the intellect and the down-and-dirty spectrums that each of us enjoys. Nothing is all academic and nothing is all practical. Marrying the two yields rich returns.

Sina: Joel and I approach the food supply from two different perspectives. He's a farmer who is deeply connected with the land, and who knows how to grow foods that heal – foods that are in harmony with nature. I'm a scientist who understands how the body becomes diseased and how to reverse that process. Both perspectives are equally important for your healing journey. Like Joel said, we're better together.

Joel: My greatest hope is that Sina and I can free you from the prison of inadequacy. So that you realize you are completely capable of nurturing yourself and the ones you love.

Sina: You already have the instincts and the tools you need to thrive. You just have to tap into your innate abilities. By the end of our journey together, we hope you will have gained enough knowledge and trust in yourself to be able to discern any new labels that appear in your grocery store or any new diet advice you may encounter.

Joel: Okay, let's be gentle here. We're going to move you from kindergarten through high school and by the end of this book, we're going to be taking you through graduate school. Once we're done, you won't want to shop for your food in grocery stores.

Remember, we're taking small steps as we coach you toward greater health, happiness, and freedom. In novels, this is called foreshadowing. Here, we're calling it knowing some fundamentals of the game before we move along a continuum of skill. I hope that's fair. Sina, are we missing anything before we begin our healing journey together?

Sina: Nope. Except, if you're interested in learning more about our stories or how Joel and I met, jump ahead to the Appendix. Otherwise, let the fun begin!

SECTION 1:

Your Roadmap To Health, Happiness & Freedom

CHAPTER 1

Meet Your Roadmap

Sina: Whether I'm presenting at a conference or working with a client, the most common question I'm asked is, "Where do I start?" People are routinely surprised when I don't immediately spout off a list of foods to eat or avoid, or labels to look for in the grocery store. While that information is helpful, it's not empowering.

The first step in your healing journey is realizing your power lies in your choice.

Health is a choice.
Happiness is a choice
Freedom is a choice.

You can choose to play a passive role in your life – to be a "victim." Or, *you can choose* to get into the driver's seat and create health, happiness, and freedom for yourself. One of the greatest gifts you can give yourself is the responsibility for your own decisions. That's where your power lies!

Joel: When you live in "Victim-land", it narrows your choices and defeats you. But the moment you adopt a personal responsibility mentality, you're freed from others' agenda, your own helplessness, and your own rut.

Sina: When you take responsibility for your own health and happiness, you set yourself free. You shift out of fight-or-flight and into a space that nurtures optimal health, heals disease, promotes happiness, and fosters freedom. Instead of living your life from a place of fear, you live from a place of love. When you take responsibility, the "impossible" becomes possible:

Optimal health and abundant energy are achievable.
Disease is reversible.
Boundaries and limitations no longer exist.
You are free!

All you have to do is *choose* - *choose* health, *choose* happiness, and *choose* freedom.

Joel: The most important first step in moving forward is *wanting* to move, and that's a choice. Inertia is perhaps the most powerful property in nature. It can make things that are stuck stay stuck - for a long time.

What we need is to start moving and then harness that inertia to carry us where we would never have imagined when we were stuck in "Victim-land". Never have people had more choice than today. A French peasant shepherd in 1300 had far less choice in life than most modern folks, especially those of us in America, the ultimate land of opportunity. Whatever your ancestry, whatever your genetics, whatever your socio-economic status, you and I have a choice. So, let's exercise it.

Your Road Map

Sina: We believe that most people want to be healthy, feel joyful and energized throughout the day, have the freedom to pursue their dreams, and trust that the food they feed their families is safe. So, we've designed a road map to help you achieve those overarching goals. (You will identify your specific goals in the next chapter).

Joel: This roadmap is an overly simplified diagram that is not perfect and is not the solution for everyone. But we use it in our daily lives. It is based on these core principles, which are located on the right side of the continuum:

- Maximal Health
- Maximal Happiness
- Maximal Freedom
- Maximal Trust
- Maximal Personal Responsibility

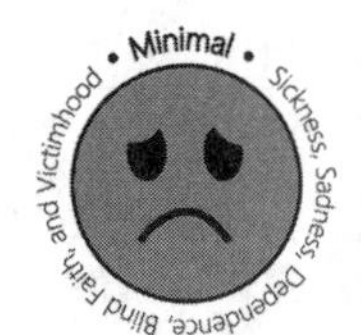

Processed Food | Higher Quality Processed Food | Store Bought Whole Food | Locally Grown Whole Food | Home Grown Whole Food

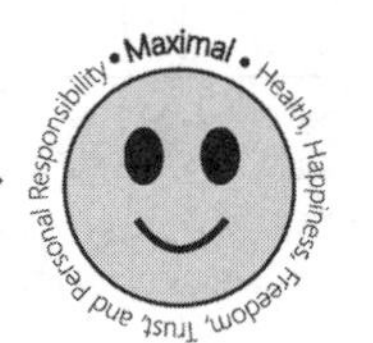

Located on the left, or minimal, side of the continuum are the opposites: sickness, sadness, dependence, blind faith, and victimhood. This roadmap consists of 5 categories, including:

- **Processed Food** – Think of food at a gas station, fast food, and anything that comes in a bag or box that contains chemicals or ingredients you cannot pronounce. Examples include: cereal, crackers, cookies, chips, T.V. dinners, pizza, lunch meat, and soda.
- **Higher Quality Processed Food** – Think of convenience foods, like those listed above, but they do not contain chemicals or toxic ingredients. Examples include: organic cereal and grass-finished, antibiotic-free meat.
- **Store Bought Whole Food** – Includes foods that are sourced directly from the ground or the animal. These foods contain no chemicals and have undergone minimal or no processing. Examples include: organic fruits and vegetables in their native state, eggs, and whole pieces of meat – think of a chicken breast with the bone and skin still attached.
- **Locally Grown Whole Food** – Includes whole foods that you purchase from local farmers.
- **Home-Grown Whole Food** – Includes whole foods that you grow.

We will explore each of these categories in detail through what we call "Practical Bites." For now, simply recognize that as you move away from processed foods and toward home-grown whole foods, you move toward maximal health, happiness, freedom, trust, and personal responsibility.

Sina: For simplicity, only food quality and source are listed on the road map. Many variables are involved in achieving maximal health, happiness, freedom, trust and personal responsibility. And, we've weaved in some of those variables throughout this book. But we are focusing primarily on food quality and food source because those are choices that you make every day, multiple times per day. In other words, shifting your quality and source of food will provide a huge return on your investment.

Joel: I think you'll quickly see that the road map outlines what you already know intuitively. You already know that eating at McDonald's® is not healthy, and that growing your own vegetables is a better option. You already know that fresh fruits and vegetables provide your body with more vitamins, minerals, and antioxidants than a box of cereal filled with artificial colors, flavors, pesticides and genetically modified organisms (GMOs).

Our goal is to help you leverage your intuition into action by making the process doable, practical and fun.

Think of the road map as a litmus test for your daily food choices. By knowing where you are currently located on the continuum and where you want to be, this map can help you make choices that will ultimately lead you to accomplish your goals.

Sina: The beauty of this road map is that *you get to choose* where you want to be. With your next bite of food, you can choose to bring yourself closer to health, happiness, and freedom or you can choose to move further away from those goals. The choice is yours.

CHAPTER 2

Personalize Your Roadmap

Sina: After recognizing that your power lies in your choice, the next step in your healing journey is to set your intention. Joel and I are coaching you toward *your* definition of maximal health, freedom, happiness, trust and personal responsibility. That means, *you* get to choose what those goals look like for you. Fortunately, they all go hand-in-hand. So, if you focus on just one of those goals, you will move closer toward achieving all of them.

In this chapter, you will identify your individual goals in each of those five areas. However, we will focus primarily on health because it's more relatable. Each Practical Bite provided in this book will move you to the right of the road map – toward *your* definition of maximal health. In the process, you simultaneously move toward maximal freedom, maximal happiness, maximal trust and maximal personal responsibility. Let's begin by identifying your individual health goal.

Choose Your Health Goal

Sina: When I work with clients, one of the first questions I ask is: What does health look like for you?

Most people don't have an answer because we take our health for granted until it's gone. Then, once we lose our health, we focus on what we don't want – fatigue, disease, being overweight, etcetera. Consequently, I commonly hear responses such as, "I just don't want to feel tired anymore," or "I just want to lose weight."

Everyone probably knows what health is not – disease, fatigue, being overweight, brain fog, etcetera. But, if you want to create health, you can't just be against disease or fatigue; you have to be "for something."

Don't focus on what you are against – poor health.
Instead, focus on what you are for – optimal health.

Joel: Sina's right. You must focus on the positive. We see this play out on the farm, as well. Every time I talk with farmers, I get a question about weeds. This weed, that weed; what are you going to do about it? In our pastures we have all sorts of plants growing. In fact, native prairie was said to have more than 40 species of plants per acre. I guarantee you, many if not most of them today would be classified as weeds.

Farmers are obsessed with weeds. Here at Polyface, we focus on creating the kind of pasture we want, not on the one we don't want. Do we always have a perfect pasture? Of course not. But if we obsess about what we have that we don't want, we'll spend all our time fighting. On the other hand, if we obsess about what we do want, then we spend all our time creating.

Interestingly, either approach changes the weed picture. One works with them and the other works against them. I've been at this business long enough to know that landscapes change, sometimes radically, from season to season. Sometimes it's a particular thing. For example, if we have a herd of 300 cows in a pasture and suddenly get 3 inches of rain overnight, probably where those cows spent the night will look horrible in the morning.

We call it pugging, where the cows stomp up the soaked ground and literally make it look like a tilled field. They mash all the vegetation into the soil and churn things up into a muddy mess. Sometimes the ground surface resembles slurry, like pudding. It's unsightly and fortunately doesn't happen very much. But we've seen this in numerous instances over the years and the pattern is always the same, under our management. The first year, that torn up patch grows nothing but weeds.

We don't spray the weeds or mow them. We let them grow and move the cows through in their normal grazing pattern. At Polyface, we move the cows every day to a new paddock, so when the cows are on that patch of weeds, they're only on it for a day. They eat some and tromp some. Those tall weeds grow long tap roots that loosen the soil and bring up new minerals.

The second year, these patches are pure clover or timothy (a succulent preferred grass). People familiar with the situation always ask us if we planted these beautiful stands of clover or timothy. We've never planted any of it. We just let the vegetation take its course, enjoyed the deep-rooted weeds, continued with the positive plan, and sure enough, healing came on the heels of contentment. Had we not been content and sprayed or mowed or fought back on those weeds, they would not have brought up the minerals and loosened the soil to make way for clover and timothy.

Sina: What a beautiful example of how you can reap unexpected benefits from working with nature, as opposed to working against it. The same concept applies to our health. What you focus your time and energy on will grow. And, what you steer your focus away from will shrink. In other words, if you focus on the extra 10 pounds you put on over the holidays, you'll be met with resistance. Hence the term, "stubborn" 10 pounds. Likewise, if you have a chronic disease and you constantly think about it and talk about it, you will find yourself getting sicker. So, let's change the pattern by taking this first step.

YOUR TURN: Take a moment and think about what maximal health looks like for you. Think BIG! Is maximal health having an abundant supply of energy throughout the day? Is it feeling younger than you did in your twenties? Or waking up every day feeling refreshed and optimistic about what adventures are in store for you that day? Is maximal health moving throughout your day with ease, joy, and unshakable peace? Or maybe it's the ability to grow your own food and cook meals that your kids love and you trust? Whatever you desire, write it down here:

____

____

____

____

Visualize & Feel Your Health Goal

Sina: Now that you have identified your health goal, you must visualize health in your mind. Creating a clear picture not only allows you to focus on what you want, so you can move toward that goal, it literally changes your body.

You're probably already aware that your thoughts can change your biology. For instance, have you ever been embarrassed and your cheeks turn red? When you went on your first date, did your hands get sweaty? Or, maybe you gave a presentation at work and were so nervous that your stomach hurt, your heart was racing, or your mouth became dry. You may have even experienced diarrhea. These are all familiar examples of how your thoughts cause physical changes in your body.

Let's apply this concept to your health goal by using another familiar example: If you walk down the street and a tiger jumps out from behind a building, your body goes into a state of fight-or-flight. It releases adrenaline, cortisol and other chemicals that are designed to help you get out of the stressful situation i.e. to either fight the tiger or run away.

Fight-or-flight is a fantastic tool to have in that type of acute situation because it can save your life. But, if you stay in fight-or-flight over a long period of time, it can lead to disease. For instance, a surge of cortisol can help you fight the tiger. But, chronically elevated levels of cortisol can lead to inflammation, which can lead to insulin resistance, autoimmune disease, heart disease, allergies, or other inflammatory condition. It also makes it more difficult to heal from disease, lose weight, or increase your energy level.

You may not think you are in a chronic state of fight-or-flight. After all, how many tigers do you see while walking down the street? But you don't have to be chased by a tiger, or under physical stress, to be in fight-or-flight. Mental and emotional stress are also viewed by your body as tigers chasing you. That means your *thoughts* and *feelings* can prevent you from healing or from achieving your health goal.

Simply thinking about a stressful situation or feeling negative emotions (i.e. anxiety, fear, or worry) can put your body in fight-or-flight. Interestingly, your body doesn't know the difference between a traumatic event that is happening in real time and you remembering a traumatic event that happened 20 years ago. In both situations, your body releases stress hormones as though the trauma is happening in that moment. In other words, your body continues to relive the trauma each time you think about it, which keeps you in a state of fight-or-flight and, ultimately, keeps you inflamed and fatigued. That's how powerful your thoughts are!

On the flip side, you can choose to use your thoughts to create health in your body. All you have to do is think it, and then see it, and then feel it. For example, research shows that new neuronal connections can be made in your brain simply by thinking about the nerves growing, visualizing it happening, and then feeling it. One of the best real-life examples of the minds' ability to rebuild the body is the story of Dr. Joe Dispenza.

In 1986, Dr. Dispenza was hit by a car while competing in a triathlon. The impact compressed six vertebras in his spine. He was told he'd probably never walk again and that radical surgery was necessary. Dr. Dispenza said no to surgery and, instead, checked out of the hospital because he believed "the power that made the body heals the body." So, he began using his mind to repair his spine. Every day, he visualized and felt the reconstruction of his spine, vertebra by vertebra. After only 10 weeks, he was back on his feet! In 12 weeks, he was training again!

That might sound too miraculous to be true. But the scientific literature is filled with examples of the body's ability to heal itself. For instance, we know that when you combine intention (i.e. thought) with elevated emotions (i.e. feelings of gratitude or joy), you can literally turn on and off your genes! And when you turn on genes that heal your body, it changes your chemistry - including your hormone levels – which changes your body, mood, perception, and every other facet of your being.

In other words, you can create healing and optimal health with your thoughts because your body will respond to your intention *as if the healing has already occurred.* In the example of Dr. Dispenza, his brain literally changed to look like the healing already happened. And, his body responded accordingly by healing itself.

That amazing healing power is inside of *you* too. And, you can access it to achieve whatever health goal you desire. All you have to do is choose to harness your power by utilizing your thoughts and feelings to create health.

When I was sick, my picture of health was enjoying a picnic lunch in the park with my husband and children. I *saw* the four of us sitting on a soft blanket, eating delicious homemade foods as we watched brilliantly colored butterflies flutter by. Then, I'd chase my children around the playground while playing a game of tag. I *felt* no pain as I moved about with ease and comfort. I could *hear* the sound of my children's laughter, *see* the smiles on their faces, *smell* the sweet scent of freshly bloomed flowers, *taste* the crisp, clean air, and *feel* the coolness of the green grass touching the bottom of my feet. I was overwhelmed by the *feeling* of love and gratitude for my health and complete healing.

When I created that picture of health, I was lying on the floor in chronic pain. I was too weak to walk up the stairs without getting winded and too tired to stand long enough to finish doing the dishes after lunch. Some days my body hurt so badly that my 6-year old son had to hold a cup to my mouth just so I could take a drink of water. But I held on tightly to my goal - visualizing and feeling it every day. And now, it's my reality.

Joel: Your story is remarkable. It illustrates the fact that managing for what we can't see, what we can only imagine, actually creates more positive movement than managing reactively to what we do see. In the ugliness of the moment, this is hard to do, of course, but Sina is absolutely right about focusing energy on where we want to go rather than on where we're stuck or where we've been. It's a powerful and profound notion, this truth that imagining our future can do more to influence its development than just about anything else. It's not just wishes and baseless hopes. It's building the future in our spirit, and that's not foo-foo stuff; it's more real than you can imagine.

YOUR TURN: Look back at your health goal. Take a few minutes to visualize what that goal looks like. Create a detailed picture in your mind. Draw your picture, cut an image from a magazine, or simply visualize it in the space provided on the following page.

Next, imagine how it feels to achieve your goal. Really feel it, deep inside of you. Allow yourself to feel the joy and the freedom that comes from achieving your desired state of health. The more senses you engage, the more likely you are to achieve your health goal. Write your answers in the space provided. It's okay to leave spaces blank. Do what you can.

1. What does it *look* like to achieve your health goal?

2. What does it *feel* like to achieve your health goal?

3. What does it *sound* like to achieve your health goal?

4. What does it *smell* like to achieve your health goal?

5. What does it *taste* like to achieve your health goal?

____

____

____

Choose Your Affirmations

Sina: In addition to visualizing and feeling your goal, you must speak it out loud.

Have you noticed how many negative comments you hear or say each day? It's estimated that you create roughly 12,000 to 60,000 thoughts per day, and the majority of those thoughts are negative! Sitting in that space of negativity will hinder your ability to achieve your health goal. So, again, don't focus on what you don't want; focus on what you do want. For example, have you ever said any of the following statements?

"I'm tired."

"I feel overwhelmed."

"I look fat."

"I just want to feel good."

"I feel alone."

"I don't want to be sick anymore."

"I have ____________ " (Fill in the blank with cancer, diabetes, heart disease, Autoimmune Disease, allergies, etcetera).

You don't feel better when you say those statements. In fact, they keep you from achieving your health goal because when you say negative words, such as "I'm fat," every cell in your body hears those words and responds accordingly by making chemicals that result in more inflammation, which promotes weight gain. In other words, you can make yourself fat by telling yourself you are fat. Likewise, you can make yourself sick by telling yourself you are sick. You can make yourself tired by saying you are tired, and so forth.

Toxic words create a toxic environment. Every time you say something negative to yourself, imagine a bucket of toxic chemicals is being poured over every cell in your body. Those toxins make you tired, fat, and inflamed.

If you don't want to be tired, fat and inflamed then stop dumping toxins on yourself. Instead of speaking negatively to yourself, *choose* health by changing your words – speak life over your body, mind, and spirit.

Joel: We know this propensity toward negativity is normal because we call Stop Lights Stop Lights and not Go Lights. Have you ever come home announcing, "Honey, guess how many Go Lights I encountered?" We remember and dwell on what stops us far more than what makes us go. This is called "hard wired to negativity."

Sina: Exactly! And, it's so easy to fall into that trap. When I was debilitatingly sick, I focused on the disease for a long time. I was stuck in a space of fear – afraid I'd always be sick, afraid my quality of life would continue to decline, afraid the pain would never stop, afraid nobody could heal me, and afraid that I would die young and miss out on seeing my children grow up. Consequently, my inner dialogue was filled with negative statements. And, as long as I focused on the negativity, I continued to get worse. Then, one day, I learned a concept that sounds so simple, yet it profoundly changed my life:

What you believe becomes your reality.

Have you heard of the placebo effect? It's when you believe that something or someone will heal you, and so you are healed. For example, people have healed from disease after taking a sugar pill because they thought they were receiving a remedy and they believed that pill would heal them. But it was their belief that actually did the healing.

Interestingly, the placebo effect is often looked upon as a bad thing. In fact, most scientists hate the placebo effect. They try to control for it, or rule it out, when conducting studies. That's why the "gold standard" for clinical studies is called "double-blind, placebo-controlled." But the placebo effect is powerful! While scientists hate it because they can't explain it, it's a miraculous tool that you can access any time you want. All you have to do is believe.

On the other side of the coin is the nocebo effect. That's the belief that you should be sick or are going to get sick, and so you become sick. For instance, the Framingham Heart Study is the most comprehensive and influential investigation into heart disease in history. It established traditional risk factors for heart disease, such as high blood pressure and diabetes.

That study analyzed women with similar risk factors for heart disease. In theory, since they all had similar risk factors, all of the women should have developed heart disease in similar numbers. But, that's not what happened.

The women who *believed* they were prone to heart disease were nearly *4 times* more likely to die from heart disease compared with women who didn't believe they were prone to heart disease. This is a powerful, documented example of how negative belief can make you sick.

Joel: Perhaps the best illustration we've had of this principle on our farm revolves around what to call poor doer calves. With about 1,000 head of cattle, we always have some that lag behind. They might be a bit sickly, thin, rough coated. They just aren't keeping up. We used to separate them into a group that we called "The Scuzzballs." So, we had the brood cow herd, the finisher herd, the stocker herd, the bred heifers, and the scuzzballs. Bud Williams, long time cattle whisperer guru, heard Daniel and I use the condescending term and remonstrated us. "Quit using that; you're beaming negative emotions and energy at that group of calves."

We took it to heart and began calling it the Wolfpack. The idea was that these sickly calves were the ones the wolves would have gotten in natural herds. We were saving them from the wolves by giving them extra care and attention. The most amazing thing happened. Rather than fighting the problems of the scuzzballs, we began thinking about how to make life better for the wolfpack.

Our change of attitude made us examine some of our husbandry principles and eventually we made some changes to weaning dates and management. By shifting our emotions to saving the animals instead of being frustrated at their poor performance, we saw things we could change and within two years, we had no wolfpack. Today, this group does not exist because we have so few poor doers they don't even merit a separate group. We have several, of course, but we simply place them in our smallest herd and incorporate them with virtually no special care. With our emphasis on faith in performance rather than fear of failure, we came up with numerous ideas to raise the health of the whole herd. Amazing.

Sina: Wow! What an amazing example of the power of belief. You created health in an animal by changing your belief about that animal! That's powerful. And, if Joel can create health in a cow by changing his belief, you can certainly create health in your own body!

Not only can you change your health with your beliefs, you can do it instantly. For example, a study out of Stanford reported that when people were told they had a gene that protects them from being obese, their physiology changed in real time!

Researchers gave subjects a meal and then measured their leptin (a hormone associated with feeling full). A week later, the researchers told half of the subjects that they had the protective gene, and then gave them the same meal and measured their leptin again. The level of leptin in their blood was 2.5 times higher than the week before!

Here's the kicker: Not all of those subjects had the protective gene! Yet, their leptin level significantly increased! Among the subjects that did not have the gene, the *belief* that they had it caused a physiological response. In other words, the belief of the subject overrode their genes!

This finding is remarkable because researchers are continually looking for the newest pharmaceutical drug that can override our genes in an attempt to "cure" sickness and disease. But the medicine you need in order to be healthy and free is already inside of you. You are fully capable of healing yourself and achieving maximal health and wellness. It begins with belief.

Once I understood the power of belief, I realized that I was keeping myself sick. Instead of speaking life over my body, mind, and spirit, I was speaking death. So, I decided to shift my belief system away from fear and towards my goal of complete healing. For example, to let go of my fear, I raised my level of consciousness. I knew that my beliefs were creating my perception. And, it was my perception that ultimately led to fear, pain, lack of energy, and disease. So, I changed my perception by changing my word choices. I began to *choose* healing words. Every negative thought and negative statement was replaced with a positive affirmation:

"I'm tired" became **"I am full of energy."**

"I feel overwhelmed" became **"I will accomplish everything I want to get done."**

"I look fat" became **"I look amazing."**

"I just want to feel good" became **"I feel fantastic."**

"I feel alone" became **"I am loved and accepted."**

"I don't want to be sick anymore" became "**I am vibrantly healthy and whole.**"

"I have ____ disease" became **"I am fully healed."**

In the beginning, I didn't always believe the positive affirmations because I was in so much pain. But I said them out loud anyway. Every day, I repeated them over and over. Eventually, those words became my reality. In partnership with diet changes, my change in perception allowed me to become disease-free and filled with energy within one year. If you allow it, positive affirmations can help you achieve your health goal too.

YOUR TURN: What you tell yourself becomes your reality. What do you want your reality to be? Choose your positive affirmations. Write them here:

____

____

____

____

____

Every morning, greet the day by saying your positive affirmations out loud. Throughout the day, if you catch yourself choosing negative words, immediately replace them with your positive affirmations.

The Whole Picture

Sina: On your personalized road map, you now have a health goal, a visual with associated emotions, and positive affirmations. Let's complete your road map by painting the whole picture.

Joel: When I talk with folks about food provenance, I want them to visualize the place where it was produced. In terms of the beef, what did the animals look like that provided the hamburger? Do you know? How were they raised? Were they in grassy pastures or knee-deep in manure in a feedlot?

Like Sina says, we can't just be against food chemicals or animal abuse; we have to viscerally picture a beautiful alternative. Whatever ugly farm pictures you've seen, juxtapose those with the pretty ones you've seen. In your mind, create a vision of a healthy farm. What does the soil look like? The fields? The animals? The overall landscape? The vegetables? Wildlife? Biological complexity? Is the water clean?

YOUR TURN: What does trust look like to you? Take a moment to write a brief description of the kind of farm you'd like your food to come from. You can even include the kind of mindset you'd like the farmer to possess. Explain your fantasy farm and farmer here:

____

____

____

____

____

Joel: Our last category is Maximal Personal Responsibility. Every day I deal with some continuing element of abuse that happened before our family arrived on our farm. Just a couple of days ago I was cutting firewood and hit some wire fence embedded in a tree. That fence is probably a hundred years old; the tree grew around it and it ruined the chain on my saw and stopped me from working.

My first emotion, of course, was irritation and anger at whoever had nailed a fence wire to that tree a century ago. Around our farm, one way to earn everlasting punishment is to nail something – anything – to a tree. Even a tree house. We built one when the children were small and I fastened it in the tree with ropes so that no wire or nails could ever be embedded in the tree.

But after venting my negative thoughts about the situation, I smiled at my own victim mentality and realized I was ridding the farm of something sinister and vicious. The wire hurt the tree and it could have hurt me if the saw had encountered it differently. But now the farm was rid of that problem and becoming more beautiful, more functional. Nobility and sacredness in our activity go a long way to overcoming the anger and tension of day-to-day imperfections. Goodness, imperfections are all around us, from relationships to policies to computer glitches.

Aggressively visualizing and appreciating that our mindset can deal with these things either as sinister opponents or ministry opportunities can go a long way in moving us from a state of perpetual agitation to a state of ongoing service and encouragement. Even though I did not install the wire fence, it's my fence now – my responsibility.

Are you angry at factory farmers? Are you angry at farmers who feed antibiotics and encourage *C. Difficile* and MRSA in hospitals? Are you angry at the farmers who created the Rhode Island-sized dead zone in the Gulf of Mexico? What are you doing about it?

Sina: I was angry for a long time when I started learning about our food supply. I remember sitting in my room conducting research for my first book when I became so angry about the corruption in our food supply. I couldn't contain my emotions any longer, so I walked downstairs and proceeded to tell my husband all the ways in which I was angry. Because husbands love that, right?

I told my husband that I was angry with the medical establishment for not being able to help me. I was angry with the government and the food industry for not protecting our food supply. And, I was angry with the media for covering up the truth and not being honest reporters.

After patiently listening to my rant, my husband asked, "What are you *really* angry about? Because you already know the system is corrupt. That's nothing new. So, what are you *really* angry about?"

From out of nowhere I blurted out, "I'm angry because *they* made me sick!"

Almost immediately he retorted, "No. No, *they* didn't. *You* made yourself sick. *You chose* to eat the foods that made you sick. And, it was your body that eventually gave out because of the choices *you* made."

How well do you think that went over? I was so angry with my husband. For the first time in our marriage, I felt like he abandoned me. But, as I calmed down, I began to wonder if there was some truth behind his comments. So, I prayed about it, and I received clarity:

I did *choose* to be sick.

I didn't intentionally make myself sick. But I did *choose* sickness.

And, it wasn't until my husband called me out that I realized I perceived myself as a "victim" because instead of taking responsibility, I was still blaming the system.

It's interesting because I used to think that I took responsibility for my life. I have always stood on my own two feet. I've worked hard my whole life, and have earned everything I have. But, that's not the type of responsibility I'm talking about.

The truth is:

I *chose* to be part of a medical system that says disease is not reversible, but we can mask your symptoms with drugs.

And, I *chose* to eat the foods that got me sick. I blindly trusted the food system. I *chose* to be an uneducated consumer.

However, once I began taking responsibility for my own health - including changing my diet, lifestyle, and perspective - my healing was rapid. I was able to get off the floor in 3 days! Within 3 months, nearly all of the pain was gone. And, within one year, there were no signs of disease in my body. The autoimmune disease had disappeared!

My rapid healing began when I let go of my anger and took responsibility for my life – sickness and all.

Joel: It's okay to be angry for a moment, but the sooner we can turn that into positive activity the better we'll be. Start with something small, such as deciding what's on your "perfect plate."

YOUR TURN: Close your eyes, and ask your body which foods would be nourishing and healing for you. Steamed vegetables? Grass-fed beef? Sauerkraut? Rice? Don't stress about what you think "should" be on your plate. As we journey through this book together, you can change what's on your plate. For now, we encourage you to begin thinking about what your ideal plate might look like. Draw your "perfect plate" on the following page.

Let's take this one step further. You know what industrial farms do and what they look like, and you know what the processing facilities look like that give us compromised food. What does the good stuff look like? Where does the good stuff come from?

YOUR TURN: Take each food item on your "perfect plate," and describe what you'd like its journey to look like – from the farm to your plate. What did it look like growing at the farm? What did it look like being transported to you? What did it look like being prepared for your

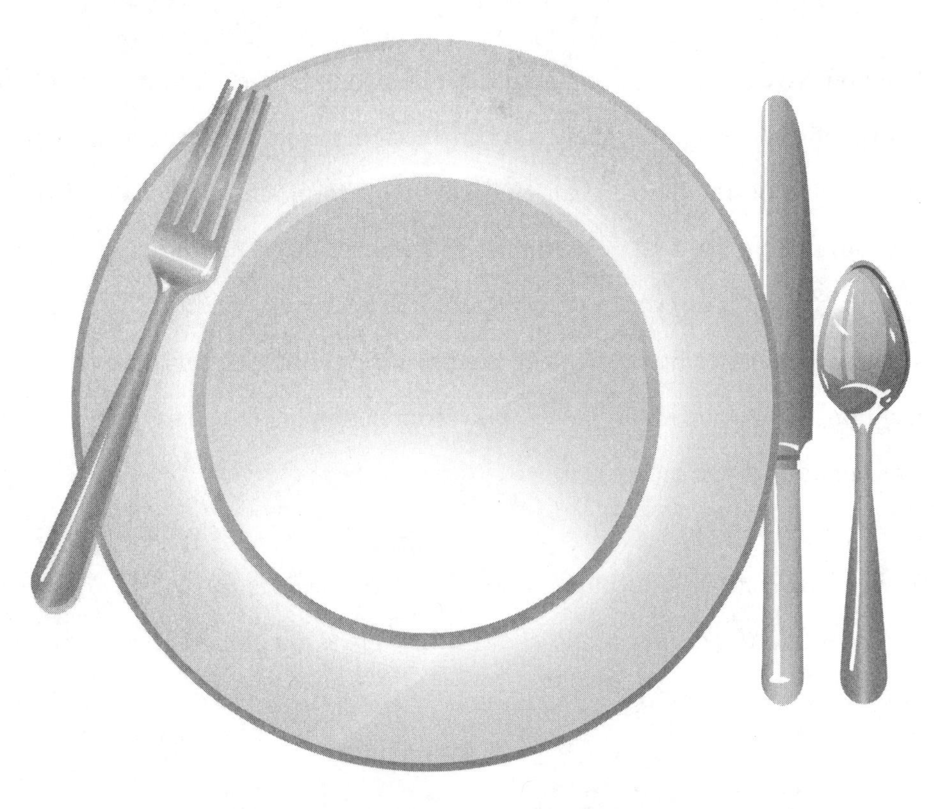

plate? Go ahead, be imaginative, and describe the journey for the different components of the meal.

Item #1 ____

____

____

Item #2 ____

____

____

Item #3 ____

____

____

Item #4 ____

____

____

Sina: You now have several different goals listed on your personalized road map. Don't allow that to overwhelm you. This exercise is partly designed to bring awareness. Again, we encourage you to focus on the health goal. And, as you incorporate the "Practical Bites" in this book, you will move toward all of your goals simultaneously – one step at a time.

Our goal is to help you turn your picture of health into reality, one Practical Bite at a time. You may still have a little way to go after reading this book, but that's okay. As we previously mentioned, there are many variables involved in moving to the right on the road map. But, at a minimum, we can help you move closer to your goal.

As we journey through this book together, remember to continuously focus on your goal, positive affirmations and your picture of maximal health. By focusing on what you want, you will be motivated to make food choices that move you along the road map toward maximal health.

CHAPTER 3

Set Yourself Up For Success

Sina: Now that you know where you are headed, it's helpful to know your starting point. We've designed a quiz to loosely gauge where you are currently spending most of your time on the road map. This quiz is not scientific. The purpose is to bring *awareness* to your current habits.

As you answer the questions, don't judge yourself. Negative thoughts and emotions will not help you achieve your goal. Besides, you're answering questions about behaviors that have already happened; they are in the past. You have the opportunity to make different choices, starting right now. So, have fun with this quiz! Think of it as our version of a Cosmopolitan® quiz, except instead of helping you find your "perfect mate," our quiz is helping you become aware of your food choices so you can find your "perfect plate."

1. **If you wanted to cook spaghetti, what would you use for the sauce?**
   A. I buy prepared spaghetti sauce from the grocery store.
   B. I buy prepared organic spaghetti sauce from the grocery store.
   C. I make the sauce using whole, organic tomatoes from the grocery store.
   D. I make the sauce using locally grown tomatoes.
   E. I make the sauce using tomatoes picked from my garden.

2. **If you wanted to eat hamburger meat, which would you choose?**
   A. Whatever is on sale at the grocery store.
   B. Organic from the grocery store.
   C. Meat from my local farmer.
   D. Meat from my own herd.

3. **When you are craving a cookie, what do you do?**
   A. Drive to the grocery store and buy the least expensive box of cookies that still looks yummy.
   B. Drive to the grocery store and buy an organic box of cookies.
   C. Make cookies from scratch.
   D. I don't eat cookies.

4. **You want to make a salad, where do you buy the lettuce?**
   A. From a grocery store.
   B. From my local farmer.
   C. I grow it myself.

5. **When reading an ingredient label, what do you try to avoid the most?**
   A. Foods high in calories.
   B. GMOs.
   C. Fat.
   D. Any ingredient I cannot pronounce.
   E. I don't read ingredient labels.

6. **When buying breakfast cereal, what do you primarily look for?**
   A. Mascot or Spokesperson (such as Toucan Sam on Froot Loops® or Michael Jordan on Wheaties®)
   B. Non-GMO or Organic.
   C. No artificial coloring or flavoring.
   D. I don't eat cereal.

7. **Pretend you plan to eat chicken for dinner. Which type of chicken do you buy?**
   A. Chicken nuggets from a drive thru.
   B. Frozen chicken nuggets from a grocery store.
   C. Boneless, skinless chicken from a grocery store.
   D. Whole chicken from a grocery store.
   E. Whole chicken from my local farmer.
   F. Whole chicken from my own farm.

8. **How do you usually eat lunch?**
   A. Sitting at my desk while working or surfing the internet.
   B. In my car.
   C. Standing in the kitchen while trying to manage the children.

D. Sitting down in a relaxed state, such as eating with co-workers while having a light-hearted discussion.

E. Sitting down while watching the news or discussing politics or other possibly inflammatory topics.

9. When eating out, which establishment are you most likely to choose?

A. Gas station.

B. Fast food chain.

C. Casual restaurant such as Chipotle® or Saladworks®.

D. Restaurant that serves locally grown or organic foods.

E. I don't eat out.

10. Your doctor tells you to stop eating red meat, but you feel good when you eat it. What do you do?

A. Stop eating red meat. The doctor knows best.

B. Post on Facebook asking your friends if they think you should eat red meat and base your decision on their opinions.

C. Continue eating red meat because your body knows what's best for it.

11. You're running errands and you get thirsty. What do you do?

A. Buy a soda.

B. Take a drink of water from a water fountain.

C. Buy a bottled water.

D. Pop into a fast food establishment to grab a fountain soda and, while I'm at it, I grab a burger too.

E. Drink my own water. I always bring filtered water with me when I leave my house.

12. Do you currently have a garden that you tend to?

A. Yes

B. No

13. Have you ever visited a farm that is local to your home?

A. Yes

B. No

Calculate your overall score by adding up the points, listed below, for each answer:

1. **If you wanted to cook spaghetti, what would you use for the sauce?**
   A. I buy prepared spaghetti sauce from the grocery store. (1 point)
   B. I buy prepared organic spaghetti sauce from the grocery store. (2 points)
   C. I make the sauce using whole, organic tomatoes from the grocery store. (3 points)
   D. I make the sauce using locally grown tomatoes. (4 points)
   E. I make the sauce using tomatoes picked from my garden. (5 points)

2. **If you wanted to eat hamburger meat, which would you choose?**
   A. Whatever is on sale at the grocery store. (1 point)
   B. Grass-fed or organic from the grocery store (2 points)
   C. Meat from my local farmer. (4 points)
   D. Meat from my own herd. (5 points)

3. **When you are craving a cookie, what do you do?**
   A. Drive to the grocery store and buy the least expensive box of cookies that still looks yummy. (1 point)
   B. Drive to the grocery store and buy an organic box of cookies. (2 points)
   C. Make cookies from scratch. (3 points)
   D. I don't eat cookies. (4 points)

4. **You want to make a salad, where do you buy the lettuce?**
   A. From a grocery store. (1 point)
   B. From my local farmer. (3 points)
   C. I grow it myself. (4 points)

5. **When reading an ingredient label, what do you try to avoid the most?**
   A. Foods high in calories. (1 point)
   B. GMOs. (2 points)
   C. Fat. (1 point)
   D. Any ingredient I cannot pronounce. (2 points)
   E. I don't read ingredient labels. (0 points)

6. **When buying breakfast cereal, what do you primarily look for?**
   A. Mascot or Spokesperson (such as Toucan Sam on Froot Loops® or Michael Jordan on Wheaties®) (0 points)

B. Non-GMO or Organic. (1 point)
C. No artificial coloring or flavoring. (1 point)
D. I don't eat cereal. (2 points)

7. **Pretend you plan to eat chicken for dinner. Which type of chicken do you buy?**
A. Chicken nuggets from a drive thru. (0 points)
B. Frozen chicken nuggets from a grocery store. (0 points)
C. Boneless, skinless chicken from a grocery store. (1 point)
D. Whole chicken from a grocery store. (2 points)
E. Whole chicken from my local farmer. (3 points)
F. Whole chicken from my own farm. (4 points)

8. **How do you usually eat lunch?**
A. Sitting at my desk while working. (0 points)
B. In my car. (0 points)
C. Standing in the kitchen while trying to manage the children. (0 points)
D. Sitting down in a relaxed state, such as eating with co-workers while having a light-hearted discussion. (3 points)
E. Sitting down while watching the news or discussing politics or other possibly inflammatory topics. (0 points)

9. **When eating out, which establishment are you most likely to choose?**
A. Gas station. (0 points)
B. Fast food chain. (0 points)
C. Casual restaurants such as Chipotle® or Saladworks®. (1 point)
D. Restaurant that serves locally grown or organic foods. (3 points)
E. I rarely or never eat out. (3 points)

10. **Your doctor tells you to stop eating red meat, but you feel good when you eat it. What do you do?**
A. Step eating red meat. The doctor knows best. (0 points)
B. Post on Facebook asking your friends if they think you should eat red meat and base your decision on their opinions. (0 points)
C. Continue eating red meat because your body knows what's best for it. (3 points)

11. **You're running errands and you get thirsty. What do you do?**
A. Buy a soda. (0 points)
B. Take a drink of water from a water fountain. (2 points)

C. Buy a bottled water. (3 points)
D. Pop into a fast food establishment to grab a fountain soda and, while I'm at it, I grab a burger too. (0 points)
E. Drink my own water. I always bring filtered water with me when I leave my house. (5 points)

12. Do you currently have a garden that you tend to?

A. Yes (5 points)
B. No (0 points)

13. Have you ever visited a farm that is local to your home?

A. Yes (4 points)
B. No (0 points)

TOTAL SCORE: _______________

Based on your total score, determine which category you likely spend most of your time:

SCORE	CATEGORY
4-13	Processed Food
14-24	Higher Quality Processed Food
25-33	Whole Food from Grocery Store
34-42	Locally Grown Whole Food
43-49	Home-Grown Whole Food

Sina: The purpose of the quiz is to bring awareness to your eating habits, have a little fun, and introduce you to some of the principles we will discuss in the Practical Bites. So, no matter your score, don't dwell on it. Remember, while this quiz provides a rough idea of where you spend time on the road map, your exact location changes with each bite of food. That means, you have *many* opportunities throughout each day to move toward your goal. And, that's where we come in!

Move Toward Your Goal with Grace

Sina: All too often, we set goals for ourselves and never achieve them. I can't tell you how many New Year's resolutions I have broken. And, every time, I felt like a failure.

I believe we can set ourselves up to fail, in part, by establishing arbitrary deadlines. Then, we get upset with ourselves when we don't achieve the self-imposed goal within the self-imposed timeline. It's a system that constantly tells us we are "not good enough." So, we are not going to do that. Instead, we are going to set you up for success:

- We have provided 72 doable Practical Bites presented in a step-by-step approach to encourage lasting change.
- Each Practical Bite begins with a short "How" followed by a longer "Why," which provides you the freedom to choose whether or not you would like to explore our reasoning behind each Practical Bite.
- Many of the Practical Bites take 5 minutes or less to implement.
- There are no deadlines. You choose your own pace. You can pick one Practical Bite a day, one a week, or one a year! The timing doesn't matter. Choose a pace that's right for you.
- There is plenty of space for grace. The point is not to be perfect. The point is to be consistent. For instance, let's estimate that you take 100 bites of food every day. If you "slip up" at breakfast, it's okay. At your next meal, you get another chance. You still have roughly 75 bites of food left in that day. Therefore, you have 75 more opportunities to move toward your goal. Ideally, over time, more and more bites you take in any given day will be chosen with the intention of helping you shift to the right of the road map - toward your health goal.

The Practical Bites in this book will help you become more aware of your food choices. And, the step-by-step approach will help you develop healthy habits. It's those habits that will help you achieve greater health, happiness, freedom, trust, and personal responsibility.

Joel: Several principles come to bear on this issue. The first is that the tortoise wins the race, not the hare. While we don't want to be lackadaisical about things, we also don't want to get in such a big hurry that we move faster than we can metabolize the changes. Don't worry about speed; focus on direction, or trajectory. If your trajectory is right, let time be your friend and not your enemy. Go at a pace you can assimilate.

Second, remember that transition is incremental, not spontaneous. Certainly, explosions and lotteries occur, but they are not the norm. Most things are a slog, a faithful step by step movement toward a target. We're tempted too often to get impatient with transition rather than simply enjoy the transition as it unfolds. Many new farmers, for example, want to start with everything right now. Buildings, machinery, plants, animals. Next thing you know, they're in complete crisis mode.

They put the buildings in the wrong place, perhaps a wet area. They put the fences in the wrong place and the animals won't flow from field to field. They got plants that won't grow where they planted them, or animals that don't do well in the environment. A host of things can go wrong. In order to minimize the catastrophe, stop and smell the step. Enjoy the incremental movement. Sina and I hereby give you the freedom to transition at your own pace. We challenge you to do something today, but we also give you the freedom to not do everything today.

Third, persuasion also occurs one step at a time. Let's say on a scale of 1 to 10 a 1 is a person who's eating food primarily out of the gas station. A 10 is the person with a garden, feeding kitchen scraps to a couple of chickens who lay eggs for the home, grows and grinds her own grain with a mill in the kitchen to make her own bread - you get the type. When we have discussions, too often the persuader tries to move the persuadee too fast up this continuum.

It doesn't work. If the gas station junkie can just get some raw fruit at the produce department of the grocery store, that's a huge step up. Sina and I are extremely cognizant that if we don't respect where you are and if we don't appreciate your context; if we just go pulpit-pounding into the 10, so to speak, we'll lose you. That argumentation is not helpful; it's off-putting and irritating. That's why we're starting gentle, at the 1, and moving methodically toward 10.

Sina: And, it's okay if you don't want to reach 10! Not everyone wants to grow their own food and be fully independent. I'm not at 10! I grow vegetables and herbs in my garden, but I also buy food from local farmers, grocery stores, and online companies that are aligned with my principles. And, that's okay too.

We will meet you where you are. But you have to meet yourself where you are too. As we take this journey together, allow yourself the space to adopt the Practical Bites that resonate with you and to move past the ones that don't. You don't need to reach the end of the book in order to succeed. Every single step is an accomplishment!

Above all else, focus on one bite at a time. With each bite of food, refer back to the road map to see if it passes the litmus test:

1. Does it bring me closer to my health goal?
2. Does it give me more freedom?
3. Does it give me more trust in my food supply?

If the answer to any of those questions is no and you still choose to eat that food, *that's okay!* The point is not to deprive yourself or punish yourself for not being "perfect." The point is to make conscious decisions that will move you toward your goal, one step at a time, while allowing room for grace. So, have fun with it! Do what you can, and remember to visit our websites to receive encouragement and supplemental material, such as cooking videos. You're not alone! We're in this together!

www.PolyfaceFarms.com

www.HandsOffMyFood.com

SECTION 2:

Step Up Your Game With Convenience

CHAPTER 4

Shift From Low To High Quality Processed Food

Most Americans spend most of their time in this first category. In fact, the typical American consumes at least *75% of their calories from processed foods.* Generally speaking, if it's prepared and packaged, it's a processed food. Examples include: cereal, crackers, cookies, chips, T.V. dinners, pizza, lunch meat, and soda. This category also includes fast food and restaurants.

In general, processed foods represent lack of health, lack of freedom, and lack of trust. For example, these foods typically contain genetically modified organisms (GMOs), preservatives, additives, artificial or natural flavoring, artificial sweetener or hormones, pesticides, and/or chemicals that are generally recognized as safe (GRAS). All of those chemicals – in one form or another - are associated with inflammatory diseases, such as: heart disease, diabetes, cancer, arthritis, allergies, and attention-deficit/hyperactivity disorder (ADHD).

The goal of this chapter is to help you move from Low Quality Processed Foods to High Quality Processed Foods, which includes foods that are still prepared and packaged for you, but are a step up in quality. Examples include: processed foods that are organic or do not contain GMOs, pesticides, herbicides, preservatives, additives, artificial or natural flavoring or coloring, GRAS chemicals, artificial sweeteners or hormones.

By switching from Low Quality Processed Foods to High Quality Processed Foods, you still enjoy the convenience of buying prepared food from a grocery store or restaurant, while simultaneously achieving huge health gains with minimal effort.

Practical Bite #1: Harness Your Power

How? You have the power to shape your food supply into what you want it to be. All you have to do is selectively give your consent. We call it, "Feed the Good and Starve the Bad." Buy food from companies and farmers that are aligned with your principles, and stop buying food from companies and farmers that are not aligned with your principles. If you don't know who you support right now, don't worry. You'll figure it out as we walk this journey together.

Why?

Sina: This is our longest Practical Bite because it's a foundational concept that you will apply throughout the entirety of the book. So, don't worry, the other Practical Bites are quicker reads.

Let's talk about genetically modified organisms (GMOs). Every living organism is made up of DNA, which is organized into segments called genes. Those genes determine your eye color, height, skin color, and other traits that make you unique. GMOs are plants, animals, or other organisms whose genes have been permanently changed in a laboratory. For instance, scientists can take a gene from one species, such as a human, and put that gene into a completely different species, such as a pig. These combinations cannot occur naturally through breeding. In fact, scientists have already created cows that produce human breast milk and pigs with noses that light up because their genes are combined with jellyfish genes.

Since you are reading this book, you are most likely against GMOs. However, for just a moment, let's put down our pitchforks and try to be neutral. Let's forget about trying to "prove" that GMOs are "bad" or "good" because there's a bigger lesson to be learned from GMOs.

Take a moment and really think about this question: What is the job of the FDA? Write your answer down here:

____

____

____

____

Now I'll tell you the story of how GMOs were "approved" by the FDA. And, let's see if your answer changes.

Before I researched GMOs, I assumed the FDA had conducted safety studies on GMOs before approving them for us to eat. That sounds like a reasonable assumption. After all, the FDA claims to be "responsible for protecting the public health…by ensuring the safety of our nation's food supply." But I was wrong.

The FDA "presumed" GMOs to be "generally recognized as safe" (GRAS). When a chemical is declared to be GRAS, it means that chemical is not tested for safety by the FDA, nor is it regulated by the FDA. The company who makes the chemical determines if that chemical is safe for you to eat. All they need is an "expert" to declare the chemical to be GRAS. Usually the "experts" have financial ties to the company. Even worse, once a chemical is declared GRAS, the company can immediately begin adding it to your food. And they don't even have to notify the FDA! The notification process is voluntary.

Since GMOs are "presumed" to be GRAS, the FDA does not test them for safety nor do they test them for toxicity. Instead, the companies making the GMOs determine if their GMOs are safe for us to eat. Yet, most Americans eat GMOs every single day. And, they don't question the safety. Why?

Most of us assume that if GMOs are allowed to be sold in our grocery stores, they are safe. We assume the FDA has tested them for safety or thoroughly vetted GMOs during the approval process. But, they didn't. The FDA gave GMOs a free pass from the lab to your dinner plate. Again, I ask you: What is the job of the FDA?

If the FDA is not testing GRAS chemicals for safety and they are not testing GMOs for safety, then who is ensuring the safety of our food?

Joel: I'm ensuring the safety of the food I raise and sell. But that's a rarity. Essentially, government oversight is a huge cover-your-tail program for big food companies. This all goes back to Upton Sinclair's book *The Jungle* published in 1906. If you know anything about the evolution of American food policy and government oversight, you know this was the defining moment. Sinclair's book theme was about horrible worker treatment at the nation's big slaughterhouses. He was a Socialist who wanted to raise awareness about worker treatment.

But the book had an unintended consequence: sales from big food brands dropped nearly 50 percent within 6 months of the book being published. Where did people get their food? They went back to their little local butchers, back to neighborhood farms (remember at that time the U.S. had 5 times as many farms as we do today) and a more trustworthy local food provenance.

The big companies begged Teddy Roosevelt to establish a government bureaucracy that would certify them as okay and get their credibility back with the American consumer. Had Roosevelt told these companies, "You made your own bed, now lie in it," many would have gone bankrupt and the local food system would have come out on top. But he gave them the Food Safety Inspection Service (FSIS) within the United Stated Department of Agriculture (USDA). This agency worked with the big food companies to create protocols that would supposedly guarantee food safety. If a company complied with the regulations, it would receive the USDA inspected stamp of approval, known as "the blue buzz," which approved it as legal to sell.

Whenever a food-borne illness crops up, what's the first response from the CEO of the implicated brand? Does he apologize? No. Does he say they're going to do things differently? No. He calls a press conference and drones on about how "we've complied with every government food safety requirement" blah blah blah. Essentially, government inspection gives cover for companies not to have to take personal responsibility for their food. Companies hide behind the government skirts to absolve the business of liability and responsibility. It sure beats personal accountability.

Of course, these government requirements to get approval often adulterate food. Whether it's GRAS or procedures like overheating (mandatory milk pasteurization) or antimicrobial use like chlorine, many of us do not want to adhere to these protocols. You would think that we, the farmers, would have the choice to opt in or out. We don't. Interestingly, whenever I've been involved with efforts to create an opt-out possibility, one of the first arguments the well-meaning bureaucrats put forth is about liability. "We'd hate to see you lose your farm over a lawsuit because you didn't have government approval." Doesn't that sound charitable?

As you can imagine, the government standards were relatively easy for big outfits to adopt because they primarily involved paperwork and infrastructure, both of which are easier to afford if you're a big operation. This regulatory prejudice against scale, inherently discriminating against smaller outfits, is ongoing. Every time we've had a modernization of these standards, within two years we lose half of our abattoirs. Welcome to the real world of abdicating knowledge because you trust the government.

The government's truth record is not good. From hydrogenated vegetable oil to the food pyramid that put crackers on the bottom, it should give us all pause to realize we would be a far healthier nation if the government had never told us what to eat. It did, though. And people who had grown accustomed to having the government take care of their education, their retirement, their creeks and rivers and a host of other things gave over their food oversight to a fraternity that believes certain things. It believes technology cures everything. It believes food and life are fundamentally mechanical, not biological. It believes people are much smarter than nature.

The result is that as a populace, we've become incredibly ignorant about food and naively trusting whenever a credentialed government expert speaks. So, in the end, you can't trust government oversight. You have to know enough to find the right people to trust. I wish it were easy, but it's not. Just like we put attention on planning a cruise or European vacation or finding a good car mechanic, we have to put attention on planning for our food quality. And as financial guru Dave Ramsey says, we tend to be successful at the things we put attention on.

Sina: I used to spend more time looking up movie and book reviews than I did looking up what's in my food. I blindly trusted our food supply, and it got me debilitatingly sick. Now that my blinders are off, I understand that "We the People" are responsible for ensuring the safety of our own food. Consequently, it's our responsibility to hold companies accountable. This may come as a shock, but the FDA agrees with us! Here's a quote directly from an FDA document on food safety:

> "...the lack of awareness and information about the [safety] risks suggests that an inefficiently **low demand may exist** for food products that are produced using adequate measures to **prevent foodborne illnesses, adulteration, or contamination.** Because the demand for many manufactured or processed foods may not be sufficiently affected

by safety considerations, incentives to invest in safety measures from farm to fork is diminished. Consequently, **the market may not provide the incentives** necessary for optimal food safety." [emphasis added]

The FDA sees us as the solution. They are asking us to be informed consumers. Our food is susceptible to "foodborne illnesses, adulteration, or contamination" because we are not demanding safety.

Think about it: Why would a company spend money and resources on safety if the customer is not demanding it? Look at it from a company's perspective. Most negative health effects are likely to occur in the long-term. It may take 20 or 30 years for an illness to develop from a single chemical in our food. How can you "prove" that one chemical caused your illness? You can't. So, there's no real incentive for long-term safety - unless we demand it.

Joel: Good point. One of the biggest issues in testing toxicity involves the Lethal Dose benchmark, known as LD. The question all the regulators want to know is what's the dose that kills you, or a rat or whatever. In other words, once that's established, they can then back off dosages to nonlethal and it's okay. Folks, I wish I were making this up, but believe me, truth is stranger than fiction.

I well remember when Bill Wolf, founder of Necessary Trading Company, one of the nation's first large suppliers to ecologically-minded farmers, was trying to get seaweed approved as a soil amendment. Because fertilizers must carry an LD designation, companies must submit testing and paperwork to the government so a magic number can go on the label. Bill started feeding rats this kelp and they just got healthier and healthier. They wouldn't die. Finally, in exasperation, he got a bucket of water and put some kelp in it and drowned the rats so he could have some mortality to check the box. Yes, he did indeed find the LD for the label and received government approval.

The problem with LD testing is that it does not account for long-term exposure to a chemical. You have to be able to see results quickly. You can't do an LD test and wait 10 years for your test subjects to die. Science wants data right now, and of course the label needs it right now. But, as we all know, cumulative affects often take years or even decades to show toxicity.

Goodness, it took 14 years to connect DDT (a synthetic insecticide) to eagle eggs that wouldn't hatch, three-legged salamanders, and infertile frogs. We look back on that time period and wonder why in the world it took so long. But that's the nature of nature - it's pretty resilient. Which is one of the most exciting things about this book. Sina and I know that if you move along the roadmap to a place of integrity and authentic food, your health legacy can change dramatically. Once the culture abandoned DDT by being made aware of its toxicity, nature returned to normal fairly quickly. That's ultimately extremely hopeful, don't you think?

Another issue in LD testing is what is known as a cocktail. All testing is done with only one compound. But seldom are compounds used in isolation. Nobody tests what happens when you take two drugs or when a farmer mixes two chemicals. All the testing is done singularly. That particular product or pharmaceutical gets its label from testing in isolation. But, in real life, it is immediately dumped into a cornucopia of chemicals and compounds used together.

The question each of us must answer is this: who will you trust? Does the government deserve your trust? Who earns your trust? Obviously the one you can trust the most is yourself. We'll help you find others to trust, but it starts with yourself. Dear folks, if you can't trust yourself, where will you turn? You'll be stressed and feel like every tiger in the world is after you if you can't step up to enough confidence to trust yourself.

Sina: If you don't trust yourself to make good food choices right now, don't worry. By the end of the book you will! You'll gain confidence on our journey together and, who knows, maybe you'll be able to help your friends and family by sharing what you learn.

For now, it's important to understand that you are the solution. That's how the system was originally set up when the FDA was created. The system was designed for you to play an active role in ensuring the safety of the food you eat. So, how do you engage in the system? How do you become the watchdog you were meant to be?

You harness your power.

Our Republic was built on the premise that all power lies within the people. According to the Declaration of Independence, "Governments are instituted among Men, deriving their just powers from the consent of the governed." The key word is "consent." That means, each of us has the power to restore the integrity of the food we eat and reclaim the freedoms we have lost by taking back our consent.

Your consent is what gives government and industry authority and influence over your food supply. To change your food supply, you simply need to selectively give your consent. But, how do you selectively give your consent?

You are already giving your consent. Each time you spend money at a grocery store, fast food restaurant, vending machine, or hot dog stand, you speak with your dollars. For instance, when I used to drink Mountain Dew®, I was saying that I was okay drinking a flame-retardant. And, when I ate Doritos®, I was consenting to allow scientists to change the unique genetic make-up of our plants and animals.

Every day, the food industry and the government hear your message loud and clear. They hear you through your dollars. You are voting for your food supply with your dollars. And, that's an amazing opportunity sitting right in front of you because it means that you help create your food supply. It's a reflection of how you spend your dollars. Consequently, you have the ability to shape your food supply into what you want it to be. You don't need government or industry to fix the problem. The power lies within the people.

So, what will you do with your power? What will you stand for?

I used to stand for the Pillsbury Doughboy®. But, one day, I flipped over the box of cake mix and read the ingredient label. I realized that he stands for propylene glycol, which is used to make antifreeze and paint and may be toxic to the central nervous system in the long-term. He also stands for xanthan gum, which is an emulsifier that can change your gut microflora. And, the Doughboy stands for BHT, which is used in embalming fluid and jet fuel and can promote tumor growth and damages DNA, in the long-term.

If I don't want to stand for toxic, synthetic chemicals in my cake mix, what can I do about it?

I can send a message to the government and the food industry by not buying that cake mix. But, standing for your principles doesn't mean you can't have your cake. It means you support companies aligned with your principles. I call it "Feed the Good & Starve the Bad."

For instance, there are cake mixes currently on the market that do not contain synthetic, untested chemicals. You can eat cake while standing for your principles by supporting those companies.

Joel: At this point, Sina, the temptation is to throw up our hands in hopelessness and helplessness. As we've gone through this explanation of the real world, for some people, their whole support structure, their whole world just crumbled.

I can hear the response coming back through these pages, "But I don't have time to vet my food. I don't have time to ferret out better provenance. It's too complicated. I don't know enough. I work a job and come home and have to fix supper and I already get up an hour before the kids to get them some breakfast before sending them off to school and and and .... It's just too much."

I get it. And that's why we're coaching you on a continuum of Practical Bites at a pace you choose so you'll be able to pat yourself on the back for doing one, but you'll also be challenged that another one awaits your accomplishment. It's like a huge treasure hunt, and the treasure is your personal and our corporate planetary health. That's a pretty awesome treasure, and worth going after, don't you think?

Sina: I do! And, the hardest part about harnessing your power is usually taking the first step. But, rest assured, every time you selectively give your consent, you will make a difference! That's the beauty of standing for your principles; we know it works! We have the data to prove it. For instance, in 2014, carrageenan was removed from Silk® soy milk, Silk® coconut milk, and Horizon® organic flavored milks. Why? According to the company, "Our consumers have expressed a desire for products without it and we are listening!"

In 2015, General Mills Inc. removed artificial flavors and colors from their cereals. Why? According to the company, "Our cereal team is always listening to consumers about how we can improve our cereals and make them better. In recent years, we've heard that artificial ingredients aren't what you are looking for in your bowl. So today...we are committing to remove artificial flavors and colors..."

I can continue listing free market wins all day long. But I'll share just one more because it's my favorite example. In 2016, Campbell's® pledged to label their products containing GMOs. Why? According to the company, "We are operating with a 'Consumer First' mindset. We put the consumer at the center of everything we do. GMO has evolved to be a top consumer food issue reaching a critical mass..."

That's the key – a critical mass. We need to reach a tipping point if we want to move the market. And, it doesn't take as many people as you might think. For example, Jeffrey Smith, founder of the Institute for Responsible Technology, estimates it will take **5% of the population to get GMOs out of our food supply.** That's a minority!

We can be that minority! We don't have to wait and hope that the government fixes our food supply. We don't have to wait and hope that the food industry fixes our food supply. "We the People" can fix it. All you have to do is harness your God-given power. And, it's as easy as "Feed the Good & Starve the Bad."

Joel: So, the cool thing is we don't have to be victims. We don't have to trust smoke and mirrors. We don't need a law and we don't need a new government agency. Collectively, all of us food buyers determine what's available in the marketplace and how farmers farm.

I was talking with a farmer friend the other day about an initiative in his county to outlaw Concentrated Animal Feeding Operations (CAFOs), commonly known as factory farms. His neighbor has a poultry CAFO and like most farmers, he's a decent guy, honest, hardworking. He's not evil or sinister. He doesn't want to pollute the river or give somebody *C. diff.* But he's raising chickens this way because it's what the market demands. The day the market demand changes, we won't have CAFOs. We won't have GMOs. It's really that simple.

I'm reminded of the old proverb where a boy has two identical puppies and asks his Grandpa which one will grow bigger. Grandpa wisely responds, "the one you feed." That's the way markets are; the ones we patronize are the ones that grow.

A while back, the administrator of the dining services at a college contacted me about putting our pork in one of the dining venues on campus. I asked him why he called me. People like that don't call farmers. His answer was profound: "The students asked for you."

Sometimes just for fun I play an imaginary game. What would the world look like if everyone spent money the way I do? You know how it is: each of us is the center of the universe, or at least that's kind of the way we view things. What if everybody bought what I bought and didn't buy what I don't buy? That's a fascinating exercise.

Be forewarned, I'm really a maverick. So, I don't have a TV. Imagine the world without TVs. The laptop works very fine, thank you. No lottery tickets, ever. No gambling, ever. (Goodness, I spoke at a conference in Las Vegas. I was there for 36 hours, ate nothing, purchased nothing, went nowhere except my speaking gig. I wonder if that's some sort of record?) No Kardashians. No chemical fertilizers, pesticides, or herbicides. No McDonald's®, Burger King®, or Wal-Mart®. Boy, this "world accordin' to me" is an interesting place, don't you think? No designer clothes, no automobiles more than $30,000. No coffee. No Caribbean cruises. Okay, enough. As ridiculous as this sounds, though, you know as well as I do that if everybody spent their money this way, all the things I DON'T buy would soon cease to exist.

The truth is that, for many people, if beer is in the fridge, the NFL is on the TV, and the sofa is holding together, life is good. That defines the level of consciousness for most people, unfortunately. But you aren't most people. As Dr. Seuss would say, "you are you." And never underestimate how few people actually make the rules. You can be a rule maker for a food make over.

Back in my newspaper reporter days before I returned to the farm full time, I would cover lots of public meetings and hearings. I always left those meetings amazed at how few people actually determine what happens. When you make your views known, when you make noise, it creates awareness and movement. Never underestimate the power of one.

Sina: So, harness your power. With every bite of food, you send a message to your body. You are determining your health by changing your gut microbiome, hormones, level of inflammation, and gene expression. But, with every bite of food, you also send a message to the food industry and the government. You tell them what you want your food supply to look like.

So, what message will you send today? What message will you send your body? And, what message will you send to the food industry and our government?

Practical Bite #2: Find A Buddy

How? Find a friend or family member who is encouraging and supportive, and connect with them on a regular basis. Have fun with your buddy and keep it positive! If you dwell on the negative, you will bring each other down instead of lifting each other up.

If your buddy is willing to join you on the journey, you can swap recipes, cook a meal together, and even have gatherings where you serve foods that are aligned with your principles. However, if your buddy does not want to take the journey with you, that's okay too. They can still support you.

For instance, you can go for a walk with your buddy and share how you are overcoming challenges in your journey (verbalizing challenges is healing but, again, focus on the solutions and not the problem), or simply call your buddy to share your exciting moments, like when you cook a homemade meal that your spouse *and* children love. Now that's something to celebrate!

Why?

Joel: It's lonely swimming against the current. When your friends have a birthday party at McDonald's®, what are you going to do? We are social beings and partnerships always survive longer, do more, and are more creative than individuals. A team of two makes one plus one equal three. That's social arithmetic, and it's been working like that since the beginning of time.

Your support buddy probably won't be a member of your family or even a member of your current social circle. When people ask me how I've stayed enthusiastic against orthodoxy's push back for so many years, I always say "customers." Our support group has not been friends, neighbors, or family; it's our customers who love us and encourage us.

Being successful often requires teaming up with someone you may not ordinarily befriend. A co-conspirator collaborator is invaluable when you're trying something new. Looking back over our farming experience, Teresa and I realize that we've never both been down together. If I'm down she's up and if she's down I'm up. I don't know if that is a subconscious response to need, or if we just have a pretty decent marriage, but I know going it alone is difficult.

You tend to become like the people with whom you spend time. If you spend the bulk of your time with naysayers and antagonism, you'll soon start believing that story line. But if you spend more time with encouragers or at least sympathizers, you'll find wind in your sails that will carry you on your journey to a better place.

Sina: Absolutely! It's easier to make diet and lifestyle changes when you have a support system. And, it doesn't have to be a large community. Having one person in your corner can mean the difference between achieving your health goal or returning to old habits.

If you've ever joined the gym, you know how much easier it is to actually go to the gym if a friend or trainer is meeting you there. They hold you accountable, while providing support at the same time. Interestingly, the scientific literature shows that people who feel supported tend to be healthier and live longer. In my experience, the people who feel supported are more likely to successfully reverse a disease, compared with people who don't have support.

During my health journey, I did not have a buddy. In fact, some of our family members were pretty nasty to us, essentially cutting us out of the family. It was rough. I had to overcome a lot of hurdles on my own, such as: how to find recipes that adhered to my food sensitivities, how to locate the food (not as easy as it sounds), how to make it taste good so my kids will eat it, how to attend a social gathering without offending anyone with my food choices, what to feed my son's friends at his birthday parties because the food is so expensive, etcetera.

But it was the emotional hurdles that were the most difficult because I didn't have anyone to talk to, or anyone who could relate. It was a very lonely road to walk. But I was fortunate, because the disease held me accountable. I can't tell you how many times I said to my husband, "If it weren't for the disease, I would not be eating this way." Why? Because the lifestyle I had chosen was too isolating, and I knew it wasn't healthy to feel alone.

Eventually, I found a buddy and it changed everything! She doesn't eat the way I do, but she accepts me the way I am and I accept her. We share recipes and websites. She even became my taste-tester for new recipes I create! We also talk about how to overcome challenges, and she provides suggestions on how to approach social gatherings or deal with family members. Having her in my corner has given me confidence and greater resolve. It's amazing how one person can make such a huge difference in your life.

So, find yourself a buddy. Find one person who will support you, even if they don't want to make changes to their diet. You just need someone in your corner for those days when you need a boost.

Practical Bite #3: Say No To Antibiotics When Eating Out

How? Here are some easy steps you can take to stop eating antibiotics when dining out:

- ❖ Eat at food establishments that do not source meat or poultry from animals that were given antibiotics. Call, send an email, or ask the manager if the meat or poultry was sourced from animals given routine antibiotics. If they weren't, support that establishment with your dollars. If they contains antibiotics, tell them you want meat and poultry produced without the routine use of antibiotics and, until they change their policy, spend your money at an establishment that is aligned with your principles.
- ❖ Use the Consumers Union scorecards to find a food establishment that is actively trying to get antibiotics out of their meat and poultry. Every year, the Consumers Union teams up with other organizations to rank the antibiotic policies of the 25 largest fast food and fast casual chains in the U.S. In their 2017 report, Chipotle® and Panera® came out on top while Domino's Pizza® and Arby's® were among the chains that earned an "F" for having no antibiotic policies in place. As of 2018, the Consumers Union began releasing a second score card that specifically ranks the top 25 burger chains. BurgerFi® and Shake Shack® received "A" grades while Wendy's® received a "D-minus," and all other burger chains received an "F," including: Sonic®, Burger King®, McDonald's®, In-N-Out®, and Carl's Jr®. Feed the companies that scored high and starve the companies that have not committed to reduce antibiotic use. You can find the scorecards online (consumerreports.org).

Why?

Joel: Far more drugs, by total volume, are used in livestock than in humans. You are what you eat, and if what you eat is doing drugs, then you're doing second-hand drugs, just like second-hand smoke.

Sina: That's exactly right, Joel. And, it's the main reason that antibiotics aren't working as well as they used to. The Centers for Disease Control and Prevention (CDC) has declared antibiotic resistance to be "one of the biggest public health challenges of our time" with more than 2.8 million people getting antibiotic-resistant infections each year, and 35,000 people dying from those infections. But those deaths are preventable!

Antibiotic resistance stems largely from our chronic exposure to antibiotics in our food. In fact, when it comes to unnecessarily using antibiotics, the worst offender is the industrialized food system. Roughly 70% of all *medically-important* antibiotics sold in the U.S. are fed to livestock and poultry. Consequently, you can help your body avoid developing antibiotic resistance by not eating antibiotics in your food.

Joel: We all know the miracle of antibiotics changed the game on infections. From pneumonia to that nasty infection when you cut your finger, antibiotics are certainly a foundational stamp on the technological advancements and life expectancy of the modern world. I don't know anybody who would prefer a world without antibiotics.

Sina and I are not demonizing antibiotics and we certainly aren't advocating their prohibition. We appreciate the positives they've brought to modern life. That said, though, our tendency is to overuse things or abuse things that we discover. Whether it was Conquistadors slaughtering indigenous people or bankers making risky loans because they know the government will bail them out, we humans seem to have a propensity to overrun our headlights, as my dad used to say.

Animals raised in Concentrated Animal Feeding Operations (CAFOs), known as chicken factories, have lots of infections because they are crowded together and usually stay in the same place all the time. A farmer friend of mine asks visitors to her farm, "Where would you like to eat breakfast? How about we float the plate on an unflushed toilet and eat it there. Would that be a good place?" Of course, visitors wrinkle up their noses and some nearly wretch at the idea. Her point is this: "in CAFOs, that's where animals eat."

They can never get away from their excrement, so they eat on their toilet, literally. This is not innuendo or exaggeration. As repugnant as it is, it's the truth. In these CAFOs, which of course are the standard of cheap food and externalized costs, fecal particulate hangs in the air. Animals poop and then stir it, walk in it, lie down in it, and as it dries it dusts into the air. The animals can't get away from it. It's on their skin, in their hair, their eyes, in their ears, and most importantly, in their nostrils. They breathe it in.

Welcome to antibiotics. The fact is that most animals, raised in overpowering fecal particulate conditions, experience numerous low-grade infections. They might not be visible to the naked eye because most are internal, but they are there nonetheless. And they exact a toll on performance, or productivity.

Antibiotics literally made it possible for animals to be crowded and ingest copious amounts of fecal particulate without getting sick. That was the breakthrough. And that's why the cheap food industry has fought tooth and nail to preserve antibiotic use. They use it subtherapeutically – administering antibiotics when everything appears healthy.

Actually, nobody knows whether antibiotics, had they never been used subtherapeutically, would have created the resistant superbugs we have today. We can't go back and unring that bell. What we do know is that routinely using antibiotics creates what are called superbugs. These are the survivors. The infectious microbes never all die; most do. But the survivors are more powerful than the originals. Remember, in the microbial realm, a whole life - from birth to reproduction to death - occurs sometimes in as little as a few hours. The ability of these fast-reproducing beings to adapt to their new environment - one with antibiotics - is hard to imagine. In one human day, sometimes a microbial species can go through several lifetimes. Amazing.

Sina: And, those superbugs become a problem for us because if the animal is hosting a superbug, the meat from that animal may also contain the superbug. If that occurs, that superbug can infect you when you eat the meat. And, because they are resistant to most antibiotics, you can die from a superbug infection.

But superbugs are not the only issue you face when eating meat and poultry that comes from animals routinely given antibiotics. Those foods likely contain antibiotic residues, which you end up eating. Those residues could lead to antibiotic resistance in *your* body, making it much more difficult to treat future bacterial infections that you may acquire. In fact, it's believed that antibiotic resistance could soon cause *hundreds* of human diseases that are currently curable to become deadly.

In addition, eating antibiotic residues can kill beneficial microbes that live in your gastrointestinal tract. We'll dive into the details later, but the bottom line is that you need those beneficial microbes to be healthy. In fact, antibiotics have such a profound impact on your microbiome that consuming antibiotics can actually decrease your life expectancy. The Office of National Statistics predicts how long we will live based on advancements in medicine and science. In 2017, for the first time, they predicted a decrease in our life expectancy due to antibiotic resistance.

Pause and let that sink in: We are causing ourselves to die at an earlier age because of the antibiotics we consume – largely through our food!

The situation is so bad that the World Health Organization has asked farmers and the food industry to stop giving antibiotics to healthy animals.

Joel: Fortunately, some farmers are moving away from subtherapeutic use. But this is the loophole the industry constantly and consistently uses to continue using them. "We only use them when animals are sick" becomes a nice big catch-all to use them nearly all the time because in those conditions, the animals exhibit sickness in many different ways.

Interestingly, one of the big chicken companies figured out a way to inject a slow-release antibiotic into the unhatched chick, when it was an embryo still in the egg. They labeled this chicken as if it was not given antibiotics, and a competitor took them to court. The chicken company doing the procedure argued that since the chick was still in vitro, it wasn't really a chicken yet and so whatever happened to it happened prior to being a chicken. The suing company argued, of course, that since the antibiotic was being released throughout the chicken's life, it was indeed given antibiotics during its life.

The court ruled in favor of the plaintiff and the defendant company had to quit using the "no antibiotics administered" on its logo. I have two takeaways from this story. First, please appreciate the level of clever speak and deception used by the industry in its labeling and advertising. Most folks, like you and I, can't even imagine this level of word-parsing and questionable ethics. Secondly, when I read about this, I couldn't help but see the irony in this obvious relation to the human abortion/sanctity of life debate. Apparently, an unhatched chick is more alive than a human baby. Fascinating, no?

To be sure, some antibiotics used in livestock are less human-critical than others. Some are not used in humans at all while others are used in both animals and humans. The crossovers are the ones that are being targeted first and most aggressively by the "get-the-antibiotics-out" movement.

Sina: The good news is that most of the top 25 chain restaurants have stopped serving chicken raised with "medically important antibiotics." They are still likely fed some type of antibiotic, but at least they are not routinely given antibiotics that are used to treat infections in humans. Beef, on the other hand, is a different story.

The majority of fast-food joints and restaurants source beef from animals that are routinely treated with antibiotics, including medically important antibiotics. Overall, the beef industry currently uses 43% of medically important antibiotics, according to Consumer Reports. But you can change that. All you have to do is "say no to antibiotics" when you eat out. It's easy to do and the gains add up quickly.

For example, if you eat out three times a week and you switch to a food establishment that serves antibiotic-free meat, you just cut out three potential doses of antibiotics, or their residues, in one week! That's a huge win for your microbiome and, subsequently, your overall health and longevity!

You're also helping to move the market when you "feed the good" food establishments and "starve the bad." For instance, McDonald's® is the largest buyer of beef in the U.S. and fast food chains purchase approximately 1/4 of all chicken. If those top buyers switched to antibiotic-free meat and poultry, it could change the entire food supply! So, how do you get them to switch?

By speaking with your dollars.

Remember, you vote for your food supply with your dollars. Think about that for a moment: The single decision of "saying no to antibiotics" in your fast food could help shift our entire food supply and bring antibiotic resistance in humans to a halt. Now that's harnessing your power!

Joel: With all that said, of course, we desperately need true blue convenience food establishments - call them fast food if you'd like - for additional options. Precious few exist, and so far, not a single one has rivaled the big fast food places like McDonald's® and Burger King®. I say somebody needs to take on this project so that on every hamburger alley and every interstate exchange, a truly grass-finished antibiotic-free option exists. I love hamburgers. There's absolutely nothing wrong with a good hamburger.

This discussion is not about demonizing meat. On the contrary, it's all about eating consciously and conscientiously so we feed the dog we want to grow and starve out the dog we don't. By the end of the book, we'll get you to left overs. Now that's the ultimate fast food.

Practical Bite #4: Look For The 100% USDA Organic Label

How? When looking for processed food in the grocery store, look for the USDA Organic Seal, as well as the words "100% Organic."

Why?

Sina: Eating organic food is one of the most important dietary changes you can make if you want to optimize your long-term health because organic means you are eating foods closer to the way God intended you to eat – without synthetic chemicals, toxins, genetic modification, and radiation.

All of those adulterants I just mentioned - in one form or another - are associated with inflammatory diseases, such as: rheumatoid arthritis, heart disease, diabetes, cancer, Alzheimer's, allergies, and attention-deficit/hyperactivity disorder (ADHD). Consequently, getting those toxins out of your diet can dramatically improve both your immediate and long-term health. An easy way to accomplish that goal is to look for the USDA Organic label.

The USDA Organic label means the ingredients in your processed food are not allowed to contain GMOs, be grown using most pesticides, herbicides, or synthetic fertilizers, or be irradiated. It also means sewage sludge is not allowed to be applied to the soil where the ingredients were grown.

Sewage sludge comes from the sewer system. The exact composition is unknown because it's made up of whatever goes into the sewer system – including human waste and any chemicals dumped down drains. That may include synthetic chemicals used by industry, hospital waste, and any detergents or chemicals you put down the drain.

The sludge is treated and processed in a treatment facility, and the residuals (aka biosolids) are recycled and applied as fertilizer on some conventionally grown crops. According to the Environmental Protection Agency (EPA), biosolids are applied to conventional crops in all 50 states. The government claims biosolids are safe to use on crops. However, some organizations, including the Environmental Working Group, have expressed concerns over the presence of toxic chemicals in the sludge, including: heavy metals, phthalates, pesticides, and dioxins.

You can reduce your exposure to those chemicals by reaching for the USDA Organic label.

Joel: Sina, you know we've struggled probably more on this Practical Bite than any in the book. And you know I love you. For the sake of folks reading our conversation, I have to explain that our farm, Polyface Farm, is not certified organic. Are you shocked? We say we're beyond organic.

For some background, let me give some credentials. When the biological farming community first started talking about organic certification, I was past president of the Virginia Association for Biological Farming (VABF), an organization that is still alive and thriving today. Nearly every state today has some sort of nonprofit organization devoted to biological, ecological, sustainable, regenerative farming. Use your favorite word; I don't care. We all know in principle what we're talking about.

As the issue gained popularity, a majority in the VABF wanted to begin certifying organic. We were a loose-knit group of radicals growing stuff with compost and eschewing chemicals. We were almost a church in some sense. Like any group, we had die-hard true-blue folks and we had tire kickers and we had a couple of folks that seemed to be interested only because they could charge higher prices. So how do we police our brand integrity? Ah, start a certification program.

I was adamantly opposed to it but saw the winds against me and decided to make the best of it. So, I made the enabling motion to begin certifying, but I did it with a built-in sunset clause that automatically terminated certification in one year UNLESS the organization voted to continue it. I was confident that in one year the "in" folks and the "out" folks would create such a schism in the organization that we would quit the whole thing.

They appointed me to the certifying committee and the policing began. At our first meeting we reviewed each applicant's paperwork and voted either pass or fail. Interestingly, the prominent and well-liked folks in the organization passed but the more fringe or radical folks failed. It was so political that I immediately resigned. Unfortunately, my prophecy was right but the timing was off. It took several years for VABF to get out of the certifying business, but it finally did and now the organization doesn't have the schisms and hard feelings from those years.

I tell that story to help people understand that my experience tainted my view of government certified organics. Yes, eventually the government took over all certification either directly or with contracts through approved organizations. And then came the compromise. Today, it's gotten so bad that numerous private add-on certifying efforts, like the Real Organic Project, are now trying to build some integrity into the label.

From dairy cows and chickens raised in Concentrated Animal Feeding Operations to hydroponic vegetables and input loopholes, the organic certification program is in real jeopardy of losing integrity. Many would say it already has.

But when I go to Kroger®, I buy organic bananas.

And that, Sina, is our point here. We're early in the book. We're going to take you beyond this, way beyond. But for now, for today, on the continuum to food paradise, today you can buy organic at the supermarket. That's not your final vote, I hope, but it's a solid vote for a different approach. Are you getting exactly what you think you are? Maybe not, but vote for the idea even if it's not perfect. Don't let perfection preclude you from starting with better.

Sina: I agree. No label is perfect. And, the USDA Organic label certainly has loopholes and shortcomings. For instance, animals raised on a concrete slab can still be considered "organic," which we will discuss in Practical Bite #10. Another issue with the label is hydroponics. I recently spoke with Dr. Linley Dixon, associate director of The Real Organic Project, who informed me that hydroponically grown plants are allowed to be certified as "organic" even though the plant never touches soil, and the major hydroponic growers feed the plants genetically modified soy byproducts.

These issues are deeply concerning and they do compromise the label. However, you have to meet yourself where you are. If you are shopping in the grocery store, you are limited by the labels. But, those labels are also your main tool for helping you make food choices. And, switching from conventional to organic is a fantastic step toward reducing your toxic load.

We are starting with processed foods because the majority of the American diet consists of processed foods. Consequently, replacing all of your conventional processed foods with their organic counterparts will dramatically reduce your toxic load. If you are not ready to swap out all of your processed foods, that's okay. Start with the processed food you eat the most. Then, once you've adjusted to that change, pick the next most commonly consumed processed food and swap it for the organic version. Utilize this strategy until every processed food in your house is organic.

Having said that, looking for the USDA Organic label can be confusing because there are actually four different categories of organic products:

1. **100% Organic** – All of the ingredients must be certified organic. The product may include the USDA Organic Seal and/or the 100% organic claim.
2. **Organic** – Up to 5% of the ingredients can be non-organic or conventional. The product may include the USDA Organic Seal and/or the organic claim.
3. **"Made with" organic ingredients** – At least 70% of the ingredients must be certified organic, which means 30% of the ingredients can be non-organic or conventional. The USDA Organic Seal cannot be used, but the product can claim "made with" organic ingredients.
4. **"Specified organic ingredients"** – If less than 70% of the ingredients are certified organic, the USDA Organic Seal cannot be used and the product cannot display the word "organic." However, the certified organic ingredients can be listed on the package along with the percentage of organic ingredients.

So, when you're at the grocery store, you can't just find the USDA Organic Seal and call it a day. If you want to eat food that is 100% organic, you must first look for the USDA Organic Seal and then look for the words "100% organic." However, "100% organic" is not always easy to find and is not always included on the package. So, for me, it's quicker to first look for the USDA Organic Seal and then read the list of ingredients. If every ingredient is listed as organic, it's a winner. The exception is salt, which cannot be listed as organic.

Joel: That's great advice, Sina. The words that come to mind are effort and vigilant. You can't get to a different place without some effort and you won't find your way there unless you're vigilant.

I would add one more warning: don't be enamored with fancy. Fancy labels and fancy packaging are expensive and hard to develop. I heard one guy say he would never buy food from anyone who advertises on TV because, by definition, he knows whoever does that is too big for his britches. Kind of an interesting litmus test.

Marketers all say, of course, that bright pretty packaging is key to everything. But on our farm, we've elected to use extremely plain packaging and labeling. All of our labels simply say "Polyface." They make no claims and bear no additional endorsements. All of those things like "grass-finished" embroil you in bureaucratic paperwork. Every additional letter must meet certain pica standards and placement credentials. And four-color printing is extremely expensive.

When our eggs went into a Whole Foods® store, we used (and still do) a simple plain cardboard carton. It has our farm name printed on it but we use only one color of ink (green, for grass) and make no claims. We don't even claim Grade A or size, like large, medium, etc. Know why? If we make a claim like that, we must have a certified processing room, which requires yet another layer of bureaucratic regulatory compliance. More paperwork. So, we just call them eggs. They're Polyface eggs, to be sure, but that's the only claim we make.

The other eggs at Whole Foods® were in glitzy plastic tri-fold cartons with fancy four-color printed glossy labels and all sorts of claims, from cage-free to pasture-raised or whatever. I warned the folks in management that I didn't want to get a call in a month complaining about our packaging and they assured me that would not be an issue. The eggs sold extremely well and things were going spritely until the phone rang. "We have a problem with your cartons; they're too plain." Trust me, the conversation went downhill fast. We exited Whole Foods® about two months after entering. Lesson learned.

So, I'm admonishing you, as a simple, small, paperwork-hating, authentic farmer and not a corporate empire, don't discriminate against plain labels. In fact, I'd say the plainer the packaging and labels, probably the better the outfit. They're putting all their effort in integrity production and not assuming sales are driven by sexy labels and packaging. Just a word to the wise.

Sina: And remember, the extra cost of fancy packaging ultimately gets passed down to you, the consumer. So, I agree with Joel. Save yourself money; don't choose food based on glitz and glamour. But do look for the USDA Organic label. Despite the loopholes, it's a huge step forward in your healing journey. And, if you're not ready to switch to an all-organic diet, for whatever reason, that's okay. Take it one step at a time; start by replacing the processed food you eat the most.

What I find interesting is that most of my clients tell me they understand the value of organic food, but they don't always buy it because it's "too expensive." I get it; organic is usually more expensive. My family had to reprioritize our entire budget in order to afford organic food. However, when you peel back the layers of the onion, feeling unworthy is actually the biggest hurdle for most of my clients. In order to spend the money on organic food, you have to believe that you are worth the extra cost. Yet, most people I know can't say these three words out loud: "I'm worth it." And that brings us to our next Practical Bite.

Practical Bite #5: Mirror, Mirror

How? Find a mirror. Look into your eyes and say these words: "I love you ___ (insert your name)." If you can't say that sentence then start with "I like you" or "I am willing to learn to like you." Say those words as often as you can throughout the day, every day, for at least one week. The goal is to eventually be able to look into your eyes and say, "I love you ___ (insert your name) and I accept you exactly the way you are."

Why?

Joel: I do a lot of speaking around the world, much of it themed toward encouraging people to do things they don't think they can do. Or to do better what they're already doing, generally by doing something different. Fortunately, I grew up in a family where unconditional love was manifested. It wasn't perfect, by any means, but I knew that no matter what I did, Mom and Dad loved me, prayed for me, and wanted what was best for me. What a wonderful legacy.

But many people don't have this advantage. And even those of us who do struggle with conditional affirmation. In other words, all worth is a tradeoff. I'll like you if you do this. I'll be your friend if you do this. I'll do this for you if you do this for me. We're wired to think conditionally in our relationships.

In school, we learn quickly what behavior receives better marks from the teacher. In social settings, we learn what brings friends and what doesn't. In sports and extracurricular activities, the prescribed strategy or game plan is all about a route to success. The guidance counselor tells us what we're suited for and designs a curriculum that satisfies the objectives of the institution.

In church we learn what makes the preacher happy. In dating, we try to do things that garner reciprocal attention. Even in the best of relationships, we have expectations of performance, attitudes, and deeds that open either doors of condemnation or doors of adoration. We get a job and it's all about finding out what pleases the boss. The boss likes people that do this; he dislikes people who do that.

The point is that our lives literally immerse in pleasing others. I differentiate pleasing others from serving others. Pleasing is about doing what others want; serving is about doing what others need. A profound difference exists between the two. The point of all this is that the unencumbered infant grows into massive encumbrances about self-worth and freedom to dream.

In my business seminars, probably the most powerful moment is when I lay out this context and then tell folks: "The most important thing you can give yourself right now is the freedom, indeed the right, to dream." Life meaning does not come from someone else; it comes from being true to yourself, to your "youness." I feel like Sina and I might be getting into the weeds on this. While it seems far removed from food and farming, it's all about giving yourself license to do the most yearning desire of your soul. Most of us don't even know what that is because we've never given ourselves license to dream.

If I don't think I'm worthy to dream, I won't. Then I'm stuck. This license is never bestowed by someone else. It has to come from our own personhood, our own worth. And that is why happiness is not in things or anything external. Certainly, catastrophe and grief can hit a happiness pause button in our lives, but eventually even that cannot derail our ability to dream.

Sina: When you have that type of unshakable peace, you are connected with yourself and have stepped into your power. But, as you said, most of us are playing a role that society has told us to play. We are living our lives based on someone else's definition of success. But you can step out of that box by realizing you are worthy just the way you are. You are good enough. Right here, right now, you are "enough."

When I was sick, it was difficult for me to justify spending money on the food, medical tests, and supplements that were required to help me heal. But, when it came to helping my children, I would spend all of our savings without batting an eye. Interestingly, every Mom I know follows the same pattern of putting her family's needs before her own, even when it's to her detriment.

That double standard may stem from genetics or societal pressure. But, in my case, it also existed because I didn't feel worthy – worthy of receiving optimal health and wellness, which ultimately boils down to not feeling loved. If you don't feel loved, it's very difficult to spend money on improving your health because then you have to admit that you are worth it. Hands down, not feeling loved is the #1 root cause of illness in nearly every client I have worked with.

Have you ever said, "I'll be happy when I lose 5 pounds," or "I'll be happy when I get married," or "I'll be happy when I can retire?" "I'll be happy when ___" is just a different way of saying: "I'll be good enough when ___."

Most of us live our whole lives never feeling "good enough" or "worthy." That limiting belief pulls you out of the present moment, where your happiness lies. For instance, when conditions are placed on your happiness then happiness becomes a carrot that is never obtainable because it is rooted in the external world, which constantly changes.

I spent most of my life chasing that moving target. As a child, I thought I'd be happy once I moved out of my parent's house. When that day came, I still wasn't happy. Then, I thought I'd be happy when I graduated from college. Nope. Then, I thought I'd be happy when I got my first job. But it was never "good enough." In fact, my carrot just kept moving. As soon as I achieved one goal, I immediately moved on to the next: I'll be happy when I get married. I'll be happy when I have a child. I'll be happy when I lose the baby weight. I'll be happy when my child is out of the terrible 2's. I'll be happy when I have a second child. I'll be happy when I write my first book.

No matter how much I achieved in my life, I never felt truly happy. Sure, I would laugh and experience happy moments. But the feeling was always fleeting. Why?

My happiness was largely based on external validation. I needed to be praised by others, particularly my parents, because I was desperate for love and acceptance. So, I lived my life doing things to make other people happy. In return, I received the praise I needed in order to feel loved. But that feeling of being loved, of being worthy, only lasted a moment. So, I needed to "up my game" and achieve something even bigger to keep earning praises.

Then one day, I realized I had spent my entire life striving to obtain something that doesn't even exist. True happiness and fulfillment come from within. It comes from loving and accepting yourself exactly the way you are. You can *choose* to be happy in this very moment. All you have to do is stop seeking approval from others and start looking within. That is when you will find true joy and fulfillment. You will realize that you are "good enough" just the way you are; you are worthy of love.

As a bonus, you will discover that the power to heal yourself – physically, mentally, emotionally and spiritually - was inside of you the whole time. You see, we are conditioned, as a society, to seek healing externally – from doctors, nurses, nutritionists, pharmacists, etcetera. But they can't actually heal you. They can't take away your disease or give you back your mental health or make you happy. Only you can do that.

In fact, your health and happiness are actually a mirror of what you believe about yourself. If you are sick then perhaps you don't feel worthy of receiving the self-care that is required in order to be healthy. If you are unhappy then perhaps you don't feel like you deserve to feel joy. If you are judgmental then perhaps you don't feel loved and accepted. Whatever you believe about yourself will be mirrored in your own life – both in how you treat yourself and how you treat others.

Many of our limiting beliefs about ourselves come from how we were treated by our parents or caregivers. Consequently, we tend to treat ourselves the way our parents treated us. If we were loved and accepted then we love and accept ourselves. If we were abused or we felt unloved then we treat ourselves with that same type of conditional love, perhaps by chasing the carrot with "I'll be happy when" statements. Many of us sit in that space of limiting beliefs our whole lives and, consequently, never find true joy or optimal health.

Why not choose to be happy right now? Don't wait to feel joy until you are "perfect." If you do, you will waste your life in a futile pursuit of that moving target. Instead, choose joy, choose acceptance, choose love. When you learn to love and accept yourself exactly the way you are, your old limiting beliefs will dissolve. You will realize that you are "good enough" just the way that you are. And, you will finally be able to release the anger, the fear, the guilt, and the anxiety.

Loving and accepting yourself may sound hard to do, but it's not. An amazing woman named Louise Hay healed herself from cancer largely by learning to love herself. She believed that your power lies in the present moment. You can't change the past and you can't predict the future. But you can control your thoughts and your beliefs in this moment. So, what will you do with this moment? Will you choose to start loving yourself or will you choose to remain stuck in your old limiting beliefs?

Try doing this throughout the day, every day for a week: Find a mirror. Look into your eyes and say these words: "I love you ___ (insert your name)." If you can't say that sentence then start with "I like you" or "I am willing to learn to like you." The goal is to one day be able to look into your eyes and say, "I love you ___ (insert your name) and I accept you exactly the way you are."

This is called Mirror Work. I learned it from Louise Hay. It sounds a little corny, but it is a game changer.

When I first tried this technique, I looked in the mirror and instantly began criticizing myself. Like a reflex, judgmental thoughts filled my mind, such as: "Wow, I look old; when did that happen? My eyes look tired. I should really do something about my hair." And, when I tried to say "I love you," I couldn't. I ended up crying half way through the sentence. It felt as though life suddenly caught up with me. All of my fears, doubts, worries, and insecurities, suddenly rushed to the surface. There was no escaping the truth because it was staring right at me - I didn't love myself.

For most of us, the mirror has become our enemy. It reveals what we are most afraid of by reflecting back to us how we feel about ourselves and how we feel about life. But, if you allow it, the mirror can be your best friend. It can show you where you are stuck and what issues you can address in order to set yourself free. It is the key to developing a deep, healing relationship with yourself where you no longer chase the carrot in search of external validation. Instead, you will finally reach a state of joy that you can tap into at any moment, and that nobody can take away from you.

Every day, as often as you can, look in the mirror, stare deep into your eyes and say, "I love you ___ (fill in the blank with your name). I love you and accept you exactly the way you are."

You may not believe it at first. I didn't. But, keep saying it over and over, every day. If you stick with it, one day, you will wake up in the morning, stand in front of the mirror, and be excited to greet your new best friend.

Once you reach that point, you will begin to practice self-care on a level that's deeper and more honest than you've ever known. You will realize that you are worth it. You are worth the extra cost of organic food. You are worth the effort of preparing a home-cooked meal in the kitchen. You are worth taking the time to meditate and exercise every day.

If you allow it, loving and accepting yourself will be your game-changer on your path to maximal health, happiness and freedom.

Practical Bite #6: Switch To Organic Eggs

How? When buying eggs in the grocery store, look for the USDA Organic label.

Why?

Sina: When I decided to start eating healthier, one of the first changes I made was to leave conventional eggs behind and only eat organic. It was easy to do; it didn't require any extra time or effort. I simply reached for the egg carton in my grocery store that carried the USDA organic label. It does, however, cost more money. But it's worth it.

Conventional laying chickens can be fed GMOs, pesticides, herbicides, and antibiotics. All of those chemicals can lead to inflammation in the chicken, which means the chicken is sick. If she's sick, her eggs can also be sick. And, eating sick eggs can make you inflamed too.

In contrast, USDA Organic certified laying chickens are not allowed to be fed GMOs, or most pesticides, herbicides or antibiotics. So, eating organic eggs decreases your toxic load.

Joel: I agree. If you're buying eggs in the grocery store, get the organic eggs. They don't have all the chemicals and antibiotics in them, and for that we can be grateful. However, they are usually not raised in much better conditions than conventional laying birds.

Most conventional laying chickens are housed in tiny cages, stacked several tiers high, in Concentrated Animal Feeding Operations (CAFOs), also known as factory farms. They can't move around much, they live on wire all their lives; can't scratch, peck, or even lay in a nest box - they just squat and lay on the cage wire.

In contrast, government certified organic laying hens can't be caged, which is a huge animal welfare issue. But, remember, organic eggs are still, for the most part, produced in large factory farms. They don't have to be, of course, but most are. That means they are still in CAFOs but in loose housing; not caged, but have the run of the floor. Regardless, the environment is usually similar for both conventional and organic laying hens – they both live in feces.

The filth and stench of an industrial egg factory is hard for a normal person to grasp or imagine. Ammoniated air caused by the high nitrogen levels in chicken manure is like sand paper to sensitive mucous membranes. God gave us, and chickens, wonderful filters in our nasal passages. We have hairs and then cilia and mucous membranes to block the dust and fecal particles from entering our body. The chickens can handle some, but not too much. If the particle load is too heavy, it overruns these filters and gets too far into the body.

As the fecal particles pass through the respiratory channels, it's abrasive on those linings and makes small wounds, like bleeding sores. This is critical to understand because nature has lots of mechanisms in place to protect it from toxic and pathogenic assault.

Remember, the world and the air around us is filled with microscopic beings; most are good and some are bad. The way our (or a chicken's) respiratory system works is to offer filters (nose hairs) and the cilia and linings to protect the bloodstream from viral or pathogenic assault. But when these linings contain bleeding lesions, the protective barrier breaks down and these bugs can directly enter the bloodstream – along with fecal particles.

Once in the bloodstream, in a chicken, the bugs can find their way into the oviduct, which is the production tube for making eggs. Normally anything in the air would never get close to the oviduct and infect an egg. It would be stopped at the respiratory membrane. But when the assault is strong enough to override that protection, all systems begin to fail.

Sina: That's similar to what is currently happening in humans. We are witnessing a huge increase in the number of people with chronic or inflammatory diseases. I bet each one of us can point to someone in our family, or a close friend, who has a chronic disease such as: allergies, diabetes, cancer, autoimmune disease, Alzheimer's or heart disease. I look around and it seems like sick is the new norm. Why? It's largely because of a breach in our barrier systems.

Just like the chicken, we have barriers that protect us from the outside world. For example, we all have a single layer of cells that line most of our gastrointestinal (GI) tract. That means *one* cell separates you from your environment. That single layer of cells is held together by tight junctions, which act like VELCRO®. When a digested food particle or other beneficial nutrient needs to pass from your GI tract into your body, the tight junctions un-VELCRO® and allow the nutrient to pass through and then they reseal. It's a highly regulated process.

Just behind those tight junctions is the gastrointestinal lymphatic tissue (GALT). The GALT is a layer of immune cells that guard against any breach in your GI tract. In fact, an estimated 60-70% of your immune system originates in the GALT. In addition, we believe that 80% of the antibodies your immune system produces originate in the GALT. The combination of tight junctions and the GALT provide a strong defense against foreign invaders, which is critical for keeping you healthy.

The tight junctions can become damaged when exposed to various triggers, such as: emotional or physical stress, certain foods, toxins, prescription drugs, and pathogens. When the tight junctions are damaged, they don't work properly. The opening and closing of the VELCRO® gates are no longer highly regulated. Instead, the gates can allow large molecules and pathogens to leak into your body – that process is called leaky gut. Those molecules are not supposed to be there. Your body doesn't recognize them, so the GALT mounts an immune response, which is inflammatory. It can begin as an acute inflammatory response. But, as your body becomes overwhelmed with toxins from the environment, it can lead to chronic inflammation. Consequently, your body can become chronically inflamed.

We think this is partly why we are seeing so many food allergies in children. Have you noticed how many children have food allergies? I can't go to a public school, daycare, or Sunday school class without seeing an allergy alert on the door. It's crazy! There are even children who are allergic to pepper!

But leaky gut can lead to more than just food allergies; it can lead to chronic disease. Let's take me, as an example. I have non-celiac gluten sensitivity. So, when I ate gluten, it damaged my gut lining, causing leaky gut. When those gluten proteins leaked into my bloodstream, my body saw them as foreign invaders. In an attempt to protect me, my body mounted an immune response, which caused my body to be inflamed. If I had stopped eating gluten, my gut lining would have healed and the inflammation would have subsided. But I kept unknowingly eating gluten. So, my body kept attacking it. (See Practical Bite #39)

The gluten protein in food looks similar to other proteins located in your tissues. Over time, my body got confused; it couldn't tell the difference between the two proteins. So, it began targeting my own tissues. That process is called molecular mimicry.

We think your body targets where you are genetically weakest. In my case, it targeted my joints and I developed an advanced stage of rheumatoid arthritis *in my 30's*. If it targets your brain, you can develop ADHD, autism, or Alzheimer's. If it targets your pancreas, you can develop diabetes. If it targets your spinal cord, you can develop multiple sclerosis (MS), and so on.

There's a lot we still don't know about disease formation. But we are beginning to understand that all chronic diseases involve chronic inflammation – meaning, if you have a chronic disease, your body has been inflamed for an extended period of time (possibly decades). In fact, the link is so strong that we are now referring to chronic diseases as inflammatory diseases. As we continue to unravel the mechanisms, I predict we will reclassify most chronic/inflammatory diseases as autoimmune diseases – operating through a mechanism involving breached barriers, like the ones just described for both humans and chickens.

But, here's the really cool part: If you understand how an inflammatory disease is created then you can reverse it! Inflammation is a big piece of the puzzle. You must lower your level of inflammation in order to reverse an inflammatory or chronic disease. You do that, by removing your triggers.

We all have unique triggers. For instance, unlike me, you might be able to eat a wheat bagel without resulting in systemic inflammation. But strawberries or kale might damage your tight junctions. In addition, we each have our own tipping point. Maybe you can eat one bagel and feel fine, but two pushes you over your threshold. Meanwhile, I get sick even if I eat one crumb of a bagel.

Joel: That's exactly right. And, nobody knows where the tipping point is for humans or chickens. How much fecal dust can a chicken handle before its system breaks down? Just like people, chickens are different, and what one can tolerate, another can't. This is why the cumulative results of dietary decisions are so profound. One Coke® won't kill anyone. Sina, your immunological breakdown didn't happen in a day, did it?

Sina: No, it took decades.

Joel: It was an accumulation of lots of little things and obviously your genetic predisposition toward certain weaknesses. We all know about the 90-year old hale and hearty grandpa who smoked a pipe all his life. But that's the exception that proves the rule. Far more pipe smokers, like one of my great uncles, got emphysema and died a slow, agonizing death, gasping for air. Imagine suffocating slowly for 5-10 years.

Sina: The bottom line is: USDA Organic laying chickens predominantly live in confinement in their own filth, similar to conventional laying chickens. But, choosing organic eggs instead of conventional eggs is still a step in the right direction because it lowers your toxic load in terms of GMOs, antibiotics, pesticides, and herbicides.

Joel: I agree, it's the lesser of two bad choices. Stick with us and we'll get you to the best option, but do the easy thing first – choose government certified organic eggs over conventional eggs.

Practical Bite #7: Say No To Chlorinated Eggs

How? Nearly all eggs sold in the grocery store are disinfected with a chemical, usually chlorine. Some of that chemical enters the porous shell and arrives on your breakfast plate.

Find out which chemical is used to disinfect your eggs by visiting the Food Safety Inspection Service (FSIS) database (www.fsis.usda.gov/mpidirectory). Match the establishment number, located on your egg package, to the processing location and simply call or email with the question: "What do you use to sterilize your eggs?" Once you know the answer, give informed consent by either continuing to buy those eggs or finding different eggs that are disinfected with a chemical you are okay consuming. If you decide you do not want your eggs disinfected, skip ahead to Practical Bite #54.

Why?

Joel: Many years ago, our farm ramped up our egg production to nearly 100 dozen per day (tiny by industry standards, where a typical commercial egg farm would produce 50-60,000 dozen per day) and we wanted to reduce our processing time: cleaning, sorting, packing in boxes. I contacted a commercial egg operation at the far end of our county and asked if I could bring over about 500 dozen at a time to run through their processing line. Surprisingly, they were amenable and charged an amount per dozen.

The football-field sized chicken houses had several tiers of wire cages (called batteries) where the laying hens lived. About nine hens lived in a cage about 2 feet x 2 feet. If you do the math quickly, you'll note that's less than half a square foot per bird. If you take a piece of 8-1/2 x 11 copy paper and fold it in half, that's a little more space than each chicken enjoys. Yes, you're right to think that's not much.

Many of these batteries had a dead chicken in it in some state of decomposition. Her cellmates gradually stomped on her and over time, pushed her carcass through the floor of the cage. Of course, their beaks were cut off halfway so they could not peck each other to eliminate cannibalism. When they laid an egg, they simply squatted on the slanted wire floor and dropped it. The egg rolled down the floor to a continuous-running conveyor belt that transported the eggs into the egg processing building.

The egg washing station consisted of shower nozzles and brushes that sprayed chlorinated hot water on the eggs. A vat underneath caught the wash water, which stunk to high heaven and was filled with manure, eggshells, broken eggs and feathers. Some eggs broke; the yellow water reeked, but the chlorine made it "sanitary" according to food safety regulations.

Sina: You know some of the chlorine and filth made its way into those eggs because the shell is porous. In fact, the USDA lists egg cleaning agents as food additives, which means they expect the cleaning agent to "become a component of" the egg.

Joel: Exactly. Needless to say, we did not want our eggs contaminated with all that fecal chlorinated bath water. We decided to clean our own eggs with just warm water and mild soap, if necessary. Why wash an egg if it's clean?

Fast forward a couple of years and we got a frantic call from one of our restaurant owner-chefs. The health department had been there regarding three folks who visited the local hospital emergency room over the previous 48 hours complaining of bloody stools. The hospital cultured the stools and concluded it was salmonella contamination. The one thing all three had in common (none was seriously injured) was eating Sunday brunch at this local white tablecloth restaurant the previous day.

As the health department officials descended on the restaurant, they saw our unwashed eggs in the cooler and immediately confiscated them, threw them in the dumpster, and fingered them as the culprit. The chef called to let me know what was happening. We immediately went to the field where the chickens that laid these eggs lived, grabbed a dozen, and even took samples of the chicken manure, sending everything to an accredited lab that does this kind of testing. The culture took two weeks to mature and we got the results: nothing. Totally salmonella free. Even the manure was salmonella free.

I waited for the health department report. And waited. And waited. After three weeks I couldn't stand it and called the inspector who wrote the report fingering our eggs. "What did your culture show?" I asked. I didn't tell her we had done a test too - don't ever trust a bureaucrat. She responded: "What culture? We didn't culture anything. I saw the unwashed eggs and assumed that was the culprit." That's your food police for you, and science, folks.

I was incredulous. That kitchen had fresh shrimp, garden dirt on carrots, all sorts of things lying around that kitchen. The chef pointed out all these possible sources of the contamination to the inspector, but she wasn't interested. She had a smoking gun. When I pressed her, she finally admitted that she did not think an unwashed egg was edible. Now folks, I'm not making any of this up. The law does not require eggs to be washed. All it requires is that they be clean, which is defined as no "adhering particles." That includes manure, feathers, or straw. That's all the law requires. But she had added her own prejudice to it and decided that in her world an unwashed egg was hazardous.

When I explained what I'd seen at the commercial egg factory, with eggs bathed in manure and chlorine, I asked her if she thought eggs bathed in manure and chlorine, with porous shells, were cleaner than eggs that were clean straight out of the hen. She stuck to her guns; I've got to give her that. She wouldn't budge. It obviously didn't matter how much manure and chlorine got into the egg, as long as it was washed.

Here's the kicker. You know how sometimes you hang up the phone with a call and before you can even get the phone in the cradle, it rings? That's what happened. I answered the incoming call and it was my friend and mentor, Allan Nation, founder and editor of *The Stockman Grass Farmer* magazine (the premier pastured livestock trade publication in the world). I wrote The Pastoralist column for the magazine and we would routinely fellowship over the phone. He had just returned from France. Before I could say anything except hello, he said: "Guess what? In France, it's illegal to sell a washed egg." What are the chances of that phrase being uttered at that moment in that context? I started laughing so hard I almost fell over. I think it would be appropriate to say I cackled.

Sina: What a great story! The bottom line is to give your informed consent. If you want to shop in the grocery store then find out which chemicals are used to disinfect your eggs. Use the FSIS database to contact the processing plant (www.fsis.usda.gov/mpidirectory). Once you know the answer, you can give informed consent: If you are okay with that particular disinfecting agent then continue to buy those eggs. If you are not okay with it then find another brand that uses a disinfectant you can live with. And, if you decide you don't want your eggs disinfected then you have another option. Skip ahead to Practical Bite #54 to learn how to find locally grown, truly pasture-raised eggs that are not disinfected.

Joel: Mamas, don't let your kids eat eggs contaminated with chlorine, no matter how sterile it sounds. Very few supermarkets carry clean eggs. You have to hunt for them (Easter egg hunt, anybody?) but it's worth it to protect yourself from the industrial contamination sanctioned and encouraged by food police hired by your tax dollars. Enjoy.

Practical Bite #8: Choose Organic Chicken

How? Instead of buying conventional chicken, reach for the chicken with the USDA Organic label.

Why?

Joel: The same arguments for buying government certified organic eggs in the supermarket apply to chicken. The fact that government certified organic meat chickens (aka broilers) are not supposed to be fed feed with synthetic chemicals and given antibiotics necessitates a higher level of care.

Sina: Exactly! Choosing organic chicken instead of conventional varieties offers you greater health benefits because conventional chickens can be fed GMOs, pesticides, herbicides and antibiotics. All of those chemicals can lead to inflammation in the chicken, which means the chicken is sick. And, eating sick chicken can make you sick too.

In contrast, when you choose organic chicken, that *one* decision has a profound impact on your health and wellness. Organic chickens are not allowed to be fed GMOs or most pesticides, herbicides, and antibiotics. And, saying no to chickens fed antibiotics reduces your chance of eating a super bug on your chicken. Plus, it reduces your chance of developing antibiotic resistance in your own body.

As previously mentioned, you don't want to develop antibiotic resistance because it means that if you get sick with a strain of bacteria that antibiotics can't kill, you may not be able to get rid of your infection. In addition, when you eat antibiotics (or their residues) that can be present in conventional chicken, it kills some of the good microbes in your gut. That sets you up for dysbiosis or an imbalance of microbes, which can lead to inflammation and subsequent disease. But you can protect your microbiome by choosing organic chicken over conventional.

Joel: Again, we're dealing with the caveat "if you're buying from a supermarket" in the same way we dealt with organic eggs. Government certified organic broilers and conventional broilers are both raised in loose-housed Concentrated Animal Feeding Operations (CAFOs). So, the issue of dust and fecal particulates overpowering the chicken's filter capacity and infiltrating the body exists in both types of chicken.

I have a farmer friend who maintains three certifications. When asked his costs to maintain them, he said it's about $200,000 a year. He's an extremely large farmer who sells through Whole Foods® and to garner market share in that market climate, he probably needs all those certifications. But farmers produce a lot of great food that doesn't carry that certification price tag on it, and that's a good thing.

You might be wondering if I have some sort of fetish about government certified organic. Notice I never say just "organic" because in America today, that word is owned by government and unless I pay for the certification license, I can't use it. It's quite a shame that those of us who developed the organic-in-principle movement are now prohibited from using the language we invented.

I lived through those times and the lively discussions as people with big hearts and sincere desires crafted this "savior federal legislation." I always wondered why leaders in our movement wanted to give policing powers to the government organization that pooh-poohed organics for half a century. Isn't that like the fox guarding the henhouse? Of course, adulteration and compromise are exactly what happened, and the entry of Wal-Mart® into the market indicated that the original ideals no longer existed.

Many people don't realize what a game changer occurred when Walmart® became the world's largest purveyor of organics; not just for chicken, but all food items imaginable. It was a category 10 earthquake in craft food country, and the ripples through the non-chemical food movement had far reaching consequences. Farmers' markets flattened. Community Supported Agriculture (CSA) flattened. Direct farm sales flattened. Indeed, the sucking sound out of the nascent local food movement was Walmart®. The USDA even commissioned a study on why farmers' markets were struggling.

I admit that I despise Wal-Mart® about as much as McDonald's®; I see them both as culturally destructive icons. That's my current bias. For the record, donations to charities do not counteract the more overriding negatives of these business models. If Wal-Mart® would allow my single axle truck to back up to its loading dock during business hours and offload items from 10 miles away that did not have a bar code, then I would think differently. In the big scheme of things, the big picture does matter. I have my inconsistencies and imperfections just like everyone, but minimizing them should be a goal; not laughing them off as inconsequential. Wal-Mart® shoppers are duplicitous, unfortunately, and generally don't appreciate the whole system their patronage supports. I may be wrong, but that's what I think.

In frustration to the whole kettle of fish, I began using the term "beyond organic" and even use it on our website. Do you know the National Organic Standard Board (NOSB) police sent me threatening legal action because I wasn't licensed to use the word? I didn't say I was organic; I just said I was beyond organic, but even that warranted litigation from them. Fortunately, I was a member of the Farm to Consumer Legal Defense Fund, called their lead attorney Pete Kennedy, and he sent a scathing letter that snuffed out the legal action quickly. And yes, I still say we're beyond organic.

That, if you're paying attention, is a lot like beyond labels. Hmmm. I wonder where we're headed with all this.

Sina: The bottom line is: meet yourself where you are. If that means buying organic chicken in the grocery store then do it. Start with the low-hanging fruit first because making the decision to switch from conventional to organic chicken helps reduce your toxic load. It also has a profound impact on your wellness by giving you a voice.

When you choose organic, you are sending a message to the food industry and the government that you will not eat GMOs, pesticides, herbicides or antibiotics in your chicken. But you are also sending the message to your body that you are worth it. You are worth the additional cost of organic chicken. You are worth being heard. You are worth being loved.

Joel: This is such a great recurring theme in your encouragement, Sina, and I think you can't say it enough or emphasize it enough. It's not prideful to want to take care of yourself. People need you. Your family needs you; your friends need you; your charitable causes need you; your vocation needs you. You'll be a lot more effective serving all these needs if you're healthy and functional.

Do I care about what other farmers are doing on their land? How they're stewarding their own acreage? Of course. But if I don't take care of mine as my first priority, how can I show them a better way? My dad used to say you can't push on a string. You lead by example. And so, if our fields are prettier, our cows slicker, our chickens more robust, our pigs more gorgeous (yes, beautiful pigs are gorgeous, believe me) then we'll have credibility. People will want to know how we did this.

And so, if you move to a better more healthful place and eat with more conviction and reduce your pharmaceuticals, you'll be a more enjoyable person to be around. People will wonder what's going on; you'll be attractive in all the right ways. Is that worth it? Yes. Sina, you're right on.

And, I agree. If you're buying your chicken in the grocery store, get the organic birds. They might not be raised in much better conditions, but they don't have all the chemicals and antibiotics in them, and for that we can be grateful. Normally too, in these factory houses that are government certified organic, the space allotment per bird is higher, which reduces stress. Stress is the number one reason animals get sick.

Sina: The same holds true in humans; stress is the number one reason humans get sick. So, don't stress about which chicken to buy in the grocery store. For now, choose the organic bird and give yourself credit for taking another step forward, and for cooking a bird in your kitchen instead of relying on fast-food or casual dining.

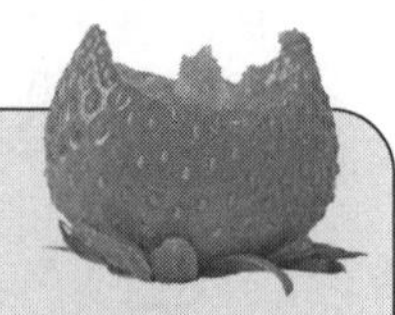

CHEW ON THIS

Have you ever wondered why the rotisserie chickens in your grocery store are so large? Many people believe it's because those conventional chickens are given hormones, but that's not true.

The USDA does not allow hormones to be given to chickens. So, if you see a label on your chicken that states "no hormones added," it doesn't mean anything. No chickens are allowed to have added hormones. In fact, if you look closely at the label, the claim "no hormones added" is legally required to be followed by a statement that reads "Federal regulations prohibit the use of hormones."

So, if chickens are not fed hormones then why are those rotisserie chickens so big? For that matter, why are chickens so much bigger than they were 60 years ago?

The short answer is genetic selection centered around hybridization. Unlike GMOs, this is simply natural mating of different breeds of chicken to create a hybrid that exhibits, hopefully, the best points of two or more strains. In the poultry industry, this developed from cross breeding a White Plymouth Rock with the Cornish, creating what is known as the Cornish Cross.

The White Plymouth Rock is a naturally tall and big-bodied bird while the Cornish is a squatty wide-breasted bird. Breeding these two disparate chickens created a large wide-breasted bird that has since been tweaked and tweaked and tweaked. The poultry industry now has strains ideally suited for deboning, others for whole broilers and yet others for breasts or other parts, even wings for that matter.

Breeding was the first and most important part of the equation. The second part was fortified feed - like high octane rations. By developing dense trace mineral recipes and vitamin packs, feed rations became denser, which enabled these birds to consume a higher nutrient ration. Will these birds die if they eat a less nutrient-dense ration, like food scraps? No, but they just won't grow nearly as fast. Which is fine if you're just raising them for yourself. But for them to perform at optimum, they need an extremely dense beak full of food every time they take a bite. These birds grow fast, then, due to selective breeding and specially formulated rations that enable the bird to ingest more energy per beak full.

Practical Bite #9: Choose Your Disinfectant On Your Chicken

How? All chicken sold in the grocery store is disinfected with a chemical, usually chlorine. Find out which chemical is used to disinfect your chicken by visiting the Food Safety Inspection Service (FSIS) database (www.fsis.usda.gov/mpidirectory). Match the establishment number, located on the chicken package, to the processing location and simply call or email with the question: "What do you use to sterilize your chickens?" Once you know the answer, you can make an informed decision. You can continue to buy that chicken or, if you don't want to eat that chemical, you can find a different chicken that is disinfected with a chemical you are okay consuming. If you decide you do not want your chicken disinfected, skip ahead to Practical Bite #53.

Why?

Sina: Like eggs, the chicken in your local grocery store has probably taken a bath in chlorine. In an attempt to kill pathogens, the United States Department of Agriculture (USDA) allows chicken to be washed in chlorine. This is often the same type of chlorine that is used to bleach paper and your clothes, disinfect swimming pools, and make certain pesticides. Interestingly, the European Union banned this practice. They will not allow American chickens to be sold to their citizens if they have been treated with chlorine. Yet, the USDA says chlorinated chicken is good enough for Americans to eat.

We all know that chlorine exposure can be dangerous at certain levels. When it comes to your chicken, the problem is that nobody knows how much chlorine residue remains on the chicken or how much ends up on your dinner plate. You might be willing to take that risk. After all, how much chicken do you eat each week? But remember, chicken isn't the only source of chlorine in your diet. It's sometimes used to bleach flours, wash salad mixes and "fresh" produce, and disinfect machinery used in industrial food processing. And, if you live in a city, chlorine is commonly added to your drinking water under the guise of "safety."

The bottom line is, there is no way of knowing how much chlorine you are exposed to on a daily or weekly basis. Nobody is tracking your cumulative exposure or assessing your overall health risk. Yet, dunking your chicken in chlorine is considered a "safe" practice in the

United States.

What's most concerning to me is the damage chlorine does to your microbiome. You have microorganisms (including bacteria, fungi, and viruses) all over your body and inside your body – they are supposed to be there. They cover your skin, eyes, nose, digestive system, and so forth. Think about that for a moment: There is an entire ecosystem of non-human cells on and in you. In fact, for every one human cell you have roughly 10 bacterial cells. That means you are more bacteria than human. Let that concept sink in: You are more bacteria than human. Isn't that mind-blowing?

Joel: It's remarkable! I remember reading a few years ago that the researchers who concluded this ratio said we're only 10 percent human. These bacteria live INSIDE our cells—can you imagine? Just like a handful of healthy soil contains more microscopic beings than there are people on the face of the earth, our microbiome contains some 3 trillion—not million, not billion, but trillion—beings. Stanford University researchers even isolated their language—yes, they talk to each other.

Whenever I pull a carrot up from the garden, wipe it off on my pants, and eat it with a few dirt spots hanging on it, I imagine these soil and intestinal microscopic critters getting together for a family reunion: "Hi, cousin, long time no see! Let me show you through the GI tract. I don't think we'll encounter an earthworm, but we might find some other worms as we go." Whenever I speak to a group, I imagine everyone like Pigpen® in the Peanuts® comic strip, with a halo of microscopic viruses, bacteria and other beings dancing and spinning around, intersecting with the group from the guy sitting in the next seat. It's like a cloud of beings and they're carrying on, having elections, teaching foreign languages. Imagination is a wonderful thing.

Sina: Let's build on your image. Can you imagine those same tiny critters wearing black tuxedos and waving batons, like conductors of a symphony, as they orchestrate all of the different functions in your body?

We used to think your human cells regulated what happens in your body. We thought your human cells controlled your metabolism, immune function, ability to repair damaged tissues, etcetera. But now we are learning that your human cells probably don't control any of those functions. It's probably the microorganisms that coordinate what's happening in your body, including: helping to digest your food, making vitamins, synthesizing essential and nonessential amino acids, regulating your immune system and your physiology, etcetera. In other words, your microbiome is largely responsible for your overall health and well-being. Thus, the secret to being healthy, happy and free is being kind to your microbiome.

That's a hard concept to grasp because you can't see your microbiome. You can't touch it, taste it, hear it, smell it, or feel it. You have to rely on your imagination. How hard is it for you to believe in something that you can't see, touch, hear, taste, or smell?

I didn't fully comprehend the importance of the microbiome until my oldest son got chronically sick. When he was 5-years old, he developed symptoms of autism. It began with sensory issues and obsessive-compulsive behaviors that grew worse over time. He preferred to spend time with animals and would not engage with children or other adults. Then he developed difficulty with verbal communication – he began to stutter and drop the endings of words. I sought help from his pediatrician who said I was "paranoid" and that "Moms worry too much in this information age." So, I brought my son to a second doctor who agreed that I was paranoid. All the while, his stuttering was getting worse.

So, I decided to test his gut microbiome. Sure enough, he had dysbiosis - an imbalance in the types of microbes growing in his gut. One type of bacteria grew to a high enough level that it was causing symptoms of autism. That's all it took - ONE type of bacteria – and my son was sick. That's crazy! But this was even crazier: The bacteria that got out of control is *normally* present in the gut. It was causing problems because there weren't enough beneficial bacteria to keep it in check. Can you imagine that? My son developed symptoms of autism because his microbiome was imbalanced. Fortunately, we were able to completely reverse the symptoms.

Joel: That story is not only incredible, it brings hope to families struggling with similar issues. There's always hope.

We've experienced something similar on the farm. One of the most dramatic nutritional therapies we ever saw was in a batch of chicks. They came in from the hatchery seemingly healthy but after about two weeks they started exhibiting problems: their toes curled up and they scooted around on their hocks. In a couple of days, they would die. Lots of them suddenly had the problem and I was beside myself as to the cause. So, I took a couple to a lab for diagnosis: curled toe paralysis, caused by a lack of riboflavin. The physical domino effect that caused the paralysis was a staph infection created by friction in the leg tendons. These meat chickens were growing so fast that their tendons couldn't keep up with the rest of their growth.

The lab suggested antibiotics, of course, but interestingly, more than half on the list couldn't be used because staph was already immune to the antibiotic. Remember superbugs? Rather than use the antibiotic, I researched where lots of riboflavin existed: liver and greens. I went to the freezer, grabbed a couple packages of liver, and fed it to the chicks. Now remember, this was a serious staph infection. Yet, within 48 hours, the birds were up and walking normally. Not only did the nutrient-dense food stop the deficiency; it even cleaned up the staph infection. Nutritional balance is a big deal.

Sina: Balance is everything when it comes to health and wellness. In fact, the connection between microbiome imbalance and disease is now well documented in the scientific literature. By 2005, scientists had already begun decoding the genome of the microbiome of humans and had found a correlation between disease formation and the type of bacteria in the gut. By 2008, scientists had made the connection between breast cancer formation and a specific type of bacteria. And, by 2014, they realized that if you lost certain types of bacteria, cancer developed.

Today we know that depression, heart disease, obesity, diabetes, multiple sclerosis, asthma, autism, allergies and other inflammatory conditions are all associated with the types and quantities of bacteria in the gut. And, we believe that diet is a critical factor in determining the diversity and numbers of bacteria that make up your unique microbiome. In other words, a poor diet can create an imbalanced microbiome, which can create disease in your body.

Consuming chemicals, like chlorine, can create an imbalanced microbiome, which predisposes you to develop a disease. Chlorine is an antimicrobial. So, it is true that chlorine will kill some of the pathogens on your chicken that could make you temporarily sick with gastrointestinal upset. But, as an antimicrobial, it also kills beneficial microbes in your GI tract – the ones you need in order to be resilient. Remember when I said that cancer can develop from loss of beneficial bacteria in your gut? Numerous studies have concluded that Americans are losing their microbial diversity – perhaps by as much as 30%. That loss in resilience is partly due to eating sterilized food – like chicken bathed in chlorine.

You need to build a balanced microbiome that is diverse in order for you to be healthy and free of disease. You can't achieve that goal by eating sterilized food. When you eat sterilized food, you sterilize your body. Remember, you are more microbe than human. So, you literally kill off pieces of yourself each time you eat chicken that has taken a bath in chlorine because the chlorine is disinfecting, or killing off, your own microbes. In doing so, you can make yourself more susceptible to disease and infection.

Joel: The over-arching problem here is equating sterility with safety. The reason the USDA wants chickens bathed in chlorine is to kill pathogens living in and on the skin. Remember, in CAFOs, or chicken factories, the birds live on their excrement. Each chicken has about a half sheet of notebook paper to live on, so they are crowded, by the thousands, into these houses. You can scarcely breathe in them without a dust mask; imagine what that does to the chickens, who are much closer to the floor than you. And they never get a mask or relief. They can't walk out the door. So, their respiratory passages, mucus membranes, feathers, eyes, nostrils, and beak are all covered with fecal particulate, 24/7. Everything is filthy coming into the processing facility and since cleaning isn't really possible since it's embedded in the skin and the meat, the easiest thing to do is bathe it all in chlorine to sterilize it.

Sina: What do you mean the feces is "embedded" in the skin and meat? The chickens are living in feces so it makes sense that the filth would be on their feathers and skin. But, how is it embedded to the point where you can't wash it off?

Joel: Errant feces rides on the exterior of the live bird and is pummeled into the skin and meat because of the aggressive plucking machines used in industrial processing. I had an amazing guy come by the farm a few years ago. He was just retiring as a quality control guy in charge of two large industrial poultry processing plants. He'd grown up in the industry from the 1950s, and he said that when they changed their picking machines from the little tub pickers like we use at Polyface to the vertical gauntlet style, it completely changed the contamination.

On our farm, we use a little tub picker. It looks like a top load washing machine without a central agitation spindle but instead a bottom that spins—the sides stay stationary but the bottom plate spins; the interior features rubber fingers that gently pop the feathers out, kind of like squeezing zits on your face. When we toss our birds into the tub picker, gravity works in our favor and the birds just do a feather strip-tease lounging on the bottom plate. When the industry shifted to shackles that run through a gauntlet of vertical cylinders covered in fingers, they lost the benefit of gravity. As a result, the picking had to be far more aggressive to pop those feathers out. That added aggression knocks anything on the outside into the skin pores.

Filthy chickens come into the processing facility from their factory houses with a lot of contamination as they enter the picking gauntlet. That contamination gets smacked into the skin and is one reason the industry has to use such high-powered sterilization agents, like chlorine, to counteract the penetration of that contamination. This quality control fellow told me that the day the industry went to the vertical gauntlets for picking was the day they started having such big contamination problems.

Sina: Once you realize how the industrial food system operates, it makes sense that sterilizing agents are required. They are a necessary evil because the chickens do not contain a healthy microbiome due to the way they are raised and processed. But I don't think most consumers know that practically all of the food in the grocery store is sterilized and that sterility has a profound impact on their health. It took me years to make that connection.

Joel: Yes, our culture's fixation on sterility denies our microbiome the bacterial and nutritional diversity it needs. Isn't it amazing that Coke® is considered safe because it's sterile, but raw milk is considered hazardous because it has living creatures in it? We'd better be happy for living creatures because without them we would not have an immune system, a digestive system, a respiratory system or any other functional system.

In the microscopic world, good bugs outnumber bad bugs by about 30 to 1, normally. Only when something upsets the immunological terrain does it flip over the other way. Nature's default position, in other words, is wellness. If it's not well, something has upset nature's balance. More often than not, the perpetrator of such upsets is the human mind that thinks it's above natural balances. On our farm, we don't want sterility; we want a habitat that encourages good bugs so they can beat the bad bugs.

Sina: That's exactly what we did to heal my son. We created an environment where the microbes kept each other in check. But, that's the opposite of how factory food is raised, hence the need for chlorine sterilization.

Joel: Exactly. Think about this for a minute: If I wanted to launch a pathogen conspiracy on a farm, what would I do? First, I'd raise only one thing. Second, I'd crowd it tightly together. Third, I'd deny it fresh air, sunshine, and exercise. Fourth, I'd house it in filthy conditions. You get the drift here. What have I just described? Modern factory chicken farming. Can you imagine a flu outbreak in the local school division and the protocol being to bring all the kids to one big gymnasium, snuggled together, with no functioning bathrooms? Can you imagine? No reasonable person would ever conceive of such a thing. And yet that is exactly what we do with commercial chickens; but no worries; we can solve everything with chlorine baths. Yum.

Sina: So, what's the solution? How can you buy chicken that has not taken a bath in chlorine?

Joel: Any chicken that carries the USDA Inspection blue seal with an establishment number will be sterilized with something. Most USDA-inspected processing plants use chlorine. But some do use alternatives such as citric acid, paracetic acid, or concentrated hydrogen peroxide (35 percent).

You can find out which chemical is used to disinfect your chicken by visiting the Food Safety Inspection Service (FSIS) website. There you will find a database containing all the inspected processing establishments in the U.S. (www.fsis.usda.gov/mpidirectory) Match the establishment number to the processing company and simply call or email with the question: "What do you use to sterilize your chickens?" Anyone using something other than chlorine will happily and eagerly tell you what they use. They'd love more calls like that.

But remember, even if your chicken is not sterilized in chlorine, it's still sterilized with some type of chemical that will kill the good bugs as well as the bad bugs.

Sina: And, the chemical alternative may be worse than chlorine. I used to buy chicken from the grocery store if I ran out of my supply from Polyface Farm. But then I followed your advice and tracked down the processing plant. I called the company and the representative was happy to inform me that their chicken is not bathed in chlorine. When I asked which chemical they use instead of chlorine, I was floored by her response. They use hydrogen peroxide, and vinegar that is derived from corn! This, of course, alarmed me because my entire family is currently sensitive to corn. So, I asked if they had data indicating if any of the corn-derived proteins from the vinegar wash remained on or in the chicken. She said, "We have no way of knowing that information. But, according to our supplier, we cannot guarantee that our chicken does not contain corn." Wow! I told her that customers need to know that information because some of us have children with allergies or sensitivities to corn. She replied, "It's not required to be labeled on the chicken package."

That didn't sound right. So, I called the USDA and they agreed with the processing plant! They said the chemicals used to disinfect chicken are not required to be listed on the label because they are "processing aids"! This is another example of how labels are failing us and why we need to go beyond the labels.

Oh, and by the way, the chicken I bought in the grocery store was organic. Yep, even organic chicken is sterilized in some type of disinfectant, which could include chlorine.

Joel: That's absolutely right, Sina. The only way you can find chicken that has not been sterilized with something is to buy from local farmers who are exempt because all chickens sold in a grocery store are legally required to be sterilized with some type of chemical.

At Polyface, we use NOTHING on most of our birds. We don't have to sterilize our birds because they are healthy, and they have a healthy microbiome. The birds we process here at the farm are exempt under PL90-492 Producer-Grower Exemption. That's why they carry such a beautiful bloom on the carcass. All of the antimicrobial sterilizing agents create a bit of off-color residual on the bird.

We do have some birds that are processed at an inspection facility. Those birds carry a USDA establishment number (called the blue buzz, because it's a round blue icon) and are sterilized using paracetic acid.

Sina: If you can avoid sterilization by exempting your birds then why bother with the federal inspection? Why not exempt all of your birds and save our microbiomes?

Joel: There are many reasons why farmers who don't like these sterilizing agents still get chickens done under USDA inspection. First, if you're shipping or selling interstate, inspection is required by law. Second, some buyers won't consider a chicken not processed under inspection due to liability. Inspection absolves the processor and seller of nearly all liability; in our litigious society, retailers, processors, and many producers desire this protection. Finally, a reseller needs inspection. An exemption exists for direct producer-consumer sales, but for second party sales, like a grocery store, inspection is required.

For the most part, pastured poultry farmers who use inspection for all or some of their birds, like our farm, do it reluctantly. We all know it does not make the chicken safer, but regulatory tolerance doesn't have enough wiggle room for much innovation. The bottom line is to appreciate that often the product is held hostage by the system and it's not a battle most farmers can fight. Until a new day dawns in which sterilization does not equate with safety, this will be the regulatory position.

Sina: And, consumers are not powerless in this situation. They can help themselves and the farmers by giving informed consent. If you want to shop in the grocery store then find out which chemicals are used to disinfect your chicken. Once you know the answer, you can give informed consent. If you are okay with that particular disinfecting agent then continue to buy that chicken. If you aren't okay with it then find another brand that uses a disinfectant you can live with. And, if you decide you don't want your chicken disinfected then skip ahead to Practical Bite #53 to learn how to find locally grown, truly pasture-raised chickens that are not disinfected.

Joel: Folks, sterilization is good in surgery and in laboratories; it's not good in our guts or the food we eat. Living food should exhibit the same vibrant biodiverse microbial ecosystem as we'd expect in any healthy and thriving natural environment. So, do your microbes a favor and take this first step. Find chicken that's not disinfected with chlorine – and preferably anything else either.

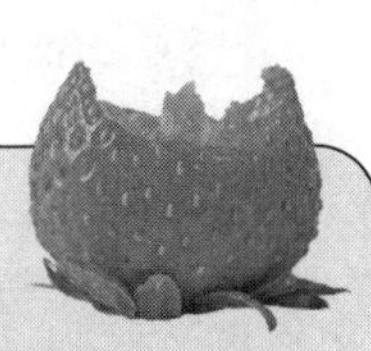

CHEW ON THIS

"Most of the salads in our supermarkets are rinsed in chlorinated water."

-Liam Fox, Secretary of State for International Trade

Practical Bite #10: Don't Waste Your Money on "Free Range" Or "Pasture Raised"

How? If you are looking for "free range" or "pasture raised" eggs or chickens in the grocery store, don't waste your money. The odds of finding true free range or pastured chickens and eggs in the grocery store is next to nil. Skip ahead to Practical Bites #53 and #54 to learn how to find true pasture raised chickens and eggs.

Why?

Sina: This is my favorite Practical Bite because before I met you, I recommended looking for the "pasture raised" label in the grocery store. Boy, was I duped!

Joel: Don't feel bad, most people have been duped. When free range poultry became a thing in consumer parlance, industrial factory farmers asked the USDA for a definition that would enable them to continue crowding chickens in confinement houses. Before I tell you what the clever industry wordsmiths concocted, stop a moment and consider what you think about when you hear the phrase "free range poultry." Stop reading for a moment and fantasize in your mind what that looks like.

Sina: I imagine chickens having the freedom to run around outside on green, lush grass while hunting for worms and enjoying the sunshine.

Joel: If that's your definition of free range then you would be wrong. The official USDA definition of "free range poultry" is actually the freedom to move all appendages to their extreme extension. I'll bet in your wildest dreams you would not have come up with that definition. Most people would have included something about outside, green grass, sunshine, pecking in the soil, chasing down some grasshoppers, and fluffing in a dirt pocket – like you did. That seems reasonable. But according to officialdom, as long as a chicken can fully extend its leg, or fully extend its wings—not necessarily at the same time, mind you—or fully extend its head above its body, that's free range. No grass. No outside. No bugs. No exercise. Only someone purposely trying to obfuscate the obvious could conceive of such a preposterous misrepresentation of the generally accepted meaning of "free range."

Sina: Wow! I used to feel good about buying organic, free-range eggs in the grocery store. I thought I was speaking with my dollars to help give chickens a better quality of life. But the "free range" label is just a marketing farce.

Joel: Yes. And, "organic" isn't any better. Organic certification requires that the chickens have "outdoor access." I remember the first time I visited an organic certified egg factory farm. The massive confinement house looked just like any other massive confinement poultry house except for one curious detail: surrounding the exterior of the house was a 3-foot strip and then a fence. The house had pop-holes every 50 feet or so, which are little 1-foot x 1-foot doors that enabled the chickens - if they ever wanted to - to step outside. Of course, the regulations that require "outdoor access" have a caveat: "weather permitting." The result? Well, today it's too hot; tomorrow it's too wet; the next day it's too dry; the next day it's too cold. Weather permitting can be used to exclude the birds any day of the year. And who wants to step onto a 3 ft. strip? It's hardly enough room to turn around.

Again, I ask the question: what do you think "outdoor access" means? Stop reading. Think about it.

Okay, I'll bet you thought about pastures and nature and exercise and soil and earthworms, maybe even a bluebird or indigo bunting flitting around. Of course. Any reasonable person would. Any person you would trust. But you see, folks, the wordsmiths and regulation police are not interested in truth or trust; they are only interested in pulling a fast one on duplicitous consumers just like you and I. We wouldn't think about playing this fast and loose with the truth, but when you're trying to pass yourself off as better than you are, and billions of dollars in sales are on the line, you become extremely inventive at clever speak.

After one of my editorials in *The Stockman Grass Farmer*, a certified organic pig producer said he didn't think it was possible to raise an ecologically-friendly hog on anything but concrete. Yes, concrete aprons—you could call them porches—are the "outdoor access" for hogs. I'm sure every consumer who reads the organic certification requirements for "outdoor access" fantasizes about concrete slabs.

The same wordsmithing has been done with "pasture raised." Pastured poultry, whether you get it local or shipped to your doorstep, is the gold standard for healthy terrain birds. But, the odds of finding true pastured chickens in the grocery store are next to nil.

Sina: So, an animal is still considered "pasture-raised" even if that animal never steps onto grass or pasture. And, an animal can be raised on a concrete slab and still be labeled as "organic." This is exactly why we must look beyond the labels to find the truth, and to protect our wallets. Keep in mind that you usually pay a premium for foods carrying those labels.

Joel: That's exactly right. I was recently in Colorado doing a food and farm conference and a guy came up to me at the after-conference meal at a local restaurant. He'd heard about me, and wanted to meet me. He produces 9,000 dozen eggs a week from 20,000 chickens in a house with pasture. He calls these pastured eggs. Now Sina, you can't have 20,000 chickens in a stationary house and have any semblance of pasture. First of all, a chicken will only walk 200 yards away from shelter. So even though you have them on 50 acres, they will never cover it all. The effective range of any chicken, no matter how free range, is only a circle 400 yards in diameter. A circle 400 yards in diameter is only 25 acres and I don't know anybody who has a circular pasture. Anyway, that's nearly 1,000 chickens per acre, which will quickly turn into a moonscape. That's a total nonrotated square footage per chicken of about 43.

In contrast, we give our 1,000 birds a quarter acre every three days, which is about 10 square feet per bird, but it's a new 10 square feet every 3 days. So, in a 240-day season, that's 80 paddock shifts times 10 square feet per, offering 800 square feet per bird. See what moving does?

I could go on in this vein for some time, but I hope by now you're starting to see a pattern of purposeful at worst, and negligent at best, clever wordsmithing to present things on labels, advertising, and sales pitches as they really aren't. No normal person could or would possibly convolute phrase meanings the way the government industrial food complex does. The first thing to understand is that words often, if not generally, have no objective meaning, especially on food labels and in food advertising. What you think from the words could be worlds different from actuality.

So, first, be aware of clever speak as a genre, as a skill. And, second, don't buy "free range" or "pasture raised" chicken or eggs from the grocery store; it's a labeling gimmick. Instead, skip ahead to Practical Bites #53 and 54 to learn how to find truly pasture-raised chickens and eggs.

Practical Bite #11: Eat 100% Grass-Finished, Organic Beef

How? In the grocery store, buy beef that is labeled 100% grass-fed and grass-finished, and USDA organic.

Why?

Joel: Beef is an herbivore. That means it eats plants but it's a bit more than that—whole plants. In other words, it does not eat just seeds; herbivores do like seeds, but just like a giraffe, they eat a few seeds or blossoms along with leaves. An herbivore has 4 stomachs and essentially a fermentation digestive system that turns cellulose into sugars and proteins. The human digestive system cannot do what an herbivore digestive system does. You and I can't go out and be content eating our lawn; a cow or sheep can. Cows are not just big humans; they're a completely different critter.

Grain is seeds. Consumed as part of a whole plant, the herbivore gets along well. For instance, when grass is in full seed, our cows go along and nip off the seed heads like candy. Is that grain? Yes, in the technical sense. But in concentrations, it creates problems. You see, our stomachs are quite acidic and cows' aren't. When they eat concentrations of grains, they become acidic. When their system is acidic, bacteria that would be killed by our acidic gut are acclimated to a higher acid environment and are NOT killed, but instead kill, or at least hurt us if we eat them on the meat.

Just remember, when it comes to deciding what to buy, you're always trying to decide between what's least bad and what's the best. Sometimes least bad is the best you can do. A baby learning to walk is not worried about how to run; it's just how to walk least bad, right?

So here we go into the store; what are we looking for?

Think about two legs propping up a decision: one leg is bad stuff; the other leg is good stuff. You want to minimize the bad stuff and maximize the good stuff. More often than not the more conventional retail interfaces, like supermarkets, will not have an "only good" option. It'll be somewhere "less bad" with "some good." That's okay; it's where you start. Even a kindergartener, learning to hold a pencil, does not shape letters perfectly. That'll come over time.

If you're really savvy, you'll look at brands and bring up their websites. Some may be "organic," others will use the word "natural" and others will use "grass-fed."

If it's government organic certified, that means at least the grain was not genetically modified, which is a good thing. But I'll take the grass-fed or grass-finished over organic and here's why.

Organic does not prohibit seed-feeding herbivores, or what is commonly known as grain-finished or grain fattening. Many brands tout their "grain-finished" beef as a good thing, but nutritionally that is the bottom of the continuum. If on their website they say things like "minimally finished on grain for just the last 100 days," that's grain-finished and nothing special. Most grain finishing is between 100 and 150 days; that's the conventional feedlot finishing phase. Better to have a plant-finished herbivore that's not certified organic than an organic one finished in a feedlot, organic or otherwise.

Sina: I agree, grass-finished is the only way to go. In fact, if the only options in my grocery store were grain-fed or grass-fed but grain-finished, I would become a vegetarian. I won't feed my family beef unless it was grass-finished, at a minimum.

Unfortunately, most beef produced in the U.S. is grain-fed. And, as Joel said, since cows are not designed to eat a grain-based diet, they can develop acidosis (too much acid), which can allow harmful microorganisms to grow, including *E. coli*. That's one reason why antibiotics are routinely given to grain-fed cows. Unfortunately, those antibiotics (or their residues) can be passed on to you when you eat the meat, which not only sets you on the path toward developing antibiotic resistance, it hurts your gut microbiome making you more likely to develop a chronic disease.

In addition, the bacterial overgrowth or gut dysbiosis that develops from a grain-based diet can lead to inflammation and numerous health problems in the cow, like metabolic disease, which also effects the quality of the meat you eat. The bottom line is that meat from grain-fed cows is often sick. And, since you literally are what you eat, consuming sick meat can make you sick. That's why I only eat grass-fed, grass-finished beef.

Studies have shown that cows fed their natural grass diet for their entire lives are healthier than grain-fed cows. For instance, compared to meat from grain-fed cows, meat from grass-finished cows can contain more omega-3 fatty acids, conjugated linoleic acids, B-vitamins, minerals, and some antioxidants, including vitamin E. Consequently, grass-finished beef is associated with a reduced risk of heart disease, diabetes, cancer and weight gain when compared to grain-fed beef.

In the grocery store, it can be tricky to identify the higher quality beef because of the labeling guidelines. "Grass-fed" means the cow ate grass for some period of time. So, if the label only states "grass-fed" without any other qualifiers then the cow may have received grains. In contrast, "grass-finished" means the cow ate grass for its entire life, including when it was at the feed lot. Does that sound backwards to you too? It's confusing. But if you want to eat meat from a cow that was raised solely on grass then look for the words "grass-finished" or "100% grass-fed" on the package.

But there's a catch: "Grass-fed" and "grass-finished" claims are not effectively regulated by the USDA. For instance, in 2016, the USDA withdrew their definition of "grass-fed," along with the accompanying standards. Consequently, if a company wants to claim "grass-fed" on their label, the USDA no longer verifies the applicant's claim to the standards because there are no real government standards. Instead, the company submits paperwork to the USDA asking for "approval" to use the word "grass-fed" on their label. There are no inspections of the farm. The company just checks the boxes and the USDA trusts that the answers are true and accurate. Consequently, the claims "grass-fed" and "grass-finished" are subjective and open to interpretation.

Joel: Yes, "grass-fed" doesn't mean anything - officially the industry says that if a cow has had one blade of grass in her life, she's "grass-fed". All of them do, of course, because nobody calves in a feedlot. That's why many of us began using grass-finished, but then you have the cheaters saying if they're on grass during finishing, that's fine. So, they feed corn on grass and that's grass finishing. You can't make this stuff up. So, we come back to know your farmer; know your food.

Sina: Yes, your best bet is to buy from a local farmer you trust. Since I don't know the farmers who sell meat at my local grocery store, and since there is uncertainty in the grass-fed and grass-finished labels, I increase my level of trust in the meat by looking for these two statements on the package: "100% grass-fed" *and* "grass-finished." Combining those two statements increases the odds of eating beef that was fed a grass diet and finished on a grass diet.

Joel: Someone could chide us for not putting any faith in labels, but the other side of that is equally true: do we really want to not put ANY trust in labels? Both of those seem extreme from a practical sense. As you continue on in the book, you'll find doable alternatives to the store; but at this point in our discussion, if you're buying in the store, at least buy from folks who are thinking enough to put it on a label or explain their protocols on a website.

Sina: Labels are complicated and, as you can see, are filled with loopholes and subjectivity. However, those labels are the tool you have at your disposal to help you find the best food in the grocery store. So, meet yourself where you are, and work with the tools you have.

When in the grocery store, I also look for the word "organic" on the label. So, when buying from a grocery store, my first choice is 100% grass-fed (and grass-finished) organic beef. I look for both of those terms on the label because each term contains gaps. For example, "organic" means the cow was not fed GMOs, given hormones, or exposed to most antibiotics, pesticides and herbicides. However, the cow can still be fed grains, as Joel mentioned. On the other hand, if the beef is 100% grass-fed (and grass-finished) but *not* organic, the cow can be given hormones and antibiotics. In addition, the grass the cow ate could have been sprayed with pesticides, including glyphosate, which is one of the active ingredients in Roundup®. I avoid glyphosate at all costs because we know it can contribute to cancer, autoimmune disease, sleep disorders, depression, infertility, autism, thyroid disease, and other ailments.

I want to be clear; I'm not saying 100% grass-fed cows eat pesticide-sprayed grass or are always given antibiotics and hormones. But according to the definition of 100% grass-fed (or grass-finished), it's possible. And, unless you contact the farmer, you don't have any guarantees; you are trusting the label. So, I account for the gaps in both labels by combining them i.e. I buy organic beef that is 100% grass-fed (and grass-finished).

My second choice in the grocery store is beef that is labeled as 100% grass-fed (and grass-finished) with "no antibiotics or added hormones." In this case, we've made sure the cow was not fed grains and was not given antibiotics or hormones, but the grass the cow ate could have been sprayed with pesticides. If I'm craving beef and this is the only option available then I will sometimes buy it. In that event, I make sure to drink plenty of water and sweat to help my body detox from possible exposure to pesticides.

Joel: What you don't want is something that only says "natural." That word is completely meaningless.

Now the next question is proximity. For most of us trying to eat better, local sourcing is on our radar. So, what if I have local organic versus New Zealand grass-finished? That gets tricky, and I wouldn't fault you either way. One is more herbivore-respectfully produced; the other is closer to your plate. Toss a coin and choose. That's okay.

Sina: Another issue is the increased cost. When I upgraded my meat, I was in sticker shock. But I knew the health benefits for both my family and the animal so I wanted to make the change.

One way to decrease your cost is to go beyond the label. If there's a grass-finished option that is less expensive than the grass-finished, organic option then contact the company.

Joel: Absolutely. You can tell a lot by going on brand websites, and I suggest you do it. If you don't want to take the time to do it on your smartphone in the grocery store, just make a note of the brands you're interested in and research them when you get home. It'll be more fun than watching a movie and very quickly you'll start getting savvy about phrases.

You'll be able to match phrases with pictures. As what I call your "sussing out" skill increases, you'll be able to make a better decision.

Sina: Exactly. And, if you don't find the information that you're looking for on the company website then call or email to ask questions, such as:

- ❖ Are your cows fed a 100% grass diet and are they 100% grass-finished?
- ❖ Are your cows given antibiotics?
- ❖ Are your cows given any hormones?
- ❖ Is the pasture where your cows graze sprayed with any type of pesticide or herbicide?

Joel: As a general rule, the supermarket option will always be primarily a "less bad" option, but that's a great place to start. As you progress through the steps in this book, we'll coach you to a point where you'll be able to go to the "only good" option. That's where we're headed, so buckle up. Start now where you shop, but enjoy the journey to Paradise.

Practical Bite #12: Eat What You Can Pronounce

How? When choosing processed foods, read the ingredient label - out loud. If you cannot pronounce an ingredient or you don't know where it comes from, how it's made, and the possible health effects then don't eat that food.

Why?

Joel: I consider unpronounceable ingredients shackles. We haven't talked about freedom much, but I think it's appropriate here. These things you can't make in your home, where it takes a Ph.D. in chemistry - Sina, you could make this stuff! - and a million-dollar lab is advertised as freeing us from the bondage of our kitchens. These unpronounceables - kind of a new take on munchables, huh? - guarantee longer shelf life, better color, perfect mouth feel, and all sorts of characteristics that make our kitchens unnecessary.

In reality, however, these unpronounceables shackle us to nutrient deficiency, irritable bowel syndrome, inflammation and a host of maladies we haven't even discovered yet due to symptom lag time. In effect, they shackled us to doctors and pain and fatigue. Isn't it interesting that in promising to free us from kitchen duties, the industry concocts ingredients that shackle us to a whole litany of establishment dependency?

Wendell Berry, perhaps the greatest voice of eco-literacy this century, writes that what is wrong with us creates more gross domestic product (GDP) than what is right with us. If you eat terrible food and stay sick and lose your marriage and your job, you now have two houses where one was before, and you have doctor visits and drugs and surgeries. All of this economic activity registers on the GDP ledger as an asset. But if you grow your garden, eat your own food, stay married and well, you don't need all that economic activity. It's not a conspiracy; it's simply what fills the vacuum when we abdicate thought acuity.

Sina: You are right that unpronounceable ingredients keep us shackled. But, once you realize what's in the majority of processed foods and you stop eating them, it can feel like you're deprived or in a prison with a new set of shackles.

I remember when my husband used to walk around Costco® every Friday afternoon and fill up on the free food samples. He looked forward to that "event" every week. Then, one day, I mentioned how it's common for foods to be made with chemical byproducts that are created in a laboratory, and how those chemicals are added to our foods without any safety testing or regulation by the FDA. The next Friday, he came home from his weekly Costco® trip and said, "Thanks a lot! You've ruined Costco® for me!"

Instead of blindly eating the free samples, my husband had picked up each box of food and read the ingredient list. He was shocked to find numerous chemicals in those foods that didn't even sound like food; chemicals such as: maltodextrin, cellulose, polysorbate, malic acid, and xanthan gum. Some ingredients he couldn't even pronounce (and he's a chemical engineer!). Since he didn't know where those ingredients came from, and he knew that nobody was testing them for long-term safety, he couldn't bring himself to eat the free samples.

We joke about it now, but in that moment, my husband did not feel free. He felt deprived. The life he knew and loved was changed in an instant. Now he's grateful because knowing the truth has set him free. He feels better than he did in his 20s! And, one of the first steps in his healing journey was removing all of the ingredients from his diet that he either couldn't pronounce or didn't want to take the time to look up. Yep, laziness can pay off!

It's crazy when you stop and think that most of us eat chemicals in our food every day and those chemicals have not been tested for long-term safety. In fact, there are roughly 10,000 chemical additives in our food supply. Most of them have not been safety tested by the FDA and most are not even regulated by the FDA. We don't know how those chemicals affect our long-term health. And, we have no idea what happens when those chemicals are combined. For instance, what happens when the brominated vegetable oil in your Mountain Dew® is combined with the disodium inosinate in your Doritos®? Nobody knows.

This regulatory loophole started in 1958 when Congress passed the Food Additive Amendment. The purpose was to test chemicals for safety before adding them to our food. What a novel concept! But that amendment contains the GRAS exemption. Remember GRAS from Practical Bite #1?

If a chemical is GRAS it's considered "generally recognized as safe." That means the chemical does not have to go through an FDA approval process. It gets a free pass from a laboratory to your dinner plate.

The GRAS exemption was meant to be a good thing. It was meant to exempt commonly used ingredients like water and vinegar. But it has turned into a loophole that affects practically everyone who eats processed food because almost all chemicals added to our food in the last decade have been added through the GRAS loophole.

When I learned about this loophole, I wondered why the FDA was not doing its job. Isn't it their job to test the chemicals in our food for safety? So, I reached out to the Government Accountability Office (GAO), which is our government watchdog. They investigate how the federal government spends taxpayer dollars and are supposed to hold other government agencies accountable.

According to the GAO, Congress messed up. When Congress wrote the Food Additive Amendment, they never declared who would be responsible for determining when a chemical qualifies as GRAS. So, the companies that make the chemicals are now deciding if their own chemicals are GRAS. What? That didn't sound right. So, I dug a little deeper and found the FDA's policy on GRAS.

It turned out to be true! The FDA issued a "guidance" document to industry with voluntary "nonbinding recommendations." In that document, the FDA reminded companies that it's their responsibility to ensure safety of the chemicals they put in our food. According to the way the law was written, the FDA believes the responsibility falls on the companies.

In that leadership vacuum, companies began declaring their own products as safe. Legally, companies need an "expert" to declare a chemical to be GRAS. So, who are these "experts?"

A 2013 study in *JAMA Internal Medicine*, revealed that the experts commonly have financial ties to the company. And, as soon as an "expert" declares the chemical to be safe, it can be immediately added to our food. There is no waiting period. And, companies don't even have to notify the FDA when they add a new chemical to our food. The notification process is voluntary!

If the FDA does not have to be notified when chemicals are added to our food, how can the FDA notify *you* if there is a problem with an ingredient, or if there's a recall? More importantly, how can the FDA ensure your food is safe if they don't even know what's in it? They can't.

But, here's the kicker: Guess who made the notification process voluntary?

The FDA!

Joel: Why am I not surprised?

The award-winning documentary *Food Inc.* profoundly influenced food buying in our country - at least for a while. It brought many issues into public awareness. I remember shortly after the movie came out, our farm store was flooded for several months with people who came saying "we saw that documentary and went home and threw out everything in the pantry. Now we want real food."

That was heartening indeed and we were glad our farm received such good footage. But by far and away my favorite portion of the documentary was toward the end when it showed business cards of what is known as the revolving door. These are people who work in the industry and then get appointed to oversight roles in regulatory agencies, and then revolve out again into the industry.

Perhaps the most egregious one was when President Obama named Michael Taylor to be his new food safety czar (why would any U.S. president use the term "czar?"). Who was this Michael Taylor? He was a king pin at Monsanto who shepherded the first GMOs onto the market. And then he gets appointed to be the supreme protector of America's food supply. How much do you think he believes in compost instead of chemicals? How much do you think he believes in pastured chicken rather than factory chicken? Grass-finished beef rather than feed lot CAFO beef? Appointments like this to watchdog agencies establish the whole food system in a mechanistic, sterile, techno-glitzy corporate fabricated unpronounceable trajectory.

Do you really trust this man to deliver safe food to you?

Sina: You know I don't! Before President Obama appointed Michael Taylor to be the Food Safety Czar, he was appointed by President Bush to be the FDA Deputy Commissioner of Policy. That's when he wrote the FDA's labeling guidelines for the first genetically engineered hormone that was introduced into our food supply – manufactured by Monsanto. It resulted in sick cows, sick milk, and sick people (See Practical Bite #20)

The point is, both sides of the political aisle have contributed to the demise of our food supply. But we can rise above it. Food crosses political lines and party boundaries. Food unifies us because we all need food – clean, healing food. And, at the end of the day, responsibility and trust are two of the greatest gifts you can give yourself. They might not come wrapped in a pretty package with a beautiful red bow on top. But they come with peace of mind, health, and freedom.

When my husband read the ingredient labels that fateful day in Costco®, he was extremely disappointed that his free sample days were over. But he reached a milestone that day; he became an informed consumer. And, that's what it all boils down to – informed consent. You have the right to choose what you want to put into your body. In order to exercise that right, you have to know your options. If you don't know where an ingredient comes from or how it's made then you cannot give informed consent. Instead, you are blindly trusting that the company or the government has tested that chemical for long-term safety. Chances are, they haven't.

So, set yourself free by allowing yourself to receive the gifts of responsibility and trust. Start small and work your way up. Pick up one item in your refrigerator or pantry and read the ingredient label. If there's an ingredient you don't know, look it up. Once you know how it's made, where it's sourced, and if there are any known adverse health effects associated with that ingredient then you can make an informed decision about whether or not you want that chemical to become part of your body.

Practical Bite #13: Avoid Artificial & "Natural" Flavor

How? Read the ingredient list on every food item in your pantry, refrigerator and freezer. If "artificial flavor" or "natural flavor" are listed, do not buy those foods again. To avoid feeling overwhelmed, start with your favorite food and then slowly move through your entire kitchen – picking one food to analyze each day or one each week.

Why?

Sina: Have you noticed how many processed foods contain flavorings? If you check the ingredient labels of your favorite foods, you'll likely find the words "artificial flavor" or "natural flavor." Even organic foods can contain "natural flavor." Why do so many of our processed foods contain flavoring?

When whole foods are processed, the flavors are often destroyed. So, manufacturers have to add flavors back to your food to make them taste good again. That may sound harmless, but the added flavors are not "natural" – they are artificial and are made in a laboratory by a chemist.

In fact, one flavoring can be made up of nearly 100 chemicals. And, companies don't have to tell you which chemicals they are using. They are often considered industry trade secrets, which is good for the company because if you knew which chemicals were added to your favorite foods, you'd probably stop eating them. For instance, the strawberry flavoring used in some shakes contains methyl anthranilate, amyl valerate, and ethyl methylphenylglycidate. If you only ate what you know, could you drink that shake?

It may sound like I'm an alarmist because I don't want to put flavoring chemicals in my body. After all, those chemicals *have* to be safe for us eat. Surely, the FDA or EPA or USDA or some government agency has tested them for safety, right?

Wrong.

Let's look at acetaldehyde, as an example. It's a flammable liquid that was designated as a carcinogen by the International Agency for Research on Cancer. That means acetaldehyde is believed to cause cancer. Yet, it is an "approved" flavoring that can be added to your food. If it can cause cancer, how did it get "approved?"

Flavorings are considered generally recognized as safe (GRAS). Remember GRAS from Practical Bite #12? GRAS means the government does not test the chemical for safety. Instead, they rely on the company to determine if the chemicals they are adding to the food are safe for us to eat. The company also determines *how much* of the chemical is safe for us to eat.

When it comes to flavorings, it gets more complicated because the Flavor and Extract Manufactures Association (FEMA) was formed as an industry solution to the FDA's hands-off approach to flavorings. FEMA sidestepped the government by creating their own GRAS determination process. Since 1960, they have declared over 2,600 chemicals to be GRAS.

FEMA consists of roughly 120-member companies. Those companies submit GRAS applications to FEMA's "expert" panel. Once approved, FEMA notifies the FDA of their GRAS determinations. At first glance, FEMA sounds pretty great. After all, it's a third-party organization that independently certifies a GRAS list.

But FEMA created their own guidelines when determining if a chemical is safe. For instance, when determining if a chemical causes cancer, FEMA's attorney and senior science advisor stated, "Whether a food ingredient is GRAS depends on general recognition of safety, not on safety *per se*...a substance that causes tumors in laboratory animals at high doses is nevertheless GRAS under conditions of intended use in human food..."

Using that guideline, FEMA has approved chemicals for us to eat that have been shown to induce cancer. For instance, FEMA declared isoeugenol to be GRAS even though a 2-year study conducted by the National Toxicology Program determined it to be carcinogenic in rats. I want to be clear on this point: The National Toxicology Program is part of the U.S. Department of Health and Human Services, which also houses the FDA. In other words, our own government declared isoeugenol to cause cancer, but FEMA said it was safe for us to eat. So, who won the debate?

FEMA.

FEMA said the cancer risk "is not relevant to humans who consume isoeugenol at low non-toxic levels." But nobody actually knows how many of these GRAS chemicals you eat on a daily basis because nobody tracks GRAS chemicals – not the government, not the companies, and not the individual. You can't even track your consumption if you wanted to since industry doesn't have to list every flavoring chemical on the label! Usually the ingredient list only states "natural flavoring" or "artificial flavoring."

So, while we don't know how much isoeugenol you are eating, we do know there is "widespread human exposure" to isoeugenol because it's now found in baked goods, chewing gum, and non-alcoholic drinks.

If companies won't tell us which chemicals make up flavorings, and the FDA does not test those chemicals for safety, and industry organizations create flawed guidelines when determining their safety, can we trust those foods?

I don't trust "natural" or artificial flavors. There's too much secrecy, too little accountability, and no way for me to give informed consent when I can't even find out which chemicals are used to create those flavors.

Joel: Words are interesting, aren't they? "Beauty is in the eye of the beholder" certainly appreciates inherent ambiguity. When I look at a well-done pile of compost, I think it's as beautiful as money. Yes, beauty is in the eye of the beholder. What is big, small, long, short—it's kind of subjective, isn't it?

Perhaps no industry better leverages word crafting, sometimes called clever speak, than the food and farming sector. For example, when food irradiation first hit the mainstream a few years ago, food processors decided it would be more palatable to consumers if they called it "cold pasteurization." Most people know what milk pasteurization is, and it's widely accepted within the culture. Using the phrase cold pasteurization for irradiation cleverly disguised the actual process. And of course, irradiating something is quite different than simply heating it, like a pan on a stove. It involves applying ionizing radiation to food. But food sales wordsmiths don't worry about misleading; they only want consumer acceptance.

Next, realize that well produced and unprocessed food does not need artificials. One of the most common exclamations from customers eating our pastured chickens is: "My, this chicken doesn't need spice or sauce; it actually has taste!" Why? Because junk chicken is bland. One spring we had a lot of extra eggs and I tried peddling some to diners around town. Normally, upscale restaurants are our customers, but with an overage, we decided to dip down into the cheaper diners. One cook tried one of our eggs and exclaimed: "Our customers don't want eggs with taste!" Another restaurant owner told me: "Our customers just want crap.

They don't care about quality." By the way, these establishments have received regional food awards; they are not dives. If the farmer does the job right, and it's not reduced to mush in processing, food doesn't need any enhancing.

One of the most poignant lessons on this, for me, was dessert at iconic local food gourmand Alice Waters' Chez Panise restaurant in Berkeley, California. After the meal, I was prepared for some sort of extravagant and exotic pastry dessert. But no, it was clementines from Michael Ableman's farm nearby. And when I ate one, I realized nothing, absolutely nothing, could have improved on that exquisite fruit.

Michael is a master orchardist and gardener; Alice had enough confidence in his clementines to offer them unmolested at arguably one of the top foodie hubs of the world. That's real food. And you can enjoy that quality too. But it starts by knowing what you've got. It starts by being dissatisfied, perhaps even gob struck, by your own duplicity in the conventional food space. Don't worry, you didn't get here overnight and you won't get out overnight. But awareness turned to disgust will do a lot to set your emotional and mental trajectory on a healing path. Welcome.

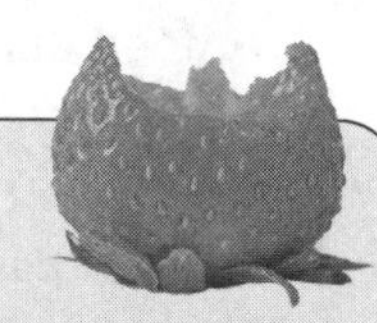

CHEW ON THIS

It is legal for your food to be exposed to radiation in the form of gamma rays emitted from radioactive elements, x-rays, or electron beams. The radiation exposure can be equivalent to 30 million chest x-rays, according to *Natural News*. And, that level of radiation is known to create chemicals in your food, called radiolytic products, that may be associated with cancer.

The government actually considers irradiation of your food to be a food additive. Consequently, you may never know if your food has been treated with radiation because individual ingredients that have been radiated do not have to be labeled. Only irradiation of a final product requires labeling. That means, if 99% of the ingredients in your frozen pizza were irradiated, but the final product wasn't, you wouldn't know.

The FDA has approved irradiation for the following foods: beef, pork, poultry, eggs, fresh fruits and vegetables, crustaceans, shellfish, spices and seasonings. Radiation for dinner, anyone?

Practical Bite #14: Choose Preservative Free

How? Read the list of ingredients on every food item in your pantry, refrigerator, and freezer. If preservatives are listed, do not buy those foods again. It can be tricky knowing which ingredients are preservatives. So, here's a good starting point: When looking at the ingredient list, the word "preservative" is often listed in parenthesis following the ingredient. You can also look for the words "no preservatives" or "preservative free" on the food package.

Why?

Joel: Think of preservatives as embalming agents. The whole point of preservatives is to slow down decay, or decomposition. Nature has some extremely beneficial preservatives like fermenting (wine, sauerkraut, kimchi) and drying. Excluding air through dehydration or pulling a vacuum, like canning, is also a way to preserve. None of these are artificial in the non-pronounceable sense. They are all permutations of natural systems.

On our farm, we feed the soil with aerobic compost. We make mountains of it using pigs to do the turning. The entire biological process revolves around life, death, decomposition, and regeneration. That circle goes around and around and around. We don't want to put anything on the soil that won't rot; if it won't rot, it won't feed the soil. We don't want anything in that compost that will inhibit decomposition. Goodness, we don't even want anything in it that won't decay, like glass, plastic, aluminum or metal.

I saw one of the greatest demonstrations of this principle in California at a school farm. Incorporated into the curriculum of the entire school system, this 3-acre farm gave students lots of opportunities to interact with plants, animals, and the soil. The two ladies running the farm program had a large worm box. Made of wood, it measured about 8 feet long, 3 feet wide, and 3 feet high.

One of the first assignments for the students was to bring some food to class. Students brought Twizzlers®, Oreo® cookies, gummy worms, marshmallows and squeezable cheese. The teachers brought an orange, apple, lettuce and a green bean. The students put all their contributions in the worm box on one end and the teachers put theirs in on the other end. The next week the students ran to the box, opened the lid, and found all their contributions sitting there untouched.

The teachers' contributions, on the other hand, were completely gone. Digested. As the students puzzled over this phenomenon, the teachers made their point: "why would you want to eat something worms won't even eat?" Wow! The point is, what drives life is death and decomposition. If it won't rot, it won't decay. If it won't rot, it won't digest.

Any artificial chemical added to a food to prevent decay or decomposition will inhibit digestion in our gut. It follows as surely as day follow night. Do you want to put the equivalent of plastic into your systems? Do you want to put digestion inhibitors in your system? Really? This is not hard to figure out.

Sina: Most of us have heard the argument that some preservatives are associated with the development of disease. For instance, propyl gallate is commonly found in microwave popcorn, frozen dinners, soup mixes, chewing gum, and other foods containing fats. It's a synthetic antioxidant that helps prevent fat from turning rancid. But studies have shown propyl gallate can kill human endothelial cells, damage DNA, elicit allergic reactions, and mimic estrogen. Yet, it's considered GRAS, so it's freely added to your processed foods. Then there's nitrite, which is often found in processed meats and is probably best known for giving hot dogs their red coloring. But nitrites are associated with certain types of cancer.

Now Joel, we could spend the entire day rattling off examples of various chemical preservatives that are associated with various diseases. But that's old news and, frankly, I find it boring. I'm interested in a concept that is so simple, it's often overlooked: I think preservatives are leading to micronutrient deficiencies, which can lead to chronic disease.

Check this out: Preservatives are added to foods to prolong shelf-life. Some preservatives work by preventing the food from being broken down, or eaten, by microorganisms like mold, bacteria, fungi, or yeast while it sits on the grocery store shelf. But remember, you have microorganisms in *your* gastrointestinal tract that *you* need in order to break down *your* food. So, if preservatives can prevent bacteria from eating food that is sitting on the grocery store shelf then can't those preservatives also prevent the bacteria in your gut from eating that very same food? And, if your bacteria can't eat the food then how can they help release the nutrients from that food so your body can absorb and use them? Plus, if your bacteria aren't being fed by that food then how can they make the vitamins and other nutrients that you need in order to be healthy and well?

The truth is, nobody definitively knows what happens when you eat preservatives in your meal. But we do know that micronutrient deficiencies are becoming common once again. It's estimated that every American is deficient or inadequate in at least one nutrient. And, sometimes, it only takes one nutrient deficiency to develop a disease. For instance, some autoimmune diseases can develop if you are deficient in vitamin D. Insulin resistance can result from a chromium deficiency. And, lack of magnesium can result in high blood pressure.

But here's the kicker: we know that an individual can take a multivitamin and mineral on a regular basis, but still develop a disease from nutrient deficiencies. Sounds crazy, right? But that's exactly what happened to me.

I took a high-quality multivitamin and mineral every single day, yet I developed deficiencies in 15 different nutrients. Two of the deficiencies were so severe that I was diagnosed as borderline for both beriberi and pellagra. Both of those diseases can lead to death. And, both were eradicated in the United States in the early to mid-1900s. Yet, we are seeing a resurgence of these types of nutrient deficiency diseases. Why?

I contend that one reason is the consumption of preservatives in our processed food. Think about it: Processed foods already contain less nutrients than whole foods, and the nutrients are less bioavailable because they are often man-made or synthetic. Then, chemical preservatives are added that may prevent your microbes from adequately digesting that food and accessing those nutrients, as well as hinder their ability to create the nutrients your body needs for optimal health. It's a recipe for disaster.

Plus, we know that some preservatives used in our foods are actually chelators, like ethylenediaminetetraacetic acid (EDTA), for example. If someone has high levels of heavy metals in their body, EDTA can be used to help lower that toxic burden. It's a chelator, so EDTA binds to heavy metals or minerals such as lead, mercury, and arsenic. That's a good thing when you have too many heavy metals in your body. But, EDTA can also pull out beneficial minerals like calcium and iron. If too much is pulled out, it can increase your risk for nutrient deficiencies. That's why, when people undergo chelation therapy, practitioners typically recommend large doses of beneficial minerals to help the patient avoid becoming deficient in micronutrients.

The problem with eating EDTA in your food is that nobody knows how much you eat on a daily basis because nobody is tracking it. Why?

You've probably already figured it out - EDTA is considered GRAS. Consequently, it is widely used in the food industry, finding its way into many processed foods, such as: some breakfast cereals, cereal bars, processed fruits and vegetables, packaged meat, and fortified grains.

So, what happens if you're a typical American who consumes nearly 75% of their calories from processed foods that contain these types of preservatives? Nobody knows. But, doesn't it seem logical that it could contribute to you developing a nutrient deficiency?

Joel: Yes. The whole point of preservatives is to stop the natural cellular development in the biological system. The cells in the food are virtually identical to the cells in our bodies. They look the same; they have the same parts; they function the same way. You don't have to be as smart as Sina to know that putting cellular disrupters into your microbiome is probably not a good idea. And none of us knows our tolerances.

Of course, we all know the junk food junkie who seems to get along fine. One smoker gets throat cancer at 45 and another one lives to 95 seemingly unfazed. But which one are you? How do you know? Do you want to play the game and find out?

I like the fable about the king who needed to hire a chauffeur. To get to the castle required navigating a narrow road on a mountain precipice. The first candidate came in and the king asked him how close he could drive to the edge of the precipice and still feel safe. "About 5 feet, m'lord," replied the first candidate. The second candidate, receiving the same question, responded "I can get within 3 feet, your majesty."

The third candidate received the same question and answered "I have no idea, Sire. I would stay as far away from it as I could." To which the king quickly replied, "You are my new chauffer." The point is, you don't want to fool around with chemicals that shut down your cells. Why this is so hard to understand I have no idea.

Sina: That's exactly my point. And, I'm not saying that preservatives are the one and only reason behind nutrient deficiencies. Clearly, there are multiple factors involved. But, what if something as simple as not eating preservatives could help prevent you from developing a nutrient-deficiency disease? Isn't that worth the effort of looking for the words "no preservatives" when you buy processed food?

Joel: This steady desire for shelf stability is a direct result of long transportation distances from field to plate and long warehousing. Have you ever noticed the sell by dates on some packaged food items? I'm not talking about canned stuff or freeze dried or dehydrated. I'm talking boxes of mac-n-cheese. Our supermarket system screams for massive inventories, which requires mega-warehousing. That long chain requires a lot of time to be built into the system.

If one classification of artificial food additives proves the industry's paradigm toward sustenance is primarily mechanical and not biological, it is the preservative business. Injecting chemicals into our food that are fabricated to stop perishable deterioration - rather than freezing, fermenting, or creating a vacuum - is food adulteration in its most obvious form.

Practical Bite #15: Don't Fear The Fat Label

How? If you count fat grams or eat low-fat foods, ask yourself why. Give yourself the space to really search your soul for the answer. Maybe you were told fat is "unhealthy" or that eating fat would make you fat. Or, maybe eating low-fat is how you were raised so you are simply following the example set by your parents. Figure out why you avoid fat so that you can begin listening to your own body instead of making food choices based on fear or inherited habits.

Why?

Sina: Do you remember the low-fat craze?

Joel: Anyone who lived pre-2000 remembers this. Goodness, Crisco® was in every cupboard and hydrogenated vegetable oil was the ultimate culinary partner. And then margarine came along, with the "It's not nice to fool mother nature" commercials because it was so close to the real thing, supposedly, that even Mother Nature couldn't tell. And remember Blue Bonnet's® jingle: "Everything's better with Blue Bonnet on it."

Sina: I remember choking down low-fat cookies and low-fat muffins. Those things tasted horrible! But I ate them because I was taught that they were "healthy." Do you remember learning about the Food Guide Pyramid in school?

Joel: That was 1979; I'm a little older than you and that was the year I graduated college. But yes, the Food Pyramid made a huge societal splash because for the first time Americans had an official recipe for what and how to eat. It was an aggressive and unprecedented intervention into the American food marketplace.

Sina: It's fascinating because the Food Pyramid seems like a harmless diagram; it's just a picture on a piece of paper, right? But that pyramid is part of the governments Dietary Guidelines. And, those guidelines are a federal document that tells all Americans, over the age of 2, which foods they should eat and which foods they should minimize or avoid. And, according to the government's own data, Americans dutifully follow those guidelines.

You might not think you abide by those government guidelines because most of us don't consciously think about them or discuss them with friends over coffee. But many of us were taught the Dietary Guidelines in elementary school, and they are ingrained in our subconscious. For example:

- ❖ Do you feel bad when you eat a cheeseburger instead of chicken or fish?
- ❖ Do you think you should remove the skin from your chicken before you eat it?
- ❖ Do you think saturated fat causes heart disease?
- ❖ Do you think red meat increases your cholesterol?

Those beliefs all stem from the government's Dietary Guidelines.

Joel: When I was in elementary school, we were practicing atomic bomb drills and hiding under our desks. At that time, it was the Russians we were supposed to fear. By the time you were in elementary school, the Russians were history and the new fear was fat. My, how things cycle. Instead of atomic bombs, it was these saturated fat bombs in our blood vessels, so we had to hide traditional foods like butter and lard.

Sina: When I step back and think about it, what's really crazy about the low-fat story is that it all started with *one* man. One man changed the course of our history. He changed the way we *think* about food. In doing so, he changed the way we eat. And, consequently, he changed our health – for the worse. His name was Ancel Keys.

Keys was able to convince President Eisenhower, the USDA, the premiere medical institutions, and the American people that fat, especially saturated fat, causes heart attacks. In fact, Keys was so successful at demonizing fat, that the U.S. Dietary Guidelines are based on his hypothesis.

It's because of Keys that the low-fat label exists. In fact, it's because of Keys that we have government-sponsored Dietary Guidelines, which are intentionally designed to nudge your food choices. They even appear right on your packaged food! Flip over the box of your favorite cookies and you'll find the "Nutrition Facts" panel. That exists because of the Dietary Guidelines. We use that information to help us decide which foods we "should" eat. Have you ever looked for the total fat grams or the amount of saturated fat on the Nutrition Facts label?

Joel: Oh yes. I've watched a lot of fat people eating stuff that doesn't have any fat in it. Strange how that works. All of this paralleled the urbanization of America. Without ties to Grandma's garden or Grandpa's milk cow, millions of people for the first time in human history grew up with no relationship to farms or actual food production. This ignorance has only accelerated today, especially with modern screen time and the entertainment cult. What was considered food because people knew how to grow things suddenly held no frame of reference in the collective psyche.

If you've never seen a cow, never felt her breath, or felt her warm muzzle nuzzle into your jacket on a January morning, it's much easier to believe some expert who demonizes butter. Without relationship, marginalizing is infinitely easier. The reason we have 15,000 visitors a year at our farm is not because we want our farm invaded by people; it's because we know that something magic happens when a person smells, touches, sees—viscerally connects with animals and plants. Watching kids climb up into mulberry trees and pick the fresh fruit, smearing their faces and hands with the red juice (caught red-handed—that's the background of that phrase) and watching their faces glow with the participatory exercise creates memories for a lifetime. They will never forget that interaction.

Demonization of foodstuffs is easy when they're just packages and the choice is this over that. But if you've interacted personally with the tomato plant or the cow or the pig whose sacrifice enabled that bacon or cheese or salad (and yes, plants are sentient too), then disrespecting them as being fundamentally bad is a lot harder to swallow. The gentle warmth and softness of a cow compels us to question whether or not she is an enemy of good health. If our only relationship with food is this package or that one, we don't attach any morality to it, any livingness, any emotion. It's just academic pieces to be parsed out based on data points.

I think one of our greatest protections against duplicity in this food sphere is to walk with the animals, talk with the animals, pull weeds in the beans and stake up a tomato. These procedures shelter us from buying into group think and categorical demonization of nutritious real food. The reason a Food Pyramid would have never been possible a hundred years ago is because sterile packages out of context didn't exist. Everyone churned butter, or bought butter from someone who did. Everyone participated in the family hog killin' at Thanksgiving and watched the lard being rendered. It was part and parcel of life and created an informed context to reasoning and gullibility.

I think few of us realize how ignorant we are. We know the names of Hollywood celebrities, but have no idea the difference between a cow and a heifer, or a hen and a pullet. The problem with profound ignorance is that it makes us infinitely more gullible to lies and deception. Welcome to modern America. And what do we fear most? That which we know least about.

Sina: Exactly! The fat label itself was born out of fear – the fear that fat will kill you. And, Americans bought into that fear. Think about that for a moment: Most of us view food through a lens of fear. We believe certain foods are "healthy" and other foods, like fat, will make us sick and even eventually kill us. We adopted those beliefs largely from the government. And, as you mentioned, we are susceptible to believing *their* "truth" because we are so far removed from *our* food supply.

But what if their "truth" is wrong? What if the federal government has been telling us what to eat for decades, and their advice is actually making us sicker? What if we've been afraid of the very thing that can heal us?

Americans have dutifully followed the Dietary Guidelines for nearly 4 decades, and what do we have to show for it? We're sicker and less free.

Check this out: In 1965, heart disease and heart attacks were still rare. At that time, based on the government's own data, Americans ate a low-carbohydrate diet! Roughly 39% of our calories came from carbohydrates while around 45% of our calories came from fat. That means Americans were eating almost half of their calories from fat yet heart disease and heart attacks were rare. Then, the government got involved and drastically lowered the amount of fat we eat. Consequently, we now eat a high-carbohydrate diet and we are seeing skyrocketing rates of heart disease and other inflammatory conditions, such as cancer and diabetes.

Of course, multiple variables are involved in disease formation, such as: more chemicals in our food supply, GMOs, stress, and nutrient deficiencies - just to name a few. But the huge shift in our macronutrient profile cannot be overlooked as a contributor to inflammatory disease.

In fact, since the early 2000's, there have been a plethora of studies conducted to test Keys' low-fat hypothesis. Overwhelmingly, these studies have concluded that it's not fat that is making us sicker. We are getting sicker, in large part, from eating too many refined carbohydrates, specifically sugar. In addition, scientists have studied over 65,000 people from around the world, and none of those studies have conclusively shown that saturated fat causes heart disease.

In contrast, there is overwhelming evidence that saturated fat increases HDL – the "good" cholesterol. In fact, the famous Framingham study actually showed that eating more saturated fat *decreased* the chance of dying from a heart attack. Yet, we are still told by doctors, nutritionists, dietitians, and leading authorities to reduce our saturated fat intake.

Joel: So how much fat should we eat? Do we have to be concerned about it, or should we eat way more?

Sina: That depends on the person. We are all individuals, which means we all have different needs. And, your needs change based on many variables, including: the seasons, stress level, activity level, hydration status, nutrient deficiency status, etcetera. But, if you look at the diet of our ancestors, in addition to the available scientific studies that are not funded by Big Ag or Big Food, the implication is that eating more *healthy* sources of fat is good for most of us.

In fact, we're currently witnessing the reversal of many inflammatory diseases with help from a higher fat diet. That's one reason why the ketogenic diet has become so popular. Although, you don't have to be in ketosis to reverse disease. Diabetes, rheumatoid arthritis, anxiety, and depression can be reversed, in part, by replacing refined carbohydrates with healthy fats. The key word is "replacing." You cannot continue eating refined sugar and then add healthy fats to your diet and expect to heal your body. It doesn't work that way. To receive the healing benefits of healthy fats, you must eliminate refined sugars.

And eating a higher fat diet doesn't give you a free pass to gorge yourself on fried foods. I'm talking about getting fat in your diet from nuts, seeds, avocados, coconut oil, olive oil, grass-finished beef, and other healthy sources of fat. For instance, my "perfect plate" consists of mostly vegetables covered in healthy fat (such as avocado oil) and sprinkled with Real Salt®, with a small amount of protein on the edge of the plate – like a garnish. Of course, sometimes my body wants more fat, sometimes it wants less, and sometimes it wants no meat. By listening to my body, I tailor each meal to my individual needs. But overall, my body wants a predominantly plant-based diet filled with healthy fats.

Having said that, some people will not do as well on a higher fat diet. For example, we think that individuals with the ApoE4 gene (which is associated with late-onset Alzheimer's disease) might benefit from eating a low to moderate fat diet, especially saturated fat, because they seem to absorb fat very well and, consequently, produce higher levels of triglycerides and possibly LDL.

Consequently, I'm not promoting a high-fat diet or telling everyone to eat more saturated fat. That's a choice only your body can make (See Practical Bite #49). But I am saying that we've been following the government's diet advice and it's making many of us sicker. But, that's not surprising.

I mentioned that the Dietary Guidelines are based on Ancel Key's hypothesis that fat, especially saturated fat, causes heart disease and that now we know it's the wrong advice for most people. But, check this out: His hypothesis was never tested before it was unleashed on the American public. Nobody fed the diets to humans to see if it really could decrease your risk of heart disease!

And, that's one of the biggest problems I have with the Dietary Guidelines. Even though they are flawed and, by law, they are revised every five years, they are taught as fact - as though the governments advice is a certainty in life. For example, it's touted by our government as a "critical tool" for medical doctors, dietitians, and nutritionists. When you get a disease, the diet advice is based on the pyramid.

The Dietary Guidelines are also used to create all federal food and health policies and programs, including: school lunches, SNAP and meals for the elderly, military, and hospital patients. It determines what type of research studies will be funded by the NIH. It's used to create educational materials that are disseminated across the USA to teach us how to eat, starting as young children in the classroom. Needless to say, the guidelines are pervasive and influential in our society.

And, here's the kicker: After the low-fat recommendation was unleashed on the American public, they finally decided that the diet should be tested. So, Keys conducted a famous study with the intent to prove his theory was correct. Surprise, surprise, his study showed that he was right! The problem is that his study was not only biased, it contained major flaws and

Keys cherry picked the data in order to get the statistical outcome he wanted. In fact, when you look at all of the data he collected, his study actually supported the hypothesis that sugar is more closely linked to heart disease than fat! Yet, that study is still cited today to support the low-fat diet!

Joel: You know the worst thing about orthodoxy is how long it takes to change it. After knowing that lack of citrus caused scurvy in sailors, it took the British navy a hundred years to officially recommend citrus for its sailors, as an official dietary recommendation. Things get entrenched and it's tough to get out of that rut. Look at the notion that Africans were inferior to whites—how long did it take to dispel that horrible myth? Or that the world is flat? Or that fairies caused disease? Look at the Spanish Inquisition that burned heretics at the stake for daring to question the Roman Catholic church on salvation by grace instead of indulgences. Throughout history we've seen culture after culture get a notion in its head.

I sometimes wonder what our great-grandchildren will look back on, from our time, and shake their heads at our stupidity. Goodness, look at the orthodoxy as recently as the 1950s over breastfeeding, how that was considered barbaric and Neanderthal. If you really wanted to be hip and with it, you didn't breast feed. That was for poor people and backwards cultures. Who would have guessed that by the early 1970s we would have La Leche League, Lamaze classes, and official medical recommendation to breast feed. I've always thought that had to be the most egregious squandering of resources in the history of humankind, not using all those breasts. Tragic, just tragic. And now we're even connecting the dots to breast cancer, that mothers who breast feed are less likely to develop this crippling disease. For those of us who think more naturally, this is not a surprise, but to the average American, these revelations come as big aha! moments. Just look at what has sustained us through the millennia. Bet on that horse to win, not the horse of food scientists and industrial substance manipulators.

Sina: I bet on the wrong horse for most of my life! One of my biggest losses came from believing the big fat lie. It took time for me to see the truth and change my perception on fat. Looking back, those low-fat foods did more harm than good because when fat is removed, flavor goes with it. So, to make low-fat foods taste good, refined sugar is commonly added. And, it's sugar that is strongly linked to heart disease, as well as all inflammatory diseases.

Refined sugar is one of the most inflammatory chemicals we know of today. And, it's chronic inflammation that contributes to heart disease and heart attacks. So, while many people still point the finger at fat, the smoking gun is sugar - at least it's one of the smoking guns.

Even the American Heart Association (AHA), the leading authority on heart health, has begun back-pedaling on their long-standing advice that we should all eat a lower fat diet. For instance, the words "low-fat" no longer appear in the AHA 2006 recommendations or their 2013 guidelines. Now they recommend a "moderate-fat" diet. Although, they still demonize saturated fat, which means they think you should eat less red meat and whole-fat dairy.

The AHA also dropped the cap on cholesterol in 2013, which means egg yolks are back in fashion. Do you remember when people stopped eating egg yolks?

Joel: Oh yes, another of those egg headed (pun fully intended) notions from the folks Sally Fallon Morrel eloquently describes as "diet dictocrats." I love that phrase because it captures marvelously the elitist, tyrannical persona of experts who dare to impugn historically normal food.

Sina: I can vividly remember my Mom standing in the kitchen, cracking open an egg, and carefully removing the egg white, making sure that none of the yolk got into the bowl. Then, she'd throw the yolk in the garbage. Even restaurants added egg white omelets to their menus. And, remember Egg Beaters®? My Mom used to cook with those. Yuck! Lucky for us, as of 2013, the AHA says that egg yolks are "good for us" once again. Oh, how easily we are swayed!

The government has also started walking back their hardcore stance on both fat and cholesterol. In 2015, when the revised government Dietary Guidelines came out, the cap on total fat and dietary cholesterol were both dropped! They said cholesterol was no longer a "nutrient of concern." In addition, the "expert" committee that advises the government on the Dietary Guidelines stated, "Reducing total fat (replacing total fat with overall carbohydrates) does not lower CVD [cardiovascular disease] risk.... Dietary advice should put the emphasis on optimizing types of dietary fat and not reducing total fat."

That's a big deal! It means fat and eggs are back on the government menu! It also means that both the AHA and our government have reversed course. Low-fat and low-cholesterol have been two pillars of their dietary advice for decades. And, now they are just gone! Did you know that?

Joel: Isn't it amazing how long it takes agendas to catch up with truth? I see this same thing in agriculture all the time. Whether it's mad cow, avian influenza, or swine flu, the explanation is always a boogieman. Something's out to getcha' is the mantra of the experts selling snake oil because then they can make you afraid and sell you something that will fix it. Salesmen love victims, and I think that's really what all this comes down to. It's not a conspiracy or some evil agenda. It's just groupthink about food as inanimate protoplasm; about life as machine; about cheap as supreme; about doctors as fixers. These are all ingrained ideas so deep in our collective psyche that popping out on the lunatic fringe is really hard. And it sets you up for opposition from friends, family, and neighbors.

Sina: I know exactly what you mean. I get a lot of pushback because I eat a relatively high fat diet. It used to bother me until I realized that many people are acting out of the "collective psyche" that you mentioned, which stems from fear. It's unfortunate, but most Americans are still convinced that fat is "bad." So, they continue to buy foods labeled as "low-fat," and peel the skin from their chicken, and count the grams of saturated fat using the ill-founded, fear-based Nutrition Facts panel.

Joel: The fear runs deep. Yet, if a person would pause long enough to look at the guidelines, they would see the glaring problems. For example, the original Food Pyramid did not differentiate between Twinkies® and whole grain oats. It did not differentiate between soaked quinoa and Nabisco® crackers. Therein lay the fatal flaw of the program; not just fats, but failure to distinguish between very basic foodstuffs nutritionally.

Sina: That's so true! When the USDA first began translating the guidelines into practice around 1978, the best they could come up with was a recommendation for Americans to eat 13 slices of bread each day to meet their daily carbohydrate needs. That's your hard-earned tax dollars at work.

Joel: Why am I not surprised?

Some of it may be incompetence, but at least part of the reason why the Food Pyramid cannot distinguish between foodstuffs nutritionally is because it would have put the USDA on a collision course with Big Food, and that would have been a no-no. The government is not an unpolitical disinvolved referee; it is a political, subjective, customer-driven entity just like business. It sells information that pleases its constituency, which tend to be the folks with enough money to offer wine and cheese tastings to politicians and bureaucrats. It's a fraternity of similar-think. Why would you trust them?

Sina: I don't trust them now, but it took a while for me to open my eyes. Speaking of which, have you noticed that the "Nutrition Facts" panel does not list a percent daily value for sugar?

I recently spoke with Michelle Walrath, co-producer of the food documentaries *Fed Up* and *GMO OMG*, who believes the missing value is intentional. While conducting research for *Fed Up*, her team discovered that the sugar lobby wanted the government to establish a daily value for sugar of 25%, meaning 25% of your calories each day should come from sugar. But the World Health Organization (WHO), who sets global health standards, issued a recommendation of no more than 10% of calories from sugar per day because they concluded sugar is a major cause of chronic disease. So, the U.S. Secretary of Health and Human Services, Tommy Thompson, flew to Geneva and told the WHO that if they published their recommendations, the U.S. would withhold their $4.6 million contribution to the WHO. Consequently, the WHO removed their reduced sugar recommendation. And, today, there is still no daily value for sugar on your food labels.

Can you imagine if there was a daily value for sugar listed on every packaged food? Just like some people track their fat intake using the label, if you knew the percent of sugar in your food, you might start eating less sugar. And, that would upset the sugar lobby. As you said, the USDA cannot collide with Big Food.

Look, I'm not suggesting that all of the Dietary Guidelines are bad. Clearly, you are better off not eating doughnuts and chocolate milk for breakfast. But, do you really need the government to tell you that?

Not only did they get it wrong, we are individuals. You cannot guide an individual to health by providing a one size fits all approach. Some of us do well on a low-fat diet and some of us don't. My body loves fat and gets inflamed when I eat grains. So, if I followed the Dietary Guidelines, I would develop an inflammatory disease because they promote a large percentage of calories from grains. When it comes to diet, one size never fits all.

Joel: And in the end, that's the problem with relegating to the federal government the authority to manipulate and disseminate information. It must be average; it must be pleasing to the big power brokers. You cannot empower common man truth from the oracles of centralized power. So yes, ultimately, I have to listen to my body, eat historically normal, and realize I have much more in common with my ancestors of 5,000 years ago than with the crew of Star Trek's Enterprise.

Sina: Well said, Joel!

Folks, don't buy into the fear behind the low-fat label. If you want to eat low-fat out of preference or because your body likes it, that's great. It's your choice and only you know what's best for your body. You don't need the government or "renowned" health organizations to tell you what to eat. And, you certainly don't need them using fear tactics to nudge you to eat the foods they want you to eat. Instead of outsourcing your authority over your own body, listen to your body. It will tell you everything you need to know about how to be healthy, happy and free. Stick around and we'll explain how to listen to your body in Practical Bite #49.

Practical Bite #16: Throw Out Artificial Sweeteners

How? Read the ingredient label on every product in your pantry, refrigerator and freezer. If an artificial sweetener is listed, throw it out – or don't buy that food again. Examples include: aspartame (Equal® and NutraSweet®), sucralose (Splenda®), saccharin (Sweet 'N Low®), sorbitol, xylitol, acesulfame K® (Sunett®). Instead, use natural sweeteners - in moderation.

Why?

Joel: This is a case of the cure being worse than the disease. As a rule, artificial sweeteners are worse than sugar. Substitutes for real food often carry side issues worse than the more natural product in the first place. Sina will carry you through the nuts and bolts. We haven't had a sugar bowl on our table for decades. Honey is right there with the salt and pepper. Brown sugar and simply granulated sugar are available in the kitchen, but not out on the table. Sometimes just limiting access can help balance out usage. My favorite sweetener? Maple syrup, of course. But its expense is enough to make it sparingly used. You get what you pay for.

Sina: I long for the day when artificial sweeteners are a thing of the past. They were introduced to the market in the 1950s and now we know they can lead to health problems, including: weight gain, increased BMI (body mass index), metabolic syndrome, gut dysbiosis and inflammation, type 2 diabetes, headaches, migraines, cognitive decline, bloating, and even cardiovascular disease. In fact, a study published in 2017 in the *New England Journal of Medicine Watch Cardiology,* prompted the editor-in-chief to declare:

> "This study raises the concerning possibility that not only have these sweeteners not helped people manage their weight, but may have actually jeopardized their cardiometabolic health."

We are learning that artificial sweeteners may contribute to your body developing an addiction to overly sweet foods by retraining your taste buds to need more and more, which equates to you craving sweeter and sweeter foods.

This begs the question, if artificial sweeteners can be so damaging to your health, why are they still on the market?

One reason is the cozy relationship that has developed between industry and universities. For instance, industry pays universities to conduct research on their products. Scientists are paid by industry through corporate-endowed positions. And, scientists are paid by industry to sit on their advisory boards. Meanwhile, professors can own stock in the same companies that sponsor their research. This crony relationship has created a new era of research where study outcomes overwhelmingly fall in industry's favor. You don't need to look further than aspartame for supporting evidence.

The sweetener aspartame is a genetically engineered compound that is used in roughly 6,000 foods and drinks, in addition to over 500 prescription drugs and over-the-counter medications. It was "approved" by the FDA for use in our food supply in 1981. By 1995, nearly 165 peer-reviewed safety studies had been conducted. Roughly half of the studies found no problems associated with using aspartame. 100% of those studies were funded by the manufacturer, G.D. Searle, which was a subsidiary of Monsanto at that time. In contrast, among the other half of the studies, 92% found problems with aspartame. All of those studies were funded by independent entities. Yet, aspartame remained on the market.

Fortunately, more recent independent research is beginning to shed light on the artificial sweetener situation. In 2017, a study published in the *American Journal of Industrial Medicine* called for "the urgent need for regulatory re-evaluation" of aspartame. The researchers reviewed the data submitted to the FDA by G.D. Searle for approval of aspartame in the 1970s. They also reviewed more recent data, and concluded that aspartame is potentially a carcinogen, meaning it may cause cancer:

> "Taken together, the studies performed by G.D. Searle in the 1970s and other chronic bioassays do not provide adequate scientific support for APM [aspartame] safety. In contrast, recent results of life-span carcinogenicity bioassays on rats and mice published in peer-reviewed journals, and a prospective epidemiological study, provide consistent evidence of APM's carcinogenic potential. On the basis of the evidence of the potential carcinogenic effects of APM herein reported, a re-evaluation of the current position of international regulatory agencies must be considered an urgent matter of public health."

For now, these sweeteners are still on the market. And, you have to be diligent when checking your labels because they can be present in many types of foods and products, such as:

- Toothpaste
- Mouthwash
- Chewable Vitamins
- Gum
- Salad Dressings
- Desserts (i.e. Baked Goods and Candies)
- Breakfast Cereals
- Processed Snacks
- Zero-Calorie Drinks
- Reduced Sugar Fruit Juices
- Cough Syrup and Liquid Medicines
- Prepared Meats

Instead of using artificial sweeteners, I use natural sweeteners, such as: maple syrup, coconut sugar, maple sugar, fruit purees, dates, and raw honey. In addition, stevia has been recommended by the American Diabetes Association as a sugar substitute for diabetics or individuals with blood sugar regulation issues.

However, this does not give you a free pass to eat natural sugar all day. In the previous Practical Bite, we discussed the relationship between sugar and inflammatory disease. It's best to eat sugar sparingly. However, the average American consumes around 17 teaspoons of sugar every day, or nearly 57 pounds per year! Compare that to 1822, when the average American is estimated to have consumed only 6.3 pounds of sugar per person per year! That equates to drinking one 12-ounce soda every FIVE days! It's no wonder we're so sick!

I'll admit it; I have a sweet tooth. I used to eat nearly an entire pan of brownies in one sitting! And, I used to make desserts frequently, which taught my children that undesirable behavior. Then, my oldest son and I both developed yeast overgrowth in our gastrointestinal tracts. I knew we needed to starve the yeast by removing sugar from our diets. But we were both addicted to sugar.

So, in order to get our sugar intake under control, my family had to wean ourselves off sugar. It took some time, but we all changed our palettes. And, now, fruits taste very sweet to us. You can imagine how sweet maple syrup tastes! Some techniques we used to wean ourselves off sugar include:

- ❖ Slowly reducing the amount of added sugar to all recipes; most of my homemade desserts contain roughly half the sugar of their counterparts.
- ❖ Diluting fruit juice with water; beginning with a 50% dilution and working toward all water and no juice.
- ❖ We stopped drinking all sodas.
- ❖ We don't eat dessert after dinner.
- ❖ We don't use dessert as a reward or treat.
- ❖ For birthday parties, I make mini-cupcakes, which encourages my children to feel satiated with a smaller portion of sugar and does not lead to a sugar high (also because the cupcakes contain less sugar).
- ❖ We slowly transitioned from milk chocolate to "dark" and "very dark" chocolate or cacao; when my kids want something sweet, I sometimes hand them a small piece of dark chocolate.
- ❖ I used to make fruit smoothies, but now I occasionally make a green smoothie using a ratio of 4 greens to 1 fruit.

Practical Bite #17: Get To Know Fake Meat

How? Read the ingredient label for each fake meat product. If it aligns with your principles then eat it. If not, leave it on the grocery store shelf.

Why?

Sina: To be clear, fake meat is different than veggie or vegan burgers. Clean, plant-based burgers can be a great option for individuals who thrive eating no meat or less meat. In contrast, fake meat is a plant-based burger that is pretending to taste and feel like a meat burger, even though it contains no meat. Joel, as a farmer who raises cattle, I'm eager to hear your perspective on this topic.

Joel: Unprocessed whole foods dominate our lexicon in this book. Few things are as contradictory to both those ideas as fake meat. We don't have time or space here to explore the whole vegan movement that inevitably led to a desire for fake meat like Impossible Burger® and Beyond Meat®. Perhaps by the time we get this tome published, other brands will dominate this space. That appears to be the trajectory.

I predict that the fake meat movement will follow the trajectory of the hydrogenated vegetable oil movement. It was the credentialed orthodoxy for several decades before it finally fell into complete disrepute by around 2010. Ditto for the food pyramid. Now the cholesterol myth is falling into disrepute. Finally. Red meat and heart disease are now being disentangled as well. We're seeing a welcome return to using lard and real butter, thanks in no small part to the tireless efforts of Sally Fallon and the Weston A. Price Foundation.

Make no mistake, nutritionally, ecologically, and economically, fake meat is a real mistake. Most of the agricultural land in the world is either too rocky, too steep, too inaccessible or too hostile to profitably grow crops. Whether the primary feedstock is peas or soybeans, fake meat requires massive mono-speciated cropland. That is an environmental disaster. As we learn more and more about biomass, diversity, and soil building through perennials, our appreciation for the prairie and its regenerative capacity escalate.

Plowing up prairies was never a good idea and it still isn't, whether it's for ethanol, cattle feed, or soy-burgers. All of the data points leading toward eliminating livestock and elevating plants are based on dysfunctional production models. Unfortunately, most livestock in the world is not raised according to nature's three Ms—movement, mobbing, and mowing. Absent any one of these three, the whole system turns from asset to liability. Most animal agriculture violates not just one, but all three of these foundational natural templates. If you want to dive into this more, please read my book *The Sheer Ecstasy of Being a Lunatic Farmer.*

Nutritionally, plants cannot deliver in either quality or quantity the vitamins and fatty acids our bodies need for optimal function. Advocates for veganism glibly advise "just take B12 tablets." Folks, supplements are neither historically normal nor a regenerative foundation for health. Food is the foundation for health; not a bunch of pills.

The fake meat crowd presents this option without showing pictures of the train car loads of peas or beans being brought to their giant incubation vats. They don't show the carnage from chemicals and mono-cropping that the plants wreak on their fields. In fact, cropping kills far more lives than animal agriculture. I invite anyone to come out and sit in a pasture with the cows and me on a summer evening to be serenaded and wowed by multitudinous life: birds, pollinators, insects, wildlife. Now go sit in a pea field or a soybean field and tell me what you see and hear. 'Nuff said.

To artificially create the nuances of meat requires highly sophisticated and capital-intensive infrastructure. That is exactly the opposite direction we want our food system to go. If we want food freedom, we need to decouple ourselves from dependency on multi-national corporations and mega-money. Animals can be raised in your house; in a city lot, a tiny homestead. Try making fake meat in your kitchen. Goodness, we can't even make high fructose corn syrup in our kitchens and that's an extremely simple and single substance. Fake meat, gentle people, is a really bad idea. I hope you'll come to this truth sooner rather than later.

Sina: Nutritionally speaking, the fake meat currently on the market concerns me. For instance, the Impossible Burger® is the vegan alternative to a hamburger. However, read the ingredients:

> Water, Soy Protein Concentrate, Coconut Oil, Sunflower Oil, Natural Flavors, 2% or less of: Potato Protein, Methylcellulose, Yeast Extract, Cultured Dextrose, Food Starch Modified, Soy Leghemoglobin, Salt, Soy Protein Isolate, Mixed Tocopherols

(Vitamin E), Zinc Gluconate, Thiamine Hydrochloride (Vitamin B1), Sodium Ascorbate (Vitamin C), Niacin, Pyridoxine Hydrochloride (Vitamin B6), Riboflavin (Vitamin B2), Vitamin B12.

Referring back to Practical Bite #12, if you only eat what you know and can pronounce, can you eat the Impossible Burger®?

Let's pretend you want to eat it; the next step is to give informed consent by learning about the ingredients. For instance, the Impossible Burger® is made using genetically engineered soy leghemoglobin. Soy leghemoglobin is a protein found in soy that carries heme, which is what makes meat taste like meat – according to Impossible Foods®, the creator of Impossible Burger®. It's made by adding the gene for soy leghemoglobin to yeast and then growing the yeast via fermentation. Next, scientists isolate the soy leghemoglobin from the yeast and mix it with other ingredients to create the Impossible Burger®.

Now that you know what soy leghemoglobin is and how it's made, how was it "approved" for human consumption?

Soy leghemoglobin is GRAS! If you recall, GRAS status is achieved when a company determines their own product to be safe for us to eat; the FDA does not approve these ingredients, they simply give the company a "no-questions letter" and remind the company that it is their responsibility to determine the safety of their own product. Keep in mind that soy leghemoglobin is genetically engineered, yet the government regulation boils down to a GRAS determination.

Knowing that, how do you feel when you read this statement from Impossible Foods®?

> "Impossible Foods has received a no-questions letter from the US Food and Drug Administration, validating the unanimous conclusion of food-safety experts that its key ingredient is safe to eat...Getting a no-questions letter goes above and beyond our strict compliance to all federal food-safety regulations... We have prioritized safety and transparency from day one, and they will always be core elements of our company culture."

Let's be clear, the company is complying with federal regulations. The problem is the current system, which is a result of our lack of demand for food safety and transparency.

However, as we discussed in Practical Bite #1, we can change the system by changing our behavior:

- ❖ Now that you know about soy leghemoglobin, is the Impossible Burger® aligned with your principles? In other words, does it provide you with greater health and increased trust in your food supply?
- ❖ If yes then eat it.
- ❖ If no then don't eat it.

It's that simple.

Give your informed consent by repeating this process for each ingredient in the Impossible Burger®, or any other fake meat you are interested in eating. Regardless of your final decision to eat it or not, you are taking a huge leap forward by knowing what's in your food and making an informed decision. Now that's worth celebrating!

Practical Bite #18: Drink Soda With Intention

How? If you drink soda, drink it with intention. For example, select one or two foods that you want to consume with soda, like pizza and hamburgers. Drink filtered water with all other foods. Or, pick a certain time of the day and allow yourself to consume one soda at that time. Drink filtered water all other times of the day.

When you drink your designated soda, be intentional: make a plan for when you will drink your soda, and pay attention to how your body and mind feel. Focus on what it smells like, what it sounds like, how it tastes, how your body feels before you drink it, and how you feel a couple hours later.

Why?

Sina: Everyone knows that drinking soda is not "healthy" and that drinking clean water is a better option. So, let's not belabor that point. Instead, let's focus on suggestions for how to make the switch from soda to water.

If you're able to instantly stop drinking soda and replace it with water then go for it! And, if you're not ready for that change, that's okay too. Getting off soda can be overwhelming and challenging. So, give yourself time, space, and grace.

You've probably heard the recommendation of swapping a soda for water at a meal. That's a fine strategy, but let's aim higher because I have faith in you. Let's plan to drink soda with intention. Using that strategy, my husband and I both stopped drinking soda and remain soda-free today.

My husband used to drink soda mindlessly, just like his parents. He once told me that he drank soda all day long because he thought soda was "exactly the same" as water. He said they are both liquid and they are both consumed when people are thirsty. So, why not drink the soda since it tastes better?

Then, one day, his professor in college said that the acid in soda can "dissolve" your bones. That was the first time my husband realized that soda was not "exactly the same" as water. So, he decided to dramatically reduce his soda intake from 4-5 sodas per day to one soda per week.

His strategy was to choose certain foods that he wanted to drink with soda, specifically pizza and popcorn. Those were the only times he would drink soda. All other times of the day, he drank water. Once he mastered that, he narrowed it down to only drinking soda once per week – on a particular day. He maintained that habit for 15 years, until he gave up soda completely two years ago. The coolest part is that he doesn't even want soda anymore! I find that remarkable since he used to drink soda all day long.

My soda story is similar to my husband's. I didn't drink nearly as much soda as he did, probably because I knew from a very young age that soda was not healthy thanks to my parents drilling it into my head. But I did occasionally drink soda. So, like my husband, I weaned myself off soda by drinking with intention. What's interesting is that my husband and I both used the same strategy even though we had not met yet! So, either it's a great strategy or we are just two peas from the same pod.

My strategy was to only drink soda with pizza. I couldn't resist that savory and sweet combination. So, I didn't beat myself up for wanting a root beer with my slice of pizza. Instead, I enjoyed it. I savored every bite and every sip. Then, one day, I paid attention to how I felt after I drank the soda. My stomach was bloated, my body felt heavy and tired, and my mind was slower. Then, roughly two hours later, I felt really tired and I was craving another soda. I was experiencing a sugar crash, and I needed a chemical pick me up.

Once I knew that my body and mind were responding negatively to the soda, it was easy to make the decision to stop drinking it all together. I didn't want to feel yucky; I wanted to feel good. So, I changed my intention. I decided to stop drinking soda. And, I began to drink clean water with intention.

Joel: I agree with Sina that you need to drink soda with intention. Growing up here on the farm in a family that eschewed chemicals before it was cool, we never had soda. In fact, I don't think we ever, I mean ever, had soda in our house. Period. We had two Guernsey cows giving 4 gallons of milk a day; why in the world would we want soda?

I really like this Practical Bite because whenever I run into somebody whose life style changes are so dramatic you can see it all over them, their explanation always starts with "I stopped drinking soft drinks."

Our former and now retired delivery driver, Richard, was grossly obese for a few years before he decided to change his life. Over the next several years he shed a couple hundred pounds and then competed in half marathons and mud runs. He does talks about his journey and one of his visual aids is a glass of water and a sugar bowl. He asks the audience "I'm thirsty; do you mind if I take a drink of water?" Of course, everyone assents and then he adds "I like it sweet, so I'm going to put in some sugar. That okay?" Everyone nods.

Then he puts in a tablespoon of sugar. And another. And another. By the time he gets to about ten tablespoons, the audience begins gasping. But he isn't finished. He adds six more and then stirs it all in. While the audience responds to this repugnant potion, he moves in for the kill: "That's how much sugar is in a can of soda." It's a moment of epiphany and nobody forgets that simple demonstration.

When Richard wanted a carbonated drink, he simply put seltzer water in juice and made his own. The first time I had real carbonated juice I was doing a speech in Portland, Oregon and a local pizza place called Hot Lips Pizza catered the lunch. Another unforgettable experience. You could tell it was food. Simple set up; great stuff.

Folks, Sina and I are NOT trying to take fun out of your lives. We are trying to acquaint you with some awesome alternatives that allow you to celebrate, enjoy food, and enjoy vibrant health. You can have it all. All sorts of beverages exist; you don't have to be shackled to conventional soda. You can explore a host of interesting flavors and possibilities, from craft teas to the old haymaker's specialty, switchel, to juices, punch and kombucha. You won't regret the adventure and your stomach will love you.

In our house today, for a treat, we don't drink conventional soda but we do occasionally imbibe spritzers. They don't use any high fructose corn syrup, using natural cane sugar instead, and they don't have all the junk in them. They're a bit more expensive and the cans are smaller, but hey, it's a treat so a few pennies won't kill you.

But I think the first line of attack is to get water that tastes good. I think half of our addiction to non-water is because most water tastes terrible.

Sina: I agree! And that brings us to the next Practical Bite!

Practical Bite #19: Hydrate Your Cells

How? Nobody knows exactly how much water you need. Everyone is different, and your water requirement changes each day based on many factors, such as: activity level, fat intake, stress level, environmental temperature, and water consumption from fresh fruits and vegetables. Thus, we are providing a generalized guideline: For adults, consume a minimum of 1.5 liters per day, which is roughly 50 ounces or 6 cups of water.

If you want to calculate a specific value, a commonly used equation is half an ounce of water per pound of body weight per day. For example, if you weigh 150 pounds, that equates to 75 ounces of water per day (roughly 10 cups of water). But this estimate includes water from all sources, such as food and metabolic water.

It's easy to forget to drink water, especially with our busy schedules. So, start your day by drinking roughly 16 ounces of clean water when you first wake up, and continue drinking clean water throughout the day. Set the alarm on your phone, computer, or watch to beep every 2 hours during the day. Each time the alarm goes off, drink a glass of water. That way, you'll stay hydrated throughout the day. Eventually it will become a habit and you won't need the alarm. Don't override your instincts, but most people have to train themselves to drink water, and it often takes time.

Why?

Sina: I know, you've heard it a million times: "Drink more water." I've heard it too. I used to nod my head in agreement and then continue with my day until I learned that most of us are living in a chronic state of sub-clinical dehydration, which can make you tired, sick, and cognitively impaired.

Hydration is so important because we are made up of mostly water. We all know that you can die from being dehydrated. You may have even experienced a headache, diminished memory, or an impaired ability to think after being dehydrated for a short period of time. But, did you know that not drinking enough water can lead to chronic disease?

Asthma, depression, diabetes, chronic pain, autoimmune disease, and cancer are all associated with chronic dehydration. In fact, since dehydration can lead to inflammation, you can connect any chronic or inflammatory condition to dehydration, including weight gain, obesity, and high cholesterol. Yep, high cholesterol can be the result of dehydration!

We are learning that water plays a more dynamic role in our lives than we could have imagined. For instance, we believe your memories, thoughts, and emotions are stored in water (along with your biofield). Your energy level is also tied to the amount of water you drink. Have you ever heard of structured water?

Joel: Yes, I think you're talking about the Japanese originated stuff.

Sina: You're going to love this!

Most of us were taught that water exists in three phases:

1. Solid – Ice
2. Liquid – Water
3. Gas - Steam

But, there's actually a fourth phase of water - a structured gel phase. Think of it like Jell-O®. Your cells are roughly 70% water, but it's not liquid water; it's structured water. In other words, your cells are filled with Jell-O®!

Structured water is so important that it's now being referred to as "the fundamental determinant of health." Structured water is critical for every function of your cells, including: DNA expression, nerve conduction, muscle contraction, cell division, etcetera. It's also why you have circulation, or blood flow, throughout your body. And, when the water inside your cells becomes unstructured, or incoherent, sickness ensues.

The mechanism is complicated and not well understood, but we believe structured water creates a separation of charge across the cell membrane - like a battery. That separation of charge is required for the cell to do its job. Therefore, sickness occurs when your body cannot create the separation of charge i.e. when the structured water becomes distorted or incoherent.

For instance, cells need a negative charge around them in order to function properly. This is partly because the negative charge maintains an appropriate distance between cells – through repulsion. If those cells lose their negative charge, they clump together. We call that a tumor.

In addition, structured water binds to hormones and other chemicals in the body, which changes its conformation. That change in shape is translated into specific actions or functions by the cells. In other words, by changing shape, the structured water dictates how the cell functions. Consequently, when the structured water inside a cell becomes incoherent, the cell is said to be diseased or dead. That cell can no longer transmit signals and loses its connection to neighboring cells. This mechanism may, in fact, be the basis for leaky gut, neurological disease, allergies, and other inflammatory conditions. Allow me to explain.

We are taught in biochemistry that you break down food in your body so you can harness the energy in that food, essentially by turning it into ATP (adenosine triphosphate). The process of making ATP largely occurs in your mitochondria. We are also taught that ATP fuels the metabolic processes throughout your entire body; it makes your body go. That's why ATP is often called the energy currency of the cell.

Consequently, many researchers and health care practitioners are focusing on mitochondrial dysfunction as the "root cause" of inflammatory disease. The basic theory is that triggers, such as antibiotics and heavy metals, hinder the function of the mitochondria, which decreases ATP production. And, lower levels of ATP ultimately lead to fatigue and disease. That theory fits the conventional wisdom that ATP stores energy.

However, newer studies have shown that ATP has no more energy capacity than any other molecule! That means ATP is not the molecule that carries your energy! So, how does your body carry or transfer the energy your body needs to function? It uses water! (There are other carriers too, like native electromagnetic fields.)

ATP does play a critical role in health, but it's not what most people think. We believe ATP plays the role of heat in your body. To understand this concept, let's take a closer look at how Jell-O® is formed.

Jell-O® predominantly consists of water and protein. When heat is applied from your stove, it unfolds the proteins, which allows them to interact with the water forming a gel. If there was no heat, no Jell-O® would form because the proteins would stay tightly folded and, therefore, would be unable to bond with water.

In your cells, ATP acts as heat by binding to proteins and unfolding them, which allows the proteins to interact with water to form structured water! And, remember, it's structured water that controls the processes in your cells. Consequently, if you have an ATP deficiency, you can't unfold your proteins properly, which means you can't structure water. And, when that happens, your body doesn't work correctly.

That means, it's not the lack of ATP itself that leads to fatigue and disease. Peel back the next layer of the onion and you'll see that the lack of structured water leads to fatigue and disease. So, what causes the structured water to become distorted?

Any trigger that contributes to inflammatory disease is likely the same trigger that leads to distorted water, including:

- ❖ Ingesting water that is not clean
- ❖ Heavy metal toxicity
- ❖ Glyphosate
- ❖ Non-native electromagnetic fields (EMFs)
- ❖ Infections (viruses, bacteria, yeast, etcetera)
- ❖ Stress
- ❖ Unhealthy Foods
- ❖ Certain Medications
- ❖ Not enough time spent outside, connecting with nature, during the healing hours of the sun's rays
- ❖ Negative thoughts and emotions

In the introductory chapters of this book, we talked about the impact of negative thoughts and beliefs on your overall health. Using water, let's dive a little deeper into this topic.

We've discussed how your genes are not your destiny; you can turn on and off your genes through diet, lifestyle choices, and your thoughts. Well, it's partly structured water that determines which genes are expressed. It tells your DNA which products to make by rearranging the configuration of the DNA, as well as the proteins involved with gene expression. Ultimately, it's your consciousness that changes the DNA. And, your consciousness is expressed through your structured water.

Let's use an example to explain this phenomenon – the "Japanese originated stuff" that

Joel mentioned. Years ago, Dr. Masaru Emoto changed the way we think about the physical realm. Using Magnetic Resonance Analysis and high-speed photographs, Dr. Emoto tried to demonstrate that your thoughts and your intentions can change the molecular structure of water. For instance, when water was exposed to loving human intentions, the physical structure of the water was pleasing and ordered – structured. Likewise, when the water was exposed to fearful or angry human intentions, the water became disfigured or incoherent.

I'll add that Dr. Emoto's intention experiments are highly criticized. And, I agree they often lacked sound controls. But modern science is not yet equipped to accurately measure the process or the outcome of intention experiments, and our modern culture is not generally open to the possibility that intention can change your genetic expression, your biology, your mood, and ultimately your health and longevity. We're too focused on your biochemistry – as though the chemicals in your body determine the fate of your health and wellness. They don't.

Regardless, newer research is supporting the idea that the water inside your body can change its structure based on the thoughts you think, the words you say, the words you hear, and your intentions for life. Just like structured water can bind to hormones, it can also bind to emotions and thoughts. The binding changes the shape of the water, which alters the action of the cell. And, just like that, we're back to speaking positive affirmations and visualizing yourself vibrantly healthy and healed.

Let's take this one step further. Since you can change the structure of water with your intentions and thoughts, if you write a kind word on the outside of your water glass, your intention changes the structure of that water. That's why I drink from a glass that has the word "Love" etched on it. And, before I take a drink of water, I hold the glass in my hand and I say, "I love you water." You can choose any kind word that resonates with you, such as: thank you, love, gratitude, peace, etcetera. The point is to use the power of intention to structure the water into a more biologically useful form.

Some scientists will not acknowledge that water carries information and that the information can dictate cell function. However, those concepts have been known for centuries in other cultures. For instance, in homeopathic medicine, you can heal your body by consuming water that is carrying information. When someone is sick, they are given a remedy consisting of water that has been imprinted from plant, mineral, vegetable, or other energetic sources. The energy, or EMF, of that substance is actually imprinted into the water. And, when the sick person consumes that imprinted water, it stimulates the persons' whole being (physical, mental, and emotional) by shifting their EMF, bringing them into balance.

So, this is how I see it: Even if I'm wrong and your intention does not structure your water, what is the harm in saying something nice to your water? It essentially costs nothing, yet that simple act of kindness might change your health and wellness by structuring your water, and it will certainly improve your disposition in the moment. So, why not do it?

Okay, I've probably geeked out here a little too much! If you want to learn more about structured water and health, I recommend reading Dr. Thomas Cowan's book, *Cancer and the New Biology of Water.* It's a short, yet fascinating read.

Joel: Wow, Sina, like all topics, this one has more to it than meets the eye. And like everything we've talked about, water is not by itself; it's not an end. It's part of a multi-faceted interactive network that includes everything from toxins to emotions. It's way more than just liquid stuff.

With a farm full of animals and plants, I know how important water is. A drooping plant in the garden can literally perk up in minutes after the soil gets a drink. With animals, when we have extremely hot summer days, they become lethargic and can literally go into a heat stroke without knowing they are in trouble.

On an excruciatingly hot day, for example, we'll go up in the afternoon and stir up the broiler chickens to make them get up and get a drink of water. These fast-growing chickens spend a lot of time lounging, digesting their food. They fill up on food in the cooler morning and then lounge. On a record-breaking hot day, some can actually go into a kind of heat stupor; they don't realize they're dehydrated until they actually faint. So, on those hot days, we make sure we stir them up to get everyone up and active for a few minutes during that critical post-food pre-drink period. Their body uses lots of fluid to digest and metabolize their morning food, which puts a strain on them in the early afternoon when it's hottest.

You would think the chickens would understand they need to stand up, move around, get some water, you know, survive. But it comes on gently, slowly, insidiously and before they know it, they're in trouble. We humans are a lot like that too in our routines and we're unaware of what our routine is creating until we have a wake-up call. Or wake up dead. As a farmer, I can tell you that water is life; it's everything. So, listen to Sina.

Sina: It's true that we are a lot like your chickens. Most of us are chronically dehydrated, yet we don't recognize it because it's a low-grade, sub-clinical level of dehydration – and it's our norm. We don't know how it feels to be hydrated, so we don't know the difference. Plus, it's common to confuse thirst for hunger. Sometimes I feel hungry and it's not logical – perhaps I recently ate. When that happens, I drink a glass of water. Every time, it turns out I was just thirsty.

Joel: One of the most dramatic almost resurrection things I ever did with an animal was one oppressive hot day when we had a fairly large calf get down with heat stroke and dehydration. The rest of the herd was fine; he obviously had a weakness. Oh, that's the other thing with animals: susceptibility to this dehydration issue is extremely individualistic. In a herd or flock of 500, same day, same field, same shade, same water troughs, one or two show stress and the rest are fine. Just like us. We're all different and have different tolerances.

Anyway, I noticed this one calf, on his side, seemingly dead. Heat stroke. Fortunately, he was fairly near the water trough, which of course is near the water line, so I hooked up a couple lengths of garden hose and ran water over him and then opened his mouth and stuck the hose in. His eyes were rolled back in his head but he was breathing, very shallow. In about 10 seconds he began to respond. He swallowed a gulp of water, then another. Then he flicked his ears and opened his eyes. Within 2 minutes he lifted his head and started looking around.

As long as he was drinking, I kept the water hose in his mouth. He drank and drank and drank and drank. Within 5 minutes he stood and walked over to the rest of the herd. He was fine after that. Sometimes I wonder if he "learned a lesson" that day, like on the next hot day slurping some extra water in the early afternoon. When animals are short of water, they become extremely lethargic and listless.

Sina: I'm glad you brought up individuality. Again, nobody knows your water requirement. And, it changes based on many variables, including: how much you exercise, your stress level, and your food choices.

For instance, eating fresh fruits and vegetables helps prevent dehydration because of their high-water content, in general. Iceberg lettuce is roughly 90% water while tomatoes can be 94% water. On the other hand, processed foods like crackers, bread, and cookies contain very little water, if any. Caffeine, alcohol, and high-sugar drinks can also be dehydrating. So, the more whole foods you eat, the less water you need to drink. Hence, the guideline changes based on your diet.

Not only does food contain water, your body also creates water when it breaks down food. This is referred to as metabolic water, and is thought to be the healthiest form of water. Breaking down fats generates more metabolic water than breaking down carbohydrates or proteins. That's one reason why higher fat diets have gained popularity – they create more metabolic water than high carbohydrate or high protein diets.

Joel: Perhaps most importantly, on our farm we have good water. Really good water. In fact, anyone who visits and drinks our water has an epiphany - like my Mexican orange juice experience. My most memorable glass of orange juice was in Mexico. I was speaking down there during citrus harvest and my host stopped along the road to buy two large glasses of fresh squeezed orange juice from a fellow squatting next to his propane refrigerator. He was a gleaner. He would go along behind the harvesters and pick up the dropped fruit and squeeze it for his little roadside stand. Wow! Once you've had that, you don't even want what's typically passed off as orange juice in our grocery stores. You might as well just drink water.

The fact is, most municipal water doesn't taste good and so people tend to not drink it as much. Our farm well water is guzzling water. When people drink it, they often gush, "You guys need to sell this!"

If your water isn't guzzling water, for whatever reason, I recommend investing in some filtering and treatment technology to get it up to speed. Don't buy bottled water. Good grief. Just get your water fixed. It's cheaper and you don't have anything to throw away. I hate waste. I don't drink anything on airplanes because I can't stand all that plastic.

Sina: Yes! You need a source of good quality, clean water. Municipal water can contain prescription drugs, birth control pills, lead, arsenic, chloramines, fluoride, pesticides, and other toxic chemicals. You can check the water in your local area by going to the Environmental Working Group (EWG) website and typing your zip code into their database (www.ewg.org)

The EWG collected data from nearly 50,000 water utilities across all 50 states. They catalogued more than 270 contaminants. Some of the chemicals that were catalogued are associated with cancer, brain damage, nervous system problems, fertility issues, and hormone disruption. And, many of those chemicals have not been assigned government standards, such as an upper limit, even though some of the levels are high enough to cause concern. Specifically, more than 160 contaminants in our water supply are unregulated, according to the EWG.

Conveniently, if there's no established standard by the government, there's no government violation. So, your county can legally declare that the water "meets all government safety standards" and is "safe" to drink. But, without standards, the county is merely passing the government regulations by DEFAULT!

Joel: Again, why am I not surprised.

With modern technology, we have these wonderful vacuum water bottles that can hold water cold, even in hot conditions, for a long, long time. I don't know about you, but I really like chilled water. I know there's debate about never drinking cold water and I'm not talking about ice water, just chilled. Cool water is generally way more appealing than tepid or room-temperature water; it's more refreshing and I think even overcomes some of the taste issues. If the touch is refreshing, you're more likely psychologically to forgive imperfect taste. That's my completely unscientific analysis of water.

I'm a guzzler. Many days I drink a gallon and a half in a day. Of course, when you're sweating it's a lot easier to get thirsty. I think this whole water thing has numerous elements:

1. The more sedentary your day the less thirsty you are. Strenuous exercise and sweating stimulate thirst.
2. Taste and texture both affect our tendency to crave or seek water. Memory of the last drink bears heavily on whether we want to go back for more. If it's a chore, we don't. If it was exhilarating and tingled to our bones, we'll probably want to go back for more.
3. Availability. Where is the water? That's why I'm such a fan of the vacuum sealed water

bottle. I carry mine everywhere. It even has a big yellow cow ear tag affixed to the handle so nobody confuses it with theirs. The closer you keep water, the more likely you are to sip.

4. Drinking convenience. Water fountains are wonderful, but it's really hard to stand there and actually drink a pint of water at the fountain. People will start to stare at you. Fountains are great for a quick slurp, but if you think you can hydrate out of a water fountain, you're kidding yourself. I challenge you to take a one-quart container and see how long it takes to fill at a water fountain. Now imagine drinking that long, without losing any of the water stream. Always drink from a vessel; it's more efficient.

Sina: And, we're back to your 80/20 rule because I would never drink out of a public water fountain! The water usually comes from unfiltered municipal sources, which commonly contain toxic chemicals. But I love the vacuum water bottle suggestion.

Joel: You should get one, they're great!

You know the old rule about doing something for 56 days before it becomes a habit? I've tried that and it's actually true. If you're struggling to do something you know would be good for you and just can't seem to be consistent about it, do it religiously for 56 days. You'll be surprised how easy it is to keep doing it. Something happens psychologically. Instead of being something you have to push yourself to think about, you suddenly feel like your day isn't complete, or you've actually missed something, if you don't do it. That's when you know it's a habit.

Here is my challenge to you. Get a good vacuum water bottle. If it's a quart (32 fluid ounces) you need to drink roughly two of them a day. Drink only from that bottle all day so you can actually track what you're drinking. When you empty the first fill, refill it. Drink an additional glass or two just for good measure. This will make you accountable so you can't say "well, I think I drank enough." No, you need to measure it a few days so you develop a new normal. Secondly, your body will begin to respond when you actually hit the benchmark. Now do it for 56 days and you'll never have to think about it again.

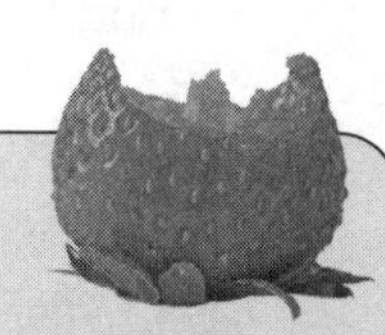

CHEW ON THIS

The fact that dehydration can increase blood cholesterol is an example of the compassion God showed when designing humans. Here's why: water is electrically charged. Those charges help keep your cell membranes in place and functioning properly. When you don't drink enough water, the cell membrane becomes less stable and doesn't work well. For example, moving nutrients into the cell and waste out of the cell becomes impaired. If you are chronically dehydrated, your liver tries to help by making cholesterol. That cholesterol gets released into the bloodstream and travels to the cell membranes where it can be used as a substitute for water in an attempt to keep your membranes functioning. Think of it as your body's last-ditch effort to keep the cell membrane glued together. In this situation, elevated blood cholesterol is not a bad thing. It's actually your body trying to help you deal with you not drinking enough water. How's that for compassion?

Practical Bite #20: Say Yes To rBGH-free Milk Products

How? Up to one-third of dairy cows in the U.S. are treated with rBGH, a genetically engineered hormone. It's primarily used by large factory farmers who supply grocery stores and restaurants with milk and other dairy products.

Labeling of rBGH milk is voluntary, meaning companies do not have to tell you if they injected their cows with rBGH. Consequently, it's important to know where rBGH can be found in your food supply, so you can avoid it.

Any dairy product could contain milk that came from rBGH treated cows, including: milk, cheese, butter, yogurt, and ice cream. In addition, milk or milk components are frequently used in processed foods. And since most Americans consume 75% of their calories from processed foods, the odds of consuming milk from rBGH treated cows is considerable.

To avoid rBGH, look for organic milk products. Organic means the milk cannot come from cows treated with rBGH because it's a synthetic hormone. If you don't want to buy organic, you can read the food label. Companies that do not use rBGH will almost certainly list it on the label. Look for a statement that acknowledges they do not treat their cows with growth hormones or rBGH (sometimes referred to as rBST).

Why?

Sina: I have a special connection with rBGH because it's the reason I began investigating our food supply. I blindly trusted our food until, one day, I read the label on my milk carton and found this statement:

> "According to the FDA, there is no significant difference in milk from rBGH treated cows and non-rBGH treated cows. FDA had determined that food products from cows treated with rBGH are safe for human consumption."

I had no idea what rBGH was or why it would be used to "treat" cows. Were the cows sick? Why were some cows "treated" and some weren't? Something wasn't right. So, I began searching the internet for information about rBGH. What I found changed the course of my life.

rBGH stands for recombinant bovine growth hormone, also known as somatotropin (rBST). It was the FIRST genetically engineered hormone introduced into our food supply. rBGH is given to cows to force them to produce more milk. Hence, it's used for economic purposes and is not intended to improve the health of the cow or the quality of the milk and meat that come from the cow. Yes, some dairy cows are slaughtered for meat in the United States.

Scientists create rBGH in a lab by combining cow genes with genes from bacteria, specifically *E. Coli.* Once the cow gene is added to the *E. Coli* gene, the new genetically engineered *E. Coli* bacteria makes a new hormone known as rBGH. The hormone is then injected into the cow. And, it works! rBGH reportedly increases milk production by 10-15%. Thus, in terms of its intended purpose, rBGH is an effective drug. However, it can make cows and people sick.

More than 20 medical conditions have been documented in cows treated with rBGH, including:

- Inability to walk due to severe hoof problems
- 40% decrease in fertility
- Blood abnormalities
- Increased mastitis
- Digestive disorders
- Shortened life span

And, sick cows produce sick milk. For example:

- Mastitis, or inflammation of the mammary gland, is one of the most common side effects of rBGH injections. It frequently leads to pus, bacteria, and blood getting into the milk that we drink. The government knew this was happening. So, how did they respond? They capped the number of somatic cells (dead white blood cells) allowed in your milk. Specifically, they allow 178 million somatic cells per cup of milk.
- Since antibiotics are required to treat mastitis, the milk likely contains antibiotics or their byproducts. In fact, the use of antibiotics in cows treated with rBGH increased so dramatically that the amount of antibiotics in the milk reached levels that were not allowed by the FDA. That's a big deal given the rise in antibiotic resistance in humans.

So, how did the FDA respond? They changed their regulations. The FDA increased the allowable level of antibiotics in our milk from 1 part per 100 million to 1 part per million. That's 100 times more antibiotic residues in our milk!

What do you think happens when you drink sick milk? Yep, you can get sick. Drinking the antibiotic residues, pus, and bacteria can wreak havoc on your microbiome. In addition, rBGH milk contains elevated levels of IGF-1 (Insulin-like Growth Factor 1). Numerous scientific studies support a strong association between elevated IGF-1 and some cancers, specifically:

- ❖ Colon cancer
- ❖ Breast cancer
- ❖ Childhood cancers
- ❖ Prostate cancer

When the FDA approved rBGH in 1993, all of this information was known. They knew that rBGH injections made cows sick, which made the milk sick and, consequently, the people sick. They knew that IGF-1 promotes the growth of cancerous cells. And, they knew that IGF-1 has been reported in the scientific literature to be "substantially elevated" in milk from cows treated with rBGH compared with milk from untreated cows. Yet, they approved the drug anyway.

Here's some additional information the FDA knew at the time of approval:

- ❖ FDA scientists repeatedly warned that rBGH could put public health in danger.
- ❖ Principled FDA employees and independent scientists who dared to question the safety of rBGH were intimidated and sometimes fired.
- ❖ The Government Accountability Office (GAO) advised against approval of rBGH.
- ❖ The primary evidence used to support the safety of milk from rBGH cows for human consumption came from two industry-sponsored rat studies.
- ❖ Employees at the FDA went on record to reveal that some of the data used to approve rBGH had been manipulated or suppressed.
- ❖ The media was silenced by Monsanto, who manufactured rBGH at the time.
- ❖ And, trusted organizations like the American Cancer Society and the American

> Dietetic Association, who advise us on diet and medical treatment, spouted industry-crafted talking points.

Yet, to this day, the FDA claims rBGH milk is safe for us to consume and that it's the same as milk from non-rBGH treated cows. Consequently, they do not require labeling!

So, you won't know if your dairy product came from a cow treated with rBGH unless the company specifically adds it to the label. Or, if a company does not treat their cows with rBGH, they are "allowed" to make that claim on the label. However, they must also add the FDA disclaimer: "FDA states: No significant difference in milk from cows treated with artificial growth hormone."

But, here's the kicker: The United States is one of the only modernized countries to allow the use of rBGH in dairy cows. Canada, Japan, Australia, New Zealand, and the European Union (made up of 28 countries) banned rBGH. Think about that for a moment: other countries won't allow their citizens to drink our milk! But the FDA says it's good enough for Americans.

All of that sounds pretty bad. But the next part of the story is what forever severed my trust in the FDA. rBGH was approved for use in our food supply in 1993, but we've been unknowingly drinking it since 1985.

Back in 1985, Monsanto was manufacturing rBGH. They conducted experiments on cows across the United States by injecting them with rBGH - the first genetically engineered hormone in our food supply. Nobody knew what would happen. Yet, beginning in 1985, the FDA allowed Monsanto to sell the experimental milk (and meat) for human consumption with *no restrictions* while the rBGH drug was still in the experimental phase of development.

Even worse, the FDA did not require those experimental products to be labeled. That means, for 8 years, some of us drank experimental milk and ate experimental meat without knowing it. And when the GAO called them out, the FDA stood behind their decision. According to the GAO:

> "The FDA does not require the labeling of food products derived from animals involved in drug treatment trials…we [the GAO] believe the public should have the right to know which food products have been produced from animals being tested with investigational drugs. Consequently, we disagree with FDA on this point."

If you knew about rBGH, you might have chosen to drink the milk anyway. That's not the point. The FDA effectively took away our choice when they decided not to require labeling of experimental foods. It's a slow erosion of our freedom.

After I learned that we were un-consenting guinea pigs in a nation-wide experiment, doubt and distrust ensued. I began to wonder, "How many other foods in the grocery store am I consuming that are coming from experimental drug trials?" "What else is in my food that is not listed on the label?" I kept asking questions and kept digging for answers.

It's crazy when I step back and think that because of ONE milk label, I have written two books, learned how to reverse disease, became a consultant, and went on a talk circuit. From that perspective, I'm grateful for the absurd FDA disclaimer on my milk carton. I should be thanking the FDA!

Seriously though, that one milk label raised a red flag, which inspired me to take off my blinders and become an informed consumer. For that, I am grateful.

Joel: How could I ever interrupt a tirade like that?

If you tried to fictionalize how bad things are, I don't think you could make up a story more outrageous than the nonfiction facts in this case. The rBGH story is perhaps the most egregious example of regulator-industry collusion in the whole food and farming sector.

The lengths to which these folks go to parse words is amazing. For example, you will never see a label that says "No Hormones" or "Hormone Free." Now all of us know what these phrases mean. But the FDA does not allow the phrase on a label because all food contains hormones. Those of us who would like to put that phrase on our food to explain that we aren't feeding artificials, injecting artificials, bathing it in artificials, we know and everyone else knows the point of the "No Hormones" phrase.

But not the FDA. No, they parse the language to the point that if it says "No Hormones" then it contains no hormones - natural or otherwise. Well, all food contains hormones. That is why you'll always see "No Hormones Added" or something to that effect on the label trying to convey what we all understand in plain English, but what the FDA word geeks tie into pretzels.

This is why you must know more than a label. A label is not enough. A label designed and regulated by government officials is not enough. It may not even be honest. And that is why I've never joined the chorus about labels. I know that by the time it passes through the collective and creative contrivances of the government industrial food complex, it won't tell you enough to be useful. Instead of the truth, the whole truth, and nothing but the truth, it's untruth, half the truth, and anything but the truth.

Now do you see why we titled this book BEYOND LABELS? When we give the lexicon of food description over to this fraternity, the resultant words simply are not trustworthy. And if you can't trust, what do you really know? And if you can't know, what do you do? Hang in there; we're going someplace.

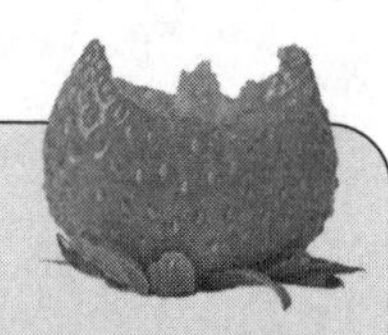

CHEW ON THIS

Many toxins, including PCBs and dioxins, accumulate in fat cells. That's fabulous news for your brain because the toxins are pulled out of your blood stream, which sequesters them away from your brain. However, it also means that some fatty foods have become delivery systems for many types of toxins, including polybrominated flame retardants. When you eat fatty foods that contain these types of toxins, they can accumulate in your fat cells, which can make you sick. In fact, some people feel fatigued and sick when they begin to lose weight (via fat loss) because the stored toxins are being released from the fat cells and enter into their blood stream. But you can reduce your toxic storage load by choosing organic when eating fatty foods, such as: milk, cheese, butter, yogurt, and meat. Organically raised livestock aren't exposed to growth hormones, GMOs, or most antibiotics or pesticides. Consequently, the fat cells of those animals should theoretically contain less toxins compared to conventionally raised livestock. Therefore, choose organic when eating animal products.

Practical Bite #21: Be Informed At Restaurants

How? The next time you eat at a restaurant or fast-food chain, ask to see the ingredient list for the food you are about to order, or look it up online. Fast-food chains and restaurants are beginning to post ingredient lists on their website.

Why?

Sina: Every day, Americans eat roughly 1/3 of their calories as fast food, according to the CDC. I bet most of us don't ask for the ingredient list before consuming those foods.

You might be surprised to learn about some of the ingredients used at restaurants and fast-food chains. For instance, a famous pizza chain uses butylated hydroxytoluene (BHT) in their pepperoni. BHT is used in embalming fluid and jet fuel. It has been shown in studies to promote tumor growth and damage DNA.

A national hamburger chain uses a famous sauce that contains propylene glycol alginate, xanthan gum, hydrolyzed soy, and high fructose corn syrup. If you only eat what you know, can you eat a sauce containing propylene glycol alginate?

And, here are just a few of the ingredients found in French toast sticks that are served at a national fast-food chain: sodium stearoyl lactylate, calcium steaoyl-2-lactylate, glycerol monooleate, polysorbate 60, polysorbate 80, arabic gum, carrageenan, soy lecithin, and calcium propionate. Yum!

Joel: We live in an unprecedented time of information. You don't have to check out a book or go to a library to do most run-of-the-mill research. All you need is the internet and you can do more research in an hour than people could do in a lifetime a century ago.

Rather than using our internet access to play video games and solitaire, we need to use that new power to ride hard on the places we eat. Places proud of their ingredients post them on their websites. Like all sleuthing, a little practice yields quick skill. I was curious about a fast food place I'd never visited but many friends recommended, so I just looked it up. The food was so bad I don't see how anybody eats there, but they're huge, nationwide, and have a tremendously loyal following. Either people don't care about provenance or they're too lazy to search.

Anyone who says this is too hard due to lack of time, think for a minute. How much time do you spend watching YouTube® or playing games? Social media? When we're talking about games or your health, which one should take precedence? With the internet, you can literally look behind the counter of almost any food establishment. There's almost no excuse for being ignorant about provenance and ingredients.

You can do most of this privately, of course, but if you're good-natured about it you can be bolder and do it in person. Don't be aggressive and discourteous about it, but with a good-humored smile and genuine interest, ask. If everyone who reads this book would do that it would revolutionize eateries. I say that not because I assume millions will read this book--although they should. I say it because it takes extremely few to get attention.

I tried to sell pork to a specialty restaurant in our area that had been featured in *Southern Living* magazine as a great place to eat. The owner and cook did taste comparisons with our pork and their industrial pork. When we put the two pieces of meat on the kitchen counter, the difference in appearance was striking. The industrial was white; ours was rose colored.

After cooking and breading and heavy spicing for schnitzel, however, the differences were hard to detect. The pork was really a conveyance of breading and spices. The owner, just as serious and matter-of-factly as you could imagine, summed up the trial with this: "Well, our customers don't care about quality anyway. All they want is junk." Thus, ended the potential sale.

I tried to get our eggs into another local restaurant, again the recipient of numerous culinary magazine awards. The cook took two eggs out of my sample carton, plopped them on the griddle (I went right after the breakfast rush), fried them sunny side up, scooped them off onto a saucer, and ate them on the spot. His eyes widened and before he even finished both of them, he said "we have to get these eggs." He told me to follow him and we marched to the end of the kitchen, took a left, and immediately were in the restaurant office.

The owner was doing paperwork, paying bills and doing what business owners do. The cook got his attention and said he'd just had the most amazing eggs ever and the restaurant needed to buy them. Without even looking up, the owner asked "are they brown?" The cook replied that they were, like real country farm eggs. Again, without ever looking up, the owner responded "we will never have a brown egg in this establishment" and summarily excused us from the office. The cook was dumbfounded. I just figured a Rhode Island red had pecked the owner's finger when he was a little boy and he was still suffering Post Traumatic Stress Disorder as a result.

I could go on in this vein for some time. One restaurant said our eggs were too big. The point is that some restaurants care and some don't. Just like people, they have perceptions and prejudices too. It's up to you and me to ferret out the mindset, temperament, and protocols of the places where we eat. To refuse is to bury our heads in the sand and wish things would get better without doing anything. I've got news for you. Nothing changes until somebody does something. You plus another somebody can create accountability, and we sure as the world need that today.

Sina: It's especially important to ask for the ingredient list if you have food allergies or sensitivities. Have you ever seen the food allergy label on processed foods sold in grocery stores? It tells you if the packaged food contains common allergens, such as: milk or peanuts. Well, restaurants and fast food chains are not legally required to list allergens on their menus.

That's crazy because all chain restaurants with 20 or more locations are now required by the government to list the number of calories contained in alcoholic beverages. Yet, there's no requirement to list food allergens; restaurants are exempt from that rule.

It's up to you to protect yourself when eating out. Again, you may be surprised at what's in your food. I recently learned that chicken from a well-known sandwich chain contains milk. Milk, in chicken? Ask for the ingredient list!

Joel: If a server or staff member is put off or acts irritated by your questions, get up and leave. Again, you don't have to be irritating to do this. I often ask if the chickens are pastured. Of course, the server assumes I've just asked if they were pasteurized. No, I clarify, I mean pastured, like out on green grass instead of in factory houses. That stumps them. Of course, it's easy for me to ask about that because I virtually never eat chicken away from home unless I know where it came from. I've had a couple of bouts with food poisoning from chicken - including at church pot lucks - so I'm pretty careful about the chicken.

I asked one server if the beef was grass-finished. "Oh, no sir, we have the finest corn-fed beef here. Only the best." I didn't order beef there.

Everyone approaches this with a different level of militancy. Do I eat stuff I'd rather not? Yes, and here's why. I don't have any food allergies and I eat really super 95 percent of the time. I have some fudge room built in. If you've been through what Sina's been through, you'll probably be more militant. And to be sure, even though you look great and feel healthy now, Sina, the chances of a relapse if you cheat is probably way higher than someone like me with a great history of clean food and a seemingly cast-iron stomach.

So, when I'm in social situations, I tuck my militancy into some diplomacy. Who wants to eat with someone who's fighting every time you get a plate of food? There's a balance here and I think most of us can fudge occasionally to keep the peace. Again, Sina, I'm willing to grant you some extra non-wiggle room because of your history. The more extreme your story, the more extreme your demeanor going forward. If you can, slice some slack. If you can't, stick to your guns.

Sina: Exactly. It's not about being "perfect." It's about giving informed consent. Knowing what's in your food before you eat it provides the opportunity to make conscious decisions, as opposed to blindly trusting the food supply. Once you see the ingredient list, you get to decide if you want those chemicals to become part of your body. If you do then go for it! If you don't then ask to see the ingredient list for another food or choose a different eatery. Either way, you will have made an informed decision.

Practical Bite #22: Look For The Duo

How? If you want to avoid GMOs when buying processed foods, look for the duo: the USDA Organic label plus the Non-GMO Project label.

Why?

Sina: One of the most dramatic changes to our food supply in the last 60 years has been the introduction of genetically modified organisms (GMOs). Without a doubt, GMOs have fundamentally transformed our food supply. One example is corn. The corn we ate as children is no longer the same type of corn we eat today. Today, most of the corn Americans eat is genetically modified (GM). And, one type of GM corn is called *Bt* corn.

To make *Bt* corn, scientists take a gene from bacteria, the *Bt* gene, and insert it into the DNA of the corn. The bacterial *Bt* gene codes for a pesticide, called *Bt* toxin. Once that bacterial gene is inserted into the corn, the *Bt* toxin is made inside nearly every cell of the corn. In essence, the corn becomes a pesticide factory. So, when a bug bites into the corn, it ingests the pesticide, which kills it by breaking open its stomach. As a scientist, that concept sounds brilliant! But the problem is, *we* eat that corn too! So, what happens when you bite into that piece of corn and ingest the pesticide?

According to the chemical companies that make the GM corn, the toxin is "safe" and doesn't affect you. They claim it only affects the bugs. But scientific studies are reporting that the toxin produced in the corn can bind to our guts, which can initiate an inflammatory immune response, and may lead to leaky gut. In other words, it may break open our guts too.

If that's true, it's bad news for us because you may not think you eat a lot of corn. How often do you eat popcorn or corn on the cob? But corn surrounds you on all sides of the grocery store aisle. Thanks to farm subsidies, corn is abundant in our food supply – and it is primarily GM corn that has been processed into cheap, synthetic byproducts that are added to your favorite foods.

It's estimated that roughly 75% of all processed foods in the grocery store contain GM ingredients – largely consisting of GM corn. You may not recognize corn on the food label. I sometimes have a hard time recognizing it because the corn has been processed into hundreds of different synthetic chemicals. Here are just a few examples of ingredients that are commonly derived from corn: vitamin E, vitamin C, dextrose, and MSG. So, if you eat processed foods, you most likely eat corn every day. And, unless you buy corn that is 100% organic, you're probably eating GM corn.

But it's not just corn that is genetically modified. Other crops have been genetically modified too, including some varieties of: soybeans, cotton, sugar beets, canola, papaya, apple, eggplant, pineapple, potato, and summer squash.

Again, the typical American eats 75% of their calories from processed foods. And, roughly 75% of those processed foods contain genetically modified ingredients. That means the typical American eats GMOs every single day. And, since Americans are getting sicker, people are asking if GMOs are safe.

The truth is that nobody definitively knows. GMOs have not been on the market long enough to definitively know how they will affect us in the long-term. And, it's very difficult to wade through the available studies because most researchers are bought and paid for by industry. Consequently, most studies on GMOs report no health risks. Fortunately, there are a few independent scientists and organizations left, which is largely why some studies actually report health risks in animals and humans fed GMOs. But the days of independent research are largely over.

Everyone has an agenda. And, in terms of your food supply, the agenda is usually not the pursuit of truth due to crony relationships between industry, academia, and the government. In fact, when it comes to GMOs, both sides have claimed that the other side has falsified data, played statistical games to get their desired outcome, cherry-picked the numbers, etcetera. Consequently, the GMO issue has become so political that we may not know the truth in our lifetime – at least not through unbiased scientific studies.

But common sense tells us that scientists are not equipped to play the role of God and that we are not designed to eat food that was created in a laboratory by transferring genes from bacteria into corn. We are better off eating the foods God gave us. Clearly, people aren't dying or getting debilitatingly sick from eating one meal of GMOs. But what's the long-term impact on our health? There may be a cumulative effect – like we see with toxins and other chemicals that enter a biological system. After all, the negative health effects, such as inflammatory disease, are usually not visible for years or even decades.

In fact, we are learning that GMOs may remain in your body, making you sick, even after you stop eating them. For example, a human feeding study revealed that the gene inserted into genetically modified soy can transfer into the DNA of the bacteria that live inside of your gastrointestinal tract. If this holds true, it means that if you eat a corn chip that was made from *Bt* corn, the bacterial gene could transfer to your intestinal bacteria and start producing *Bt* toxin – a pesticide – inside of your gut. If that happens, your intestinal bacteria will become pesticide factories that continue to make pesticides in your body, even after you have removed GMOs from your diet. In other words, eating GMOs may negatively change your microbiome for an unknown period of time.

Meanwhile, industry hires scientists to go on television and claim that "most scientists" agree GMOs are safe. Even though those scientists are often mercenaries for hire. And, industry assures you that GMOs have undergone an extensive government "approval" process. Even though the FDA never "approved" GMOs; they simply "presumed" GMOs to be GRAS.

But what about the USDA? They are in charge of agriculture, so isn't it their job to "approve" GM crops?

Shockingly, the USDA does not "approve" GM crops; they simply "deregulate" them. They look at a company's petition, and if the new GM plant "does not present a plant pest risk, the petition is granted, thereby allowing the deregulated article [plant] to be introduced into the marketplace without restriction." Yes, you read that right; the USDA allows GMOs on the market with no restrictions. And, once a product is "deregulated", it can immediately be sold in your local grocery store.

Yet, if you speak out against GMOs, they label you as "anti-science" or "anti-progress," and sometimes they try to destroy your reputation in order to silence any resistance.

Joel: Anytime somebody responds that "most scientists say" I always think about expert conventional thinking throughout history. If we start naming things that orthodox experts agreed on, it's quite an interesting list. I wonder what our descendants, a century or more from now, will consider laughably absurd in our beliefs.

Here are some things our ancestors believed strongly enough that no one could argue them into a different position:

1. The earth is flat.
2. Bad fairies cause illnesses.
3. Slavery is okay.
4. Women don't want to vote.
5. Native Americans are barbarians.
6. Pasteurization is the best way to make milk safe to drink.
7. Hitler could be appeased.
8. Hydrogenated vegetable oil is healthier than butter.
9. High fructose corn syrup is the same as maple syrup.
10. Rice Krispies® are the foundation of good health (USDA Food Pyramid).
11. Formula is superior to breast milk.

We could add numerous things to this list, but you get the picture. Every single culture, at any point in time, believes stupid things. Things that are later proved untrue. Just because people vote for it or the majority believes it does not make it true; in fact, often that's a litmus test for foolishness.

So, what about GMOs? Do you realize how many mechanisms nature has in place to make sure a GMO cannot occur? When the industry says "oh, it's just a permutation of Mendel's peas," nothing could be further from the truth. Mendel, who developed hybridization, was breeding different kinds of peas - it was peas on peas. It wasn't peas on pigs on mold on trees.

My litmus test for things that ain't right is this: when the sexual plumbing doesn't match up, it just ain't right. We humans are pretty clever, and we can invent things that we can't morally, ethically, or physically metabolize. That should give us pause when we go wading into DNA manipulation like a bunch of swashbuckling sailors, abandoning hesitation.

The precautionary principle is a scientific term for carefully appreciating potential catastrophic consequences. While we don't want to be so cautious as to never take risks, we also don't want to be foolhardy when dealing with something as anti-nature as GMOs. This technology does not speed up natural processes; it throws all-natural processes to the wind and breaks down every barrier erected by nature to protect this from happening. That should give us all pause.

Sina: The good news is that consumers are pausing! 90% of Americans want GM foods to be labeled, according to a 2015 poll. I can't remember the last time 90% of Americans agreed on anything! But, consumers are uniting on this issue. Unfortunately, government and industry are working against us.

For example, in 2016, Congress passed the National Bioengineered Food Disclosure Law, which directed the USDA to establish a national mandatory standard for labeling foods that are genetically modified. The intention was good. But, unfortunately, the standards are filled with loopholes and lack of transparency.

Specifically, companies don't have to use the word "GMO" on the label. Instead, they can provide an electronic or digital link, or a QR code. In addition, small food manufacturers or small packages are allowed to simply list a phone number or web address, which would require consumers to hunt down the information. And, even though companies do not have to comply until 2022, some companies have already met the new requirements by simply placing a circular symbol on the product that says "bioengineered." So, while the law was designed to establish a national standard for GM foods, the labeling is still confusing and only adds to the complexity of the grocery store labyrinth.

Since it can be difficult to identify foods in the grocery store that are genetically modified, a convenient and safer path is to look for the USDA Organic label, in addition to the Non-GMO Verification Label.

Buying foods that carry the USDA Organic label is a huge step forward in reducing the toxic load on your body. However, that label cannot always be trusted. For instance, the U.S. has been a dumping ground for fraudulent "organic" corn and soybean imports for years. Just recently, the U.S. purchased more "organic" grain from Turkey than Turkey can produce. Apparently, a shipment of conventional grains left Turkey and by the time it arrived on U.S. soil, it had magically turned into "organic" grain.

Joel: Ongoing issues with imported grain from the far east, most of which comes through Istanbul, casts additional doubt on organic feedstock credibility. And, in 2019, a business in Ohio that handles 5 percent of all organic grain grown in America was found to be fraudulently calling it "organic". The man who owned the company committed suicide prior to the court appearance.

This is why our farm does not use organic government certified grains; we use GMO-free from local farmers that we can visit and trust. And, our mill tests what comes in for pesticide residues, including glyphosate (Roundup®). I've decided to get my grains from farmers I know and from a mill that tests rather than relying on paperwork passed through docks around the world. It's a trust issue.

When you think about the ability to create shady deals in the global commodity network, prudence makes you wonder just what or who you can trust. Most folks don't realize that half of all organic grain consumed in the U.S. is imported from foreign countries - half.

Sina: Exactly! And, one of the reasons there is fraud is because the existing organic regulations are not being enforced by the U.S. government. The intention behind the USDA Organic label is good, but the follow-through is lacking.

I think of the USDA Organic label like a bucket filled with water. And, each time our trust in the label is broken, the bucket springs a leak. For instance, while the USDA Organic label does not technically allow GMOs, residue testing for GMOs is not required during the certification process nor is it required to maintain USDA Organic status. In addition, when certifying a processed food as USDA Organic, there is no requirement to test for the presence of GMOs. The only exception is when the certifying agent decides testing is necessary. However, according to the USDA, "The certifying agent will review ingredient purchases and production records." In other words, certification hinges largely on reviewing paperwork.

How do we know the processed foods carrying the USDA Organic label are truly GMO-free if there's no testing of the farms or the final food product? Pop! The bucket sprang a leak. And, that's where the Non-GMO Verification Label comes in – it patches the GMO hole in the USDA Organic bucket.

The Non-GMO Verification seal was created by the Non-GMO Project, which is a non-profit, independent organization dedicated to preserving and building the non-GMO food supply. They provide verified non-GMO choices that are easy to spot in the grocery store because their seal of approval is a colorful butterfly that is usually printed on the front of the package. The Butterfly has become the most trusted label available for GMO avoidance.

In order to carry the Butterfly on the package, the product must pass a third-party verification process, which typically includes molecular or immunological testing methods. And, the product must undergo a renewal evaluation each year to ensure continued compliance.

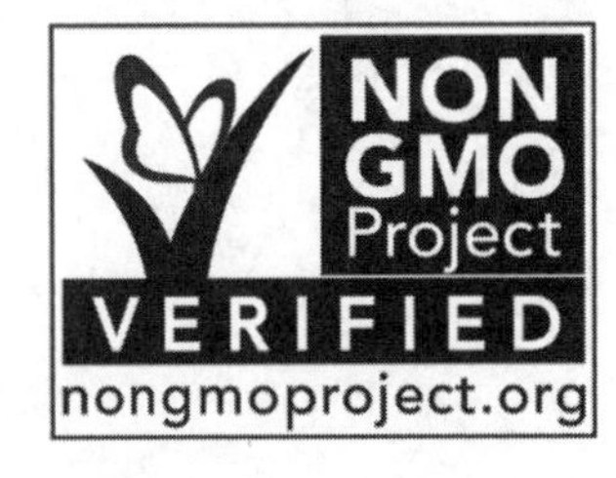

Figure 1: Image used with permission from the Non-GMO Project

The Butterfly is an easy way to take responsibility for my food choices while harnessing the power of the free market. Think about it: the government can make mistakes with its label, like allowing millions of pounds of magically "organic" grains on the market, and there's seemingly no consequences. An independent company, on the other hand, has an incentive to stay on high ground. Unlike the government, if the Non-GMO Project makes a mistake, they could go out of business. I don't see the USDA going out of "business" any time soon, in spite of its failings.

Joel: You've got that right. The bureaucracy carries on whether it's effective or not. That's why private business and non-profits have more credibility; their brand is everything.

Sina: The bottom line is, if you want to avoid GMOs in your favorite processed foods, pair these two labels together because the Butterfly fills a hole that exists in the USDA Organic label.

CHEW ON THIS

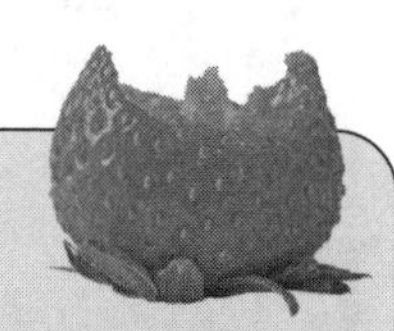

Speaking of labels, why are genetically engineered foods still allowed to be called by the name of the original food? For example, corn that is fused with bacterial genes is still called corn. But, the name "corn" comes with the expectation that all the genes in that corn are genes that belong to corn. So, when genes are added to corn and that GM corn is still labeled as "corn," isn't that false advertising?

Think about it: when plums are crossed with apricots, the new fruit is given a new name: pluot. When tangerines are crossed with grapefruit, they also get a new name: tangelo. We also have limequats, which are a cross between a lime and a kumquat. The list goes on and on. All of these fruits were renamed even though they were simply bred with other fruits, using pollen. So, why doesn't corn get a new name since it is now a cross between bacteria and corn? That corn makes a bacterial toxin inside itself. So, wouldn't it be more transparent to give this new creation a new name, like bactocorn or cornteria or cornoxin?

After all, in 2013, the Supreme Court ruled that GM corn could be patented because it contains a type of gene that is not found in nature. So, why is GM corn still called corn?

If genetically modified foods and genetically modified ingredients were given new, transparent names, there would be no need for a special GMO label. The new name would instantly let you know that the food is not in a natural state.

Practical Bite #23: Look For The Trio

How? If you want to avoid GMOs and glyphosate when buying processed foods, look for the trio: USDA Organic seal plus the Non-GMO Project seal plus the Glyphosate Residue Free seal.

Why?

Sina: Most people have heard of Roundup®. It's the weed killer commonly sprayed on yards. It's also commonly sprayed on food crops, playgrounds, parks, and school grounds. One of the active ingredients in Roundup® is glyphosate. Glyphosate can also be found in other herbicides, but Roundup® is by far the most widely used herbicide in the world.

In fact, it's so widely used that glyphosate can be found in human hair, blood, and urine, as well as drinking water, rain samples, and the food we feed our families including, for example: common breakfast cereals, snack bars, and granola. Consequently, it's no surprise that an estimated 93% of Americans have glyphosate in their bodies, with children having the highest level, according to a 2015 study by the University of California at San Francisco.

Avoiding glyphosate is one of my top priorities because it is damaging on many levels:

- Studies have shown that glyphosate can change the gut microbiome, creating an imbalance. This is partly because glyphosate is a **patented antibiotic**, which means it kills "good" microbes in your gastrointestinal tract, as well as "good" microbes in the soil. You need those microbes in order to survive. Remember, you are more microbe than human; you have roughly 10 bacterial cells for every one human cell. Those microbes help regulate every system and every cell in your body. So, if you kill them off by eating antibiotics, like glyphosate, you increase your likelihood of developing an illness or disease.
- Glyphosate can weaken the gut barrier by damaging the tight junctions, which can result in **leaky gut**.
- Glyphosate is water-soluble, which means it can travel through your blood and, subsequently, damage any cell in your body that is nourished by your blood, including your blood-brain barrier. If that happens, toxins can enter your brain, including heavy metals; it's called **leaky brain**.

- Glyphosate is an **endocrine disruptor**, meaning it can lead to adverse neurological, reproductive, developmental, and immunological effects.
- Glyphosate can **shut down the cytochrome P450 detox pathway**, which can result in toxins accumulating in your body.
- Glyphosate is a **chelator**, meaning it grabs on to certain metals, such as: iron, copper and manganese. When sprayed on food crops, glyphosate pulls metals out of the soil, making them unavailable to the plant. Without those metals, the immune system of the plant is weakened. When you eat those sick plants, you can become deficient in those micronutrients too. In addition, "good" bacteria in your gastrointestinal tract also need certain metals to function properly. Manganese, for example, helps protect bacteria from oxidative damage. So, when you eat glyphosate, your "good" bacteria can also become weaker, which can result in you becoming more susceptible to disease.
- Glyphosate was declared a "probable human **carcinogen**" by the World Health Organization (WHO) in 2015. In 2017, the state of California listed glyphosate as a known cancer-causing agent. In 2018, the world was stunned when a jury courageously declared glyphosate to be responsible for a dying man's cancer. And, in 2019, two additional juries found glyphosate guilty of contributing to cancer.
- Glyphosate **may contribute to the formation of Parkinson's, depression, anxiety, diabetes, obesity, and sleep disorders** because it blocks the shikimate pathway. Plants and bacteria use the shikimate pathway to make essential aromatic amino acids, including: tyrosine, tryptophan, and phenylalanine. Your human cells do not have the shikimate pathway, so you rely on plants and the bacteria in your gastrointestinal tract to make those essential amino acids for you. But studies have confirmed that glyphosate blocks the shikimate pathway, which inhibits the plants and bacteria from making the amino acids you need in order to be healthy.

  For instance, bacteria in your gut make tryptophan, which is converted into serotonin. In fact, roughly 95% of your serotonin is made in your gut – not in your brain, like previously thought. Consequently, if the shikimate pathway is blocked by glyphosate then you could be low in serotonin, which can lead to blood sugar dysregulation, depression, anxiety, and cognitive decline. Low serotonin can also lead to low levels of melatonin because serotonin is converted into melatonin. And, decreased levels of melatonin can lead to decreased gut motility, difficulty sleeping and sleep disorders, as well as dysregulation of the reproductive and immune systems. The bacteria in your gut also make tyrosine, which is converted to dopamine. Since glyphosate blocks the pathway that makes tyrosine, glyphosate can lead to low levels of dopamine in your body. And, low levels of dopamine have been linked with Parkinson's disease.

Those are just a handful of negative health effects associated with glyphosate. We're continually learning how far reaching its tentacles truly are. For instance, in 2019, a study published in *Scientific Reports* suggested that you can pass disease to your offspring through your exposure to glyphosate. Specifically, second and third-generation offspring suffered "dramatic increases" in diseases, such as: "prostate disease, obesity, kidney disease, ovarian disease, and parturition (birth) abnormalities," according to the study.

Think about that for a moment: the third-generation, which would be your great-grandchildren, had no direct exposure to glyphosate. Yet, they developed diseases because their great-grandparents were exposed.

This phenomenon is called generational toxicity. And, unfortunately, when regulating bodies – such as our government – determine the level of glyphosate exposure that is considered "safe," they do not take into account transgenerational impacts. In other words, nobody knows what level of glyphosate exposure will promote disease in your offspring. Yet, most of us are exposed to glyphosate every day, often without knowing it.

Joel: GMOs opened the floodgates for glyphosate, which was developed by Monsanto and is now owned by Bayer Corporation. Some GMOs, like corn and soybeans, were engineered to be immune to Roundup®. And, because they can be sprayed with impunity, they are. More is always better, right? With reckless abandon, farmers can now spray to their hearts' content. And nature is responding to that activity.

A couple of years ago I was doing a week of seminars in Australia and did the normal Los Angeles to Sydney flight. As I grabbed my bag off the baggage carousel, two women standing right next to me noticed the cow ear tag on my luggage. That's my little identification doodad to make sure I don't mistake it - or that somebody else doesn't mistake it.

They both brightened up and asked if I was a farmer. I said yes and asked them what they were doing in Australia. "We work for Bayer Corporation and we're on our way to Perth for an international symposium on Roundup-induced super weeds," they replied, as nonchalantly as if they were ordering pizza. Rarely does anyone strike up a conversation with me when I travel, and even more rare is the person who knows what a cow ear tag is. As much as these two ladies and I were on different planets in our worldviews, I enjoyed the camaraderie this far away from home.

They said farmers in Arkansas employed people with machetes to hack down these mutant super weeds ahead of the harvest combines because these gargantuan plants broke up the headers and guts of million dollar combines. Wow. The things the industry doesn't publicize. Isn't it amazing? Just like antibiotics have given us superbugs, GMOs have given us superweeds. Why would anyone wonder about the link between the two? Survivors always adapt.

Glyphosate is currently at the heart of the litigation against Bayer Corporation. Although we've had some big damage awards, nothing has actually been paid out. The first tactical ploy by the Monsanto attorneys is to ask for a trial splitting the case into two parts. First, argue the science of Roundup®. Second, argue negligence. Two completely different trials, with the second one being contingent on winning the first.

We are emotional beings. As much as we'd like to think we are data driven and empirically-minded, we all ultimately make decisions from the heart. And so, a dispassionate scientific inquiry into the question: does Roundup® cause cancer? will absolutely end in a hung jury. When I say science is subjective, academics get their pants in a wad and dismiss me as a nut. But just a couple of days ago I read an article by a scientist who had the courage to admit that science is subjective. His point was that we pick what we see.

So, in this trial, a 2010 study of 20 mice painted with glyphosate, caused 40 percent to develop tumors. Bayer scientists will show the study was epidemiologically flawed and that animal experiments don't necessarily translate to humans.

By the same token, when Bayer says its 40 years of studies and Environmental Protection Agency (EPA) bean counting has shown no association with Roundup® and cancer, the scientists on the other side will say those studies had flaws and can't be trusted. It'll be tit for tat for days as these scientists parse the meaning of "is."

Lo and behold, in 2018, a jury surprised me by deciding glyphosate does cause cancer. What apparently soured the jury on the government and Monsanto position was the despicable thread of emails showing collusion and agenda-driven science. It was too rotten to ignore.

Sina: Those emails revealed that Monsanto and the EPA have worked together to keep glyphosate on the market. Here are just a few examples of what the emails revealed:

- Monsanto wrote research papers in secret and then passed them off as written by scientists in academia. A Monsanto executive told other company officials that costs could be kept down by writing research papers themselves and then hiring academics to put their names on the papers: "we would be keeping the cost down by us doing the writing and they would just edit & sign their names so to speak."
- Scientists within the EPA disagreed over the safety of glyphosate. There was no scientific consensus that glyphosate is safe for humans. (This is an established pattern in our food supply. For instance, scientists within the government did not agree that GMOs or rBGH were safe, yet both still entered the market).
- The U.S. Department of Health and Human Services planned to conduct a scientific review of the safety of glyphosate. But senior EPA officials killed the review. According to court documents, Jess Rowland, Deputy Division Director at the EPA, sent an email to Monsanto executive Dan Jenkins stating, "If I can kill this, I should get a medal." The review was never conducted. In a separate email, Mr. Jenkins told a colleague that Mr. Rowland was planning to retire and "could be useful as we move forward with ongoing glyphosate defense." Revolving door, anyone?

All of that is bad, but here's the piece of evidence that is most revealing and damaging: Monsanto never conducted cancer studies on Roundup®. Even though Monsanto adamantly claims that Roundup® is safe for us to eat and does not cause cancer, Monsanto's lead toxicologist stated in her deposition that she "cannot say that Roundup® does not cause cancer" because "[w]e [Monsanto] have not done the carcinogenicity [cancer] studies with Roundup®."

In other words, they never tested the final product! They "tested" glyphosate by itself, but they never tested glyphosate plus all of the other ingredients contained in Roundup®, such as surfactants to help glyphosate enter the plant cells and other additives designed to extend the product's shelf life. We don't know all of the ingredients in Roundup® because they are not required to be listed. However, the final product has been reported to be more damaging than glyphosate alone.

Monsanto, of course, denies any wrongdoing.

Joel: Of course! And farmers are not juries. And most farmers certainly are not San Franciscans, where these two trials were held. And so "Farmers Stay with Bayer Herbicide" is the big headline in the Wall Street Journal after these verdicts. While shares dropped by a third after the first case, farm use appears to be holding steady.

Well, how much glyphosate gets used, anyway? On soybeans alone, 120 million pounds. On corn alone, 95 million pounds. All other uses amount to about 60 million pounds. Add all those up and you have 275 million pounds. As you know I tend to do, let's put that in perspective. A tractor trailer hauls about 50,000 pounds of freight. So that's 5,500 tractor trailer loads. A trailer is usually 48 feet long, so if you took off the tractors and just lined up the trailers end to end, that would be a line 50 miles long. Just meditate on that a moment.

Every year, every year, every year that's how much Roundup® herbicide is dumped onto the U.S. That doesn't count use in any other country. One more comparison for magnitude. Officially, 214,000 acres of organic corn are grown in the U.S. That's worth roughly $130 million. Annual sales of glyphosate are $5 billion. Talk about David and Goliath. So, all the organic corn grown in the U.S. is less than 3 percent of the value of Roundup® sales. Kind of puts things in perspective, no?

Now you know why even in the face of multi-million-dollar liability verdicts, nothing changes at the Monsanto production facility. The herbicide is ubiquitous in farmland, the toxin of choice, favorite partner to control weeds.

Those famers are complicit in this glyphosate tragedy because of their inability to think outside the box. In the Wall Street Journal article, Waverly, Iowa farmer Mark Mueller is quoted as saying he "considers glyphosate essential for sustainably farming his 1,600 acres." Did you catch the word sustainably? Like many farmers practicing no-till, he says it helps keep his soil in place. He could also keep his soil in place by growing perennial prairie, pruning it with herbivores (cattle instead of bison). However, this version of no-till as a system substituted herbicide for tillage (plowing).

In order for a crop to grow, competition must be eliminated. Just like weeds in your flower bed, aggressive and opportunistic plants choke out the one you desire in that spot. All plants emit auxins, which are hormones to retard competition. The dominant plant in any spot emits the most auxins to suppress competition. That's why controlling competition through preparing a seedbed is necessary to enable the seeds you plant to grow. Without suppressing competition, they'll get crowded out. That suppression can be done with mulch, tillage (spading, plowing, working the soil in some way) or herbicide.

In general, no-till cropping traded plowing for herbicide. Clearly, the trade reduces soil erosion. But the advantages are not as clear-cut as many might think. Pumping herbicides into the ecosystem is arguably trading the devil for the witch.

The underlying problem in this whole discussion is the assumption that corn and beans are the only viable things to grow. What is the rationale for planting so much corn and soybeans? Because they are the two highest demand crops. Corn is starch; beans are protein. Energy and protein are the two keys for nutrition. And these two crops deliver it at higher levels per acre than other crops like wheat, barley, oats and sunflowers. While it is true that corn and beans enjoy special protections in the Farm Bill (crop insurance) the primary driver of planting corn and beans is those two crops offer the greatest production per acre.

Heritage grains like spelt or amaranth simply don't have the market demand that the more common corn and soybeans do. Everything in the industrial system pushes simplification. Separating two crops in just two big grain bins is far simpler than separating three in three bins, or four or five. Industrial systems all gravitate toward simplicity and specialization rather than complexity and diversity.

Without question, a perennial prairie under excellent management can grow as much meat and milk as corn and beans, but it's much more difficult to finish a beef and make a cow milk on forages than it is on simple corn and beans. Pasture management choreography is literally a ballet whereas growing crops is more formula and recipe. Plants don't escape. They don't need daily attention. Plants are simpler than animals, so as long as farmers can survive economically with crops, they really have no incentive to switch to a more ecological animal-plant integration.

But nobody can think that far out of the box, so it continues to be an argument between herbicide and tillage. It can't be an argument between corn and grass. And that's a shame.

Back in the courtroom, apparently exasperated that its buddy Monsanto wasn't faring well in these trials, the EPA issued an order declaring that glyphosate does not cause cancer. I guess we can start putting it in lemonade.

The declaratory letter is in direct contradiction, if not rebuke, to both California and the WHO. California lists glyphosate as an official carcinogen. The WHO lists it as "probably" causing cancer.

Meanwhile, around the world, the orthodox scientific community is circling the wagons around Monsanto: Canada, Australia, the European Union, Germany, New Zealand, and Japan. Government regulators in all these countries agree with the EPA's assessment.

In yet another state-federal showdown, the EPA accuses California of a "false and misleading statement" and further claims that federal regulatory assessment should trump the states'. In other words, if a state wants to be more careful, it can't.

In the courtroom, this EPA declaration will give weight to Monsanto's position that to put warning labels on Roundup® would violate their regulatory directives. "We couldn't tell people it was carcinogenic even if it was, because federal labeling regulations wouldn't let us. How can we be held responsible for something we didn't say when to say it would have violated the law?"

Wow, that sounds like a great cover to me. Suddenly, just like that, 42,000 lawsuits vanish. Such is the machinations of the courtroom. The EPA stepping into the fray this aggressively indicates a concerted effort, at the highest levels of global chemical business, to protect Monsanto, Bayer and all their cohorts. Nobody should underestimate the resolve, the cleverness, and the power of these players to take care of each other when the fraternity is assaulted.

The way to change the system is to quit playing their game. That means eating consciously, systematically chipping away at the market share these big players enjoy.

Sina: Clearly the government is not going to protect you from glyphosate. And, while it's nearly impossible to completely avoid it, there are steps you can take to dramatically reduce your exposure. One of those steps is to buy foods with the USDA Organic label. That label means the food is not supposed to contain glyphosate. But, there's a catch – another hole in the USDA Organic bucket.

The USDA does not certify farms as organic. Specifically, the National Organic Program (NOP) develops and enforces the organic standards. And, they hire certifying agents who decide which farms and businesses meet those organic standards. According to the NOP, not all farms are tested for the presence of glyphosate. The certification process is largely "paperwork oriented." Certifying agents can request glyphosate testing during the certification process. However, it is not required. And, according to the NOP, "most certifiers" do not test for glyphosate. Instead, they rely on the rule that land cannot be certified as organic unless no pesticides have been sprayed for three years. In addition, once farms are certified as USDA Organic, the certifying agents only test 5% of the farms each year for pesticide residues.

In addition, the USDA Organic certification process does not require testing of *final* food products either. That means, your favorite box of cookies can be labeled as USDA Organic and still contain glyphosate because *final* products are not tested for glyphosate. The only exception is when the certifying agent asks for testing. According to the USDA, "it's at the certifier's discretion as to when they test for pesticide residues." Pop! The bucket sprang another leak.

The USDA does not routinely test for the presence of glyphosate on our food either. In 2017, there was a glimmer of hope when the USDA announced they would begin testing corn syrup for glyphosate, as well as its break down product, AMPA. But it never happened. A USDA spokesperson said the testing program was replaced with a different program that was "a more efficient use of resources." To this day, the USDA does not routinely test our food for glyphosate, even when those foods are carrying the USDA Organic label.

If the certifying agents only test 5% of farms for pesticide residues and they don't test for glyphosate on our food, and the USDA doesn't test for glyphosate on our food then how do we know glyphosate is not in our food? Pop! Once again, the USDA Organic bucket has sprung a leak.

As a result of these leaks, independent organizations such as the Environmental Working Group have begun testing foods for the presence of glyphosate and AMPA. Alarmingly, foods that are certified as USDA Organic are testing positive for glyphosate, including: some organic protein powders, organic rolled oats, organic beers, and organic wines. One of the brands to test positive was Nature's Path®. According to the company:

> "While organic farming certifications prohibit the use of glyphosate, organic products do not always end up completely free of glyphosate residue. While this news may come as disappointing, it is not entirely surprising. Glyphosate use has skyrocketed in the past decade, and it maintains the ability to adhere to water and soil particles long enough to travel through the air or in a stream to nearby organic farms."

This is where the Glyphosate Residue Free verification seal comes in – to patch the glyphosate holes in the USDA Organic bucket.

The Glyphosate Residue Free verification seal is a free market solution provided by The Detox Project. In order to qualify for the Glyphosate Residue Free seal of approval, a food or ingredient must pass the strictest testing – "no glyphosate or AMPA residues down to the limits of laboratory detection."

The Glyphosate Residue Free certification fills the glyphosate hole that exists in the USDA Organic label. First, all products that achieve Glyphosate Residue Free status are tested at least three times per year, in addition to being subject to spot checks. Second, the Glyphosate Residue Free verification process tests *both* the individual ingredients and the final products. That means, the ingredients in your favorite cookie are tested for the presence of glyphosate and the cookie itself is tested.

That's important because each ingredient may contain glyphosate in a small enough amount to pass USDA organic standards. However, when you add all of the ingredients together, the level of glyphosate may be higher than allowed. Without testing the final product, you wouldn't know if that cookie contains prohibited levels of glyphosate.

Figure 2: Image Used with Permission from The Detox Project

So, I hold the USDA Organic label accountable by pairing it

with the Glyphosate Residue Free seal. The Glyphosate Residue Free verification seal is a quick and easy free market solution that increases my trust in my food supply because I know a third-party has checked my food for the presence of glyphosate and its break down product, AMPA. Just like we filled the existing GMO hole in the USDA Organic bucket by patching it with the Non-GMO Project Butterfly, I fill the existing glyphosate hole in the bucket by patching it with the Glyphosate Residue Free seal.

All three of these seals complement each other; separately they are flawed, but together they are better. They are not perfect together. And, the USDA Organic bucket will undoubtedly continue to spring leaks. But this patchwork is the strongest protection we currently have when avoiding GMOs and glyphosate while shopping in the grocery store for processed foods.

Joel: I'm glad you said "grocery store", Sina, because lots of options exist outside of grocery stores. One thing you need to remember is that ALL of these certifications require mountains of record keeping, paperwork, and money. They aren't free and they aren't cheap. The outfits that dominate in their use are extremely large - you have to be able to sell in supermarkets.

A little foreshadowing of what's to come - we're hoping to eventually coach you out of supermarkets and this whole game. The caveat on this whole Practical Bite is "if you're buying at the supermarket." But if you're not, and if you've found something better, it's often a smaller organization or farm to which you have a personal link. Perhaps you go visit. Perhaps you know someone who knows the source personally.

What I'm getting at is that as you move on up the continuum, you may start finding food that doesn't have any third-party certification and scarcely a label. That would be our farm.

I can't help but chuckle over my experience in Florida a few years ago. A rabble-rousing farmer there had been selling raw dairy products to a militantly loyal clientele and the state food police raided his farm. They put police tape on the freezers and shut everything down. He was selling raw milk, butter, ice cream, yoghurt, kefir - all of it completely uninspected and raw.

The Farm to Consumer Legal Defense Fund (everyone should join - yes, you) came to his aid and worked out an arrangement with the state food police that enabled anyone to register an otherwise prohibited food item as a pet food and sell it as not for human consumption. It only cost $25 per item, so this farmer spent about $200 for pet food labels for all his illegal food and he was back in business.

This loophole of freedom launched a plethora of food craft entrepreneurs. In only one year, 12 raw milk all-grass dairies sprang into existence. But people began making value added foods, heat and eat and all sorts of pet food. I did an urban foodie speaking tour in three Florida cities and all these urban gourmands told me that they had left organic certified and all the other certifieds because they learned "if you want the good stuff, you get the pet food." People aren't stupid and if you give them choice with responsibility, they'll surprise you with their ability to find authenticity.

With all that said, Sina is right about buying at the supermarket.

Sina: So, if you are looking for an easy way to ensure the highest level of glyphosate and GMO avoidance in your store-bought processed foods, look for the trio: 100% USDA Organic plus Non-GMO Project Butterfly plus Glyphosate Residue Free.

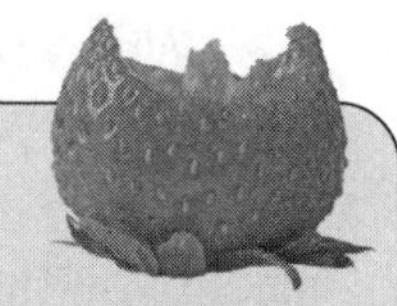

CHEW ON THIS

In 2016, the FDA began testing for glyphosate in our food. They were under pressure from the Government Accountability Office (GAO) who basically scolded the FDA for doing such a bad job of protecting our health. In a 2014 report, the GAO concluded:

- "FDA and USDA should strengthen pesticide residue monitoring programs and disclose monitoring limitations."
- "In 2012, FDA tested less than one-tenth of 1 percent of imported shipments [for pesticides]."
- "FDA does not disclose in its annual monitoring reports that it does not test for several commonly used pesticides…including glyphosate…"
- "FDA does not use statistically valid methods…to collect national information on the incidence and level of pesticide residues."
- "Limitations in FDA's methodology hamper its ability to determine the national incidence and level of pesticide residue in the foods it regulates, one of its stated objectives."

As a result, the FDA began testing some foods for glyphosate, but they would not release the results. Through the Freedom of Information Act, internal emails were obtained, which revealed that the FDA found "a fair amount" of glyphosate on nearly all of the tested foods. Fortunately, because of pressure from the GAO and consumer groups, in 2016, the FDA began including glyphosate in their annual testing program. You can find their report online: www.fda.gov/food/pesticides/pesticide-residue-monitoring-program.

While this is a step in the right direction, the report is not consumer-friendly. For instance, the most recent report concluded that glyphosate and/or its residue were found in 59.5% of all corn and soy samples. But they don't indicate which processed foods contain the adulterated corn and soy. So, if you don't want to consume glyphosate, do you stop eating all foods containing corn and soy? That would eliminate nearly every processed food in your grocery store! Therefore, at least for now, the safer and easier solution is to look for the USDA Organic label and the Glyphosate Residue Free label when trying to avoid glyphosate in processed foods.

Practical Bite #24: Look For The Quartet

How? When buying processed foods, look for the quartet: USDA Organic seal plus the Non-GMO Project seal plus the Glyphosate Residue Free seal plus the Land to Market Ecological Outcome Verified seal.

Why?

Sina: Yep, you guessed it! The USDA Organic bucket sprung another leak!

Joel: By now, your head must be spinning. So is mine.

Sina: I know! Labels are complicated. It shouldn't take the combined efforts of a farmer and a Ph.D. to navigate the grocery store! But that's the system we have. The deeper we walk into this labyrinth, the more grateful I am that Joel agreed to navigate the complexities of the grocery store with me. By revealing the strengths and weaknesses of these labels, in addition to explaining how we approach them and how we wade through the clever wordsmithing, our hope is that you can implement the same type of reasoning and line of questioning when the next label hits the market. So, let's start walking down the next path in this maze!

The USDA Organic label does not allow produce to contain GMOs, be sprayed with most pesticides or herbicides, grown using sewage sludge or most synthetic fertilizers, or irradiated. And, in terms of meat and poultry, the animal cannot be given hormones or most antibiotics and must be fed an organic diet (containing no GMOs or most pesticides or herbicides). But the USDA Organic label does not directly account for soil health. And, soil health is critical for your health. In fact, the loss of biodiversity in the soil is mirroring the loss of biodiversity in our guts. And, that's where the Land to Market Ecological Outcome Verified (EOV) seal comes into play.

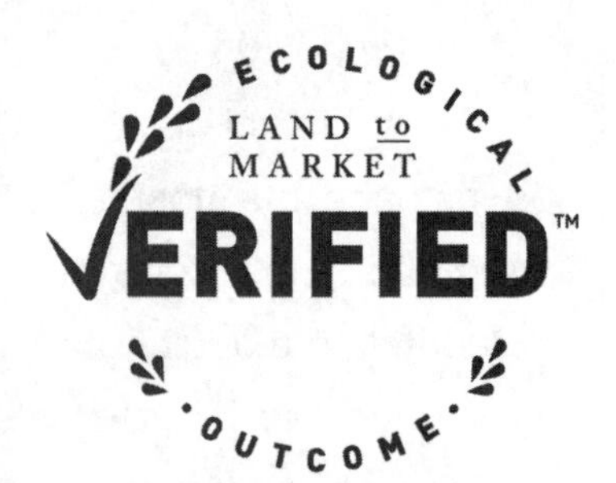

Figure 3: Image Used with Permission from The Savory Institute.

The EOV seal was created by The Savory Institute. It's a quick and easy way to identify products that contain raw materials that were grown using regenerative farming practices. The goal of regenerative farming is to regenerate, or continually improve the health of the soil, water, and ecosystem. As you know, the health of the soil is critical for the health and diversity of the microbes that live in the soil. And we depend on those microbes for our survival.

Some of the practices that can lead to regenerative outcomes include:

❖ **No tilling** - Helps prevent loss of top soil and fosters a more diverse and resilient soil microbiome.

❖ **Covering the soil with cover crops or mulch** – Fosters a more diverse and resilient soil microbiome and reduces run-off, which lowers the water requirement, and helps prevent loss of top soil.

❖ **Growing a variety of plants and animals in one location** - Adds microbial diversity and nutrient density to the soil and, consequently, to the plants and animals living on that soil. In contrast, industrial farming promotes monocultures, stripping the soil of nutrients and microbial diversity. Some organic farmers also promote monocultures. Therefore, even if your food is labeled as USDA Organic, it may be lacking a healthy microbiome, as well as an optimal nutrient profile.

The EOV seal complements the USDA organic seal, the Non-GMO Project seal, and the Glyphosate Residue Free seal. Each seal addresses a specific gap in your food supply. For instance, the EOV verification protocol evaluates the health of the land and ecosystem. None of the other seals do that. However, the EOV verification process does not require that organic practices are followed. For example, a farm can spray pesticides and potentially still qualify for the EOV verification as long as the indicators used to measure health and effectiveness of the land are trending in a positive direction year over year. So, both seals work together to close the existing gaps in your food supply.

Joel: I'm not opposed to it, but my struggle with all of these certifications and verifications is that they cater to a certain type of person. They cater to a person who loves paperwork and spending time filling in dots and measuring to a fault.

Many of us farmers, however, would rather spend that time building compost piles or making sales calls. People wonder why I don't soil test. I beg you, come out and walk the fields with me. I'll show you earth worm castings 3-inches high. You can turn your heel on those things. Their presence is nature's way of telling me the soil is rich in nutrients and diverse in microorganisms. When your soil contains worm castings, the plants germinate better, grow fast, and produce higher yields. Folks, I don't need to spend days a year filling out boxes to know I'm heading in the right direction when I have 3-inch earth worm castings. Or when our hay windrows are so huge you can't jump over them.

Every farm and every business has its weak link, and at the risk of being labeled a party pooper, I don't think for most of us these certifications are our weak link. We need to be moving the animals. Or teaching our kids how to plant a tomato. Or selling the tomato. Let me assure you that as a farmer, if I opted for these 4 labels, I would spend many days a year complying with paperwork and making educated guesses about which boxes to check. Folks, I have far more important things to do with my time.

So, the caveat remains, if you buy at the supermarket, watch for all these certifications/verifications. But remember that they cater to a certain type of outfit, and that type of outfit may not be the best for you or the planet. Knowing these farms and farmers like I do I can assure you that some of them are great and some of them are charlatans. All certifications can be manipulated.

Sina: I agree with you, Joel. On one hand, these labels represent a loss of freedom for both the farmer and the consumer. They require money, paperwork and time from the farmer, which often equates to higher prices for consumers. Plus, these labels are a reminder of how far removed we are from our food supply. They highlight our dependence on subjective measures, faulty government regulations, third-party organizations, and marketing tactics. The fact that four labels need to be combined to help protect our health is proof that we can't trust the food in the grocery store – and we know it. So yes, both farmers and consumers are shackled by the labels.

On the other hand, you have to meet people where they are. It would be fantastic if everyone bought all of their food from their local farmers instead of piecing together labels – like patchwork. But even you buy organic bananas from the grocery store because bananas don't grow in Virginia. And, I make processed foods using ingredients that my local farmer can't grow. For instance, since I don't eat grains, I bake with organic coconut flour. Coconuts don't grow in Virginia. So, I buy coconut flour from an online company. When you and I make those purchases, we are relying on the labels.

It's not feasible or practical for me to visit the coconut farms in Central America where my coconuts come from. Or, for you to visit a banana farm in Costa Rica. So, how would we know if those farms have 3-inch high earth worm castings or huge hay windrows? In these instances, you and I rely on the labels.

I agree that the EOV label is not perfect. At this point, I think we've exhaustively proven that no label is perfect. But the EOV label is the only label currently on the market that is taking the health of the soil into consideration. The USDA Organic label was designed with soil health in mind, hence no spray, but regenerating the soil is not a requirement in order to receive the government seal of approval. So, a farmer can destroy the top soil and the microbial diversity of the land, but still be certified organic. That approach puts the health of the land, plants, animals, and consumers in jeopardy.

A few weeks ago, I spoke with David Rizzo, the Chief Operating Officer of Savory Global, who explained that the Land to Market EOV seal is different than any other certification because it provides "a voice for the land." By measuring the health of the land, farmers and ranchers can better communicate with the land and, consequently, change management practices based on what the land needs. That's a lofty goal! It will take time to learn how to listen to the land i.e. to know which measurements are accurate, effective, and reproducible.

The Savory Institute understands that; hence, the protocol is updated every year. The current protocol was reported as "an effective short-term monitoring approach that ranchers could implement annually to monitor grazing lands and determine the impacts of ranch decision-making on important ecosystem indicators," according to a 2019 article in the peer-reviewed journal *Environments*.

Joel: The problem with these labels is that the farmer must farm to check the boxes, enslaved by the subjective confinements of the certifying organization.

Sina: Agreed. All of the certifications are subjective. And, as you stated, the USDA Organic seal, Non-GMO Verification seal, and the Glyphosate Residue Free seal are all check lists of what can't be done to the animal, plant, or product.

The EOV seal is unique in that regard because it's outcome-based. For instance, to qualify for the EOV seal, the producer (i.e. farmer or rancher) must show, through data, that their soil is actually regenerating. This is done by measuring indicators of the health and effectiveness of the land, such as: soil health, biodiversity, water cycle, mineral cycle, energy flow and community dynamics. The outcomes must continue to trend in a positive direction in order to receive and maintain the regenerative seal of approval. In that regard, it's different than most practice-based certifications.

Joel: Now, dear readers, I hope you understand that all of this is not cut and dried. Those of us on the front lines of these issues wrangle and wrestle and converse late into the night on some of these nuances. And we don't always agree. And you, yes you, have to put attention on it until you become satisfied with what works for you. A place where you can rest, trust, and be free from the bondage of uncertainty, toxicity, and the tentacles of orthodox assumptions.

Sina: You and I both agree that the "place" you are speaking of is not in the grocery store. Every label and every certification is based on assumptions, subjective measures, and clever wordsmithing. However, nearly everyone shops in the grocery store for food, including you. And, in that setting, labels are the primary tool at our disposal for helping us make informed decisions.

So, for now, we must choose foods in the grocery stores based on the labels currently on the market. And, when you combine all four seals - USDA Organic plus Non-GMO Project plus Glyphosate Residue Free plus EOV - you are helping to promote the health of the land, the plants and animals grown on that land, and the people who eat those products. That is, until the USDA Organic bucket springs another leak, or the next label comes out that trumps them all!

Practical Bite #25: Eat Real Salt

How? Instead of buying common table salt, purchase unrefined Real Salt® or Himalayan salt. Look for the word "unrefined" on the label. And, the ingredient list should only include salt - no other chemicals should be listed.

Why?

Joel: I go to a quack wellness coach and she recommends lots of salt intake, but not just any salt. Common Morton's® salt is highly processed, which means it is missing many of the beneficial elements contained in unrefined salt. Raw salt, like raw milk and raw honey, is full of minerals that our bodies need. Full-nutrient salt is what everyone used until very recent times. And people used a lot of it because prior to refrigeration and freezing, salt as a preservative literally permeated stored food.

Here in the U.S., the most common is salt-cured pork, especially ham. When you think about how much salt our ancestors ate and overlay that with modern aversion to salt, it's a wonder anyone survived to tell the tale. Like many things, just because it's called or labeled salt does not mean it's the same thing. The mineral balance in unprocessed salt is completely different than the ratios in refined salt, or what's commonly known as iodized salt. Get the real stuff and sprinkle liberally. This is one time not to be conservative.

Sina: Before I got sick, I never thought twice about salt. I always bought common table salt because that's what my Mom used. After all, salt is just a sodium and a chloride atom stuck together, right? How different can salt really be?

It's crazy to think about, but common table salt was keeping me sick. When I was trying to reverse the autoimmune disease, I spent a lot of time and money cooking the best grain-free, organic foods I could find. Yet, I was still sick. After nearly every meal, I'd have a stomach ache. It didn't make sense, until I learned that common table salt contains corn!

Corn-derived chemicals are used as anti-caking agents in some name-brand salts, like the one I was using. So, every day, I was unknowingly sprinkling corn all over my grain-free meals. The amount of corn in the salt is small, but it's enough for someone with non-celiac gluten sensitivity to react.

Luckily, one of my friends recommended an alternative to common table salt that does not contain corn – Real Salt®. I was reluctant to try it because it's pink with little brown flakes. I was used to salt being white, so I actually thought Real Salt® looked contaminated. But I was desperate to add flavor to my food so I took the plunge and tried it. Much to my surprise, Real Salt® tasted fantastic!

In fact, it's become my secret weapon to get my children to eat vegetables! I'm serious! They will eat almost any vegetable as long as they can put Real Salt® on it. And, they insist on sprinkling the salt on their food themselves. Even my niece loves this salt! She has always refused to eat broccoli. My sister tried melting butter on top, but she still wouldn't eat it. Then, she tried cheese on top, but my niece hated it. So, during one of my trips to California, I made broccoli for her and she loved it! All I did was steam organic broccoli, drizzle organic avocado oil all over it, and sprinkle Real Salt® on top. Now, she actually asks my sister to make her broccoli! Real Salt® has been a game changer for our entire family.

So, why does it taste so much better than common table salt. After all, salt is salt, right?

It turns out, there's more in your salt shaker than just sodium and chloride. In fact, even though sodium and chloride are naturally occurring elements, common table salt is not "natural" at all. It's roughly 97.5% sodium chloride and 2.5% added chemicals – which can include moisture absorbents, fluoride, iodine, and anti-caking compounds (to make sure it pours and flows freely). Examples of anti-caking agents are sodium aluminosilicate and magnesium oxide – both are GRAS, which means they are not tested for safety by the FDA nor are they regulated by the FDA. If iodine is added then the salt probably also contains sugar, which is used to stabilize the iodine. And, the sugar commonly used is dextrose, which is often derived from corn. As you can see, common table salt is far from "natural."

In contrast, both Real Salt® and Himalayan salt are not refined and do not contain added chemicals. Both of those salts contain sodium chloride in addition to over 60 naturally-occurring trace elements and minerals, including; calcium, magnesium, potassium and iron. Remember when I said I almost didn't try Real Salt® because it is pink with colored specks? It has color because it contains naturally-occurring trace elements and minerals! That's one reason why common table salt is white – the elements and minerals have been stripped away during the refining process.

That's also why common table salt doesn't taste as good. It's those naturally-occurring elements and minerals that create the complex and pleasing flavor profile that my children love. Plus, those trace elements and minerals are in their natural state, making them easily absorbed by your body. And, since most Americans are deficient in at least one micronutrient, consuming Real Salt® or Himalayan salt can help correct that deficiency.

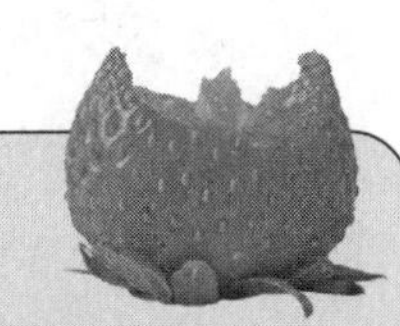

CHEW ON THIS

Sea salt is routinely used as an alternative to common table salt. But, there's a lot of confusion around sea salt. Technically, all salt is sea salt because it originated from the sea – either from dead seas, ancient sea beds, or modern oceans. However, sea salt that is sourced from modern bodies of water is susceptible to an increased risk of contamination from toxins, such as: mercury, PCBs, and dioxins. Those pollutants accumulate in the oceans and can be transferred to the salt. In fact, the majority of all sea salt producers that source their salt from modern oceans are now "refining" their salt because of the pollution. So, it's not as "healthy" as it used to be.

Practical Bite #26: Say Yes To Wild-Caught Fish

How? When selecting fish or seafood at the grocery store, look for the words "wild-caught" on the label. Avoid fish or seafood that is labeled as "farm-raised." The most common farm-raised fish are: salmon, catfish, tilapia, swai, sea bass and cod.

Why?

Joel: As our oceans struggle to stay healthy and fisheries struggle to keep up with global demand, the fish industry turns to fish CAFOs for help. Just like chicken, beef, or pig CAFOs, these fish farms have high animal concentrations, use antibiotics, and generate mountains of manure. Normally, farmers raise catfish in self-contained ponds because they live in freshwater as opposed to salt water. Ditto for tilapia.

You might wonder how salt water fish are raised in confinement. How do you keep them contained in the ocean? The answer is massive mylar boxes. Using netting too small for the fish to escape, these boxes float in the ocean like huge barns. In some areas, the manure generated from these concentrated production facilities creates overloads. The manure overpowers the ocean's ability to flush it all away.

Sina: I refer to fish farms as the industrialized farms of the sea. Because, as you've described, farm-raised fish are grown in similar conditions as industry-raised cows, chickens and pigs.

While wild-caught fish are captured from natural habitats such as lakes, oceans or rivers, farm-raised fish are typically grown in large cages that float in the water. Consequently, farm-raised fish can contain higher levels of contaminants and tend to have higher instances of disease – much like industry-raised cows, chickens and pigs.

For instance, farmed fish are grown in crowded conditions. Consequently, antibiotics are given in order to prevent disease. Sound familiar?

In addition, farmed fish are commonly treated with vaccines in an attempt to prevent infection due to the crowded conditions. Some fish farms give five vaccinations per fish! Meanwhile, studies are reporting adverse effects from the vaccines, such as: inflammation of the liver and kidney, as well as autoimmunity. One study concluded "Autoimmunity…is common in vaccinated farmed Atlantic salmon."

Farmed fish are also treated with pesticides because the farming conditions attract pests and marine insects, such as sea lice. Again, I ask you, does that sound familiar? To get rid of sea lice, farmers add pesticides to the fish feed. A commonly used pesticide is emamectin benzoate, which can cause tremors, spinal deterioration, and muscle atrophy when fed to rats and dogs.

Even worse, the pesticides used to treat the pests circulate throughout the ocean and have been shown to kill juvenile wild salmon that are migrating. In other words, industrialized sea farms are actually hurting the wild fish population.

In addition, once the pesticides used in fish farms circulate in the ocean, they can concentrate in the fat of marine life. This obviously contaminates the wild fish population. But it gets even worse. That contaminated fat is often used to feed farm-raised fish. So, the farmed fish get a second dose of pesticides. Consequently, studies have consistently reported higher levels of pesticides in farm-raised fish compared with wild-caught fish.

Even cancer-causing PCBs (polychlorinated biphenyls) have been found in farm-raised fish. PCBs are also found in wild-caught fish. But the level is typically higher in farm-raised varieties partly because PCBs accumulate in fat and the farmed fish are typically fed fish fat.

Farmed fish have also been shown to contain higher levels of polybrominated diphenyl ethers (PBDEs), which are industrial flame-retardant chemicals that can lead to learning and memory deficits in laboratory animals, as well as thyroid hormone dysregulation. Again, the higher levels are largely due to the feed given to farmed fish.

The contamination of farmed fish is a known problem. In fact, some fish farmers are trying to lower the toxin level of the farmed fish feed by replacing the fish oil with soybean and/or canola oil. That substitution will most likely lower the pollutants, but it introduces new problems, including: the natural diet of fish does not include soy and canola, those oils do not contain the beneficial fatty acid profile that fish oil contains, and those two ingredients will likely be from genetically engineered sources.

The bottom line is: Industrialized fish farms often produce sick fish. If you don't want to get sick, don't eat sick fish.

Joel: I like fish as much as the next guy. But I don't like these fish CAFOs and I sure don't want to encourage wild fisheries collapse. So, what's a solution? This is completely personal and I'm not suggesting you adhere to it, but I have a rule that I don't eat fish unless I'm within 100 miles of the ocean. Does that deny me some choice? Absolutely.

I'm thinking much bigger than just my health. I'm thinking planetary health. Not long ago a person 100 miles away from the ocean never ate fish. Or they would eat other aquatic animals like frogs and freshwater fish caught in the wild. If our rivers ran as pure as they did before Europeans arrived, we'd have a lot more fish in our rivers. I remember as a child fishing in the small river that traverses the edge of our farm. It had suckers, eels, and red eye that you could watch from the riverbank. These fish, truly abundant, offered many an afternoon's entertainment as they lounged in the river. Sometimes we caught them and ate them. I haven't seen any of those critters in the river for decades.

When you realize that 500 years ago North America was 8 percent water due to the tireless work of 200 million beavers, you can hardly imagine how many fresh water fish were available inland, away from the ocean. Today, our surface area is only 1 percent water and we've lost all that inland aquatic abundance. This is one reason I'm committed and aggressive about building ponds on farms. We have more than a dozen on our farm and they have largemouth bass, blue gills, catfish, and carp.

You might think I'm going a bit far afield here, but it's important to realize that our context as modern Americans is quite different than it was a mere century ago. Our impact on the ecology is almost beyond comprehension. Yes, this book is about our personal health primarily, but we must appreciate its tie in, its relatedness, to the whole womb in which we're nested.

Everywhere I travel, I try to enjoy the local specialty. When I was in Norway last year, I ate wild salmon like a crazy man. It was like eating butter. I've learned that it's normally so good, any attempt at duplication somewhere else isn't worth eating. Like my orange juice experience in Mexico that I shared in Practical Bite # 19, you can't beat fresh foods grown in their native land.

Sina: I agree with you, Joel. I don't routinely eat fish because of overfishing and the contaminants in our oceans. However, when I do eat fish, it's always wild-caught.

Studies have shown that compared to wild-caught fish, farmed fish have a lower protein content and higher concentrations of omega-6 fatty acids, which tend to be inflammatory. They also contain less anti-inflammatory omega-3 fatty acids when compared to wild-caught fish. In fact, wild-caught coho salmon reportedly contain 2-3 times more omega-3 fatty acids than their farmed counterpart. That's important because you can't make those fats; you must eat them from sources rich in omega-3 fats, like wild-caught salmon.

In addition, cold water fish – like salmon – are a good source of vitamin D. And, as you know, lack of vitamin D can trigger an inflammatory disease. Other micronutrients that are found in wild-caught salmon include: selenium, niacin, vitamin B12, phosphorus, magnesium, and vitamin B6. Wild-caught salmon also contain a natural form of astaxanthin, which is a very strong antioxidant.

All of these nutritional differences are largely due to diet, which reflects the environmental differences between wild-caught and farm-raised fish. For instance, salmon are carnivorous fish so they eat other fish in the wild. But farmed salmon are fed a horrendous diet of pellets that are commonly made out of fish oil, ground-up chicken feathers, chicken poop, vegetable oils, wheat, and genetically modified soy, corn and yeast.

Have you ever noticed that wild salmon are pink? Their meat is pink because they eat an antioxidant known as a carotenoid, which is naturally present in krill, shrimp and other foods salmon eat in the wild. It's similar to how the feathers of flamingos are actually grey when they are born, but they gradually turn pink because they eat a natural diet of brine shrimp and algae. But farmed salmon are not fed their natural diet, so they are not pink – they are grey or off-white. But consumers expect salmon to be pink. So, to get you to buy their fish, farmers dye the meat by adding a synthetic pigment to the fish food, such as synthetic canthaxanthin – a chemical found in sunless tanning pills.

Joel: Seems like they could offer that as a two-fer. "No need to buy tanning pills. Just eat our salmon and get tanned at the same time." What a great marketing shtick. Lots of possibilities there for an ad campaign.

Sina: And now there's a new threat to the wild fish population - genetically modified (GM) fish. Yep, the first-ever GM animal to be sold for human consumption has been approved by the government in both Canada and America.

In 2017, Canada became the first country in the world to sell GM salmon in grocery stores. The GM salmon are touted to grow to market size in half the time as wild salmon while eating 25% less food. That just sounds wrong. But the FDA has already "approved" GM salmon as "safe" for you to eat. And, as of March 2019, they lifted the import ban that Congress put in place. That means GM salmon are being grown in the US right now and will hit the grocery store shelves this year, in 2020.

And, it doesn't stop with salmon. At least 35 other species of fish are currently being genetically modified with the intention of selling them to consumers. And, soon you will have the option to buy fish made from cell lines in a petri dish! And, NONE of these laboratory creations are clearly labeled!

Joel: Is this a good place to talk about biological boundaries? My mentor Allan Nation used to explain it this way: "There's a reason why a mouse is the size of a mouse and an elephant is the size of an elephant. A mouse the size of an elephant would not be a very successful mouse, and an elephant the size of a mouse would not be a very successful elephant."

In our love affair with hubris and technology, modern western humans have pretty much decided that anything we can develop is fair game. In the classic Steven Spielberg movie Jurassic Park®, you'll recall, the creator of the park, John Hammond, and the mathematician, Ian Malcolm, watched raptors devour a cow and destroy the rigging. In an ensuing debate over lunch, the mathematician states the thesis of the movie: "Your scientists were so preoccupied with whether they could, they didn't stop to think if they should."

That is one of the most profound questions in all of humanity. Just because we can, should we? It speaks of something higher than simple mechanical invention. It speaks of natural boundaries, morals, ethics. But with amoral science, we don't ask those kinds of questions. My dad used the phrase "over running our headlights" to explain this concept. The truth is we are clever and smart. Indeed, clever and smart enough to invent things we can't spiritually, emotionally, or physically metabolize.

Years ago, I was a guest on Patrick Buchanan's radio show. It was during the early days of the Clinton administration. The big news of the day was that the Clintons had hired a chef for the White House who wanted to use free range chicken. Buchanan found me and put me on the show to talk about free range chicken. He asked me what was different about the chicken we raised on pasture on our farm, and I replied "our chickens don't do drugs."

He asked the obvious question "why do they feed drugs to chickens?" Of course, I had several threads prepared for the answer, but all I got out was "It makes them grow faster" and he interrupted me, as radio talk show hosts are wont to do. "What could possibly be wrong with making them grow faster?"

Duh. Cancer is really fast growth. Infection is really fast growth. The very notion that a supposedly smart person would ask such a thoughtless question belies the deep hubris imbedded in our culture. That somehow, we can cheat nature. We can adulterate, disrespect biological systems. That no matter what we invent, we can always get ourselves out of the jam by inventing the next generation of remedies.

I'm reminded of a statement by one of the prominent libertarian thinkers of our day who visited our farm. I'm a libertarian, but not like this. Anyway, he said during our tour "of course I'm for earth first. Use up the earth and then move on to Mars." Can you imagine someone with an ounce of sense saying something that ridiculous? It's embarrassing.

Okay, enough of the rant. Back to you, Sina, to close this Practical Bite down with your steady hand and reasonable conclusion.

Sina: The bottom line is: avoid farm-raised fish; buy wild-caught instead. And, cooking it on a grill, as opposed to in a pan, allows fat to drip from the fish, which helps remove PCBs, dioxins, and other pollutants that can be stored in the fat.

Practical Bite #27: Bring Your Lunch

How? If you eat out at lunch, start preparing your lunch at home instead. Try bringing your lunch once a week, and then slowly increase the frequency until you are packing your lunch every day. With the money you save, you can fill your packed lunch with healthy foods, such as: whole, organic fruits and vegetables and meat from truly pasture-raised chickens.

Why?

Sina: Bringing lunch to work may not seem very "cool." In a way, it's reminiscent of being back in grade school when your Mom used to pack a brown bag lunch for you to eat every day. Did your Mom do that?

Joel: No, I'm older than you so I was in school when lunches were novel. Back in those days, schools actually cooked from scratch. When I was a teenager in the early 1970s, I supplied two public schools with eggs from my hens - they actually cracked eggs and cooked from scratch. Those were early days, of course, and generally that's not done any more. I guess I was in that sweet spot between *Little House on the Prairie*, prior to schools providing lunches, and the time when to save money or offer something different parents began sending lunch as an alternative. Today, the pendulum has moved to lunch entitlement even during the summer. And a lot more than lunch. How times change.

Sina: My Mom always packed my lunch with a sandwich and crackers. So, every day, I traded my sandwich and crackers for cookies and juice boxes! I hated packed lunches. However, if you can get past the "uncool" factor, making your own lunch will save you money, and that money will allow you to more easily afford healthy foods.

A 2015 Visa survey reported that Americans spend more than $11 per meal when eating out compared with only $6.30 per meal when preparing their own lunch. That may not sound like a lot, but it adds up over time. For instance, eating out for lunch for just one week would total $77 for one person. How much healthy food can you buy at the grocery store or from your local farmer with $77?

I can buy 10 packs of hot dogs from Polyface Farm, which is 80 hot dogs (They are uncured and only contain meat and spices with no nitrites or nitrates). How many lunches can you make for yourself with 80 hot dogs?

Joel: And the savings are even more if you use leftovers for lunch. All these lunchables and snackables with their individual packaging are extremely expensive. When I worked at the newspaper, I brought a thermos full of hot stew or something left over. It literally saved thousands of dollars a year. Sina, using your math of about $70 a week savings, at 50 weeks in a year that's $3,500. How much better food could you buy if you added $3,500 to your grocery budget?

I've decided the most prominent benchmark designating folks who "get it" with food is leftovers. This is a little beyond our lunch discussion here, but it's a good place to bring up the ramifications of leftovers. By definition, leftovers mean that you did not eat single service portions. How much food today is sold in single service packaging?

The whole idea is that nobody eats together at a table. You graze when you want, opening your single service package, and then go about your business. Preparing for a family to eat together and dip out of common serving dishes not only saves mountains of plastic and packaging, but it means that usually you have leftovers you can eat tomorrow. I think that may be where I became such a fan of soups and heavy stews. I can eat a good soup any time; hearty soup is easy to take with you in a thermos, requires almost no utensils other than a spoon, no plastic wrap. I mean, what could be easier, more convenient, and better for the environment? Come on, folks, think with me here.

Sina: I love leftovers! I routinely eat them for lunch and even breakfast. It saves time and money.

Joel: And if you have two working folks in a family, which most do, the savings is $7,000 a year. How about adding that to your household grocery budget? If this is a sudden Aha! moment for you, wonderful. But goodness, what's more satisfying than an apple and a hunk of cheese? Or some nice potato salad? The best way to save money on food is to use your kitchen instead of subcontracting some else's.

Sina: That's a taste of the savings when it's just one person eating mainly at fast-food or fast-casual establishments. Think of how much you spend for a family when dining at fancier restaurants, like The Cheesecake Factory® or P.F. Chang's®. One meal for a family of 4 can easily add up to $80.

Instead of spending all of that money for one meal, apply it toward healthier options at the grocery store or the farm. For instance, for $80, you can buy 16 pounds of organic, grass-finished ground beef at Wegman's or nearly 17 dozen eggs from Polyface Farm. That's a total of 204 eggs! You can make a lot of lunches with 16 pounds of beef or 204 eggs!

Joel: Today, right now, you can purchase a world class broiler from our farm for less than boneless skinless breast conventional chicken at the supermarket.

We've already referred to the food documentary Food Inc®. The one part I still cringe every time I see it is that family that says they can't afford fresh produce. They say this as they pull away from the Burger King® drive-in window. The son pulls his meal from the bag and it's a burger and big fries and a soft drink that looks to be about a gallon. That meal cost more than two whole pounds of our premium all grass ground beef. And two pounds of our ground beef has multiple times the nutrition of that Burger King® meal.

But you have to cook it. You can't just drive up to a window and order it. Therein lies the rub. But really, how long does it take to cook a hamburger? A few minutes and a dirty skillet. Your kids can wash the dishes so they learn there's more to life than Game of Thrones® or whatever violent-game-du-jour happens to be. In the amount of time it takes to make the left hand turn into the fast food joint, speak through the ordering microphone and try to understand the garbled response, wait at the window, and pull back out into oncoming traffic, you could make your own freakin' burger at home at a third the price and know where it came from. Sounds like a good trade to me.

Practical Bite #28: Be Prepared With Snacks

How? Have ready-to-eat snacks available in your home, car, and office such as: organic fresh fruits, celery and carrot sticks, hummus, guacamole, trail mix, granola, fruit bars, jerky from grass-finished cows, dried seaweed, tiger nuts, or dried chickpeas.

Why?

Sina: This tip is simple and straight forward, but it's a game changer. Having snacks available can determine whether you achieve your goal or fall off the wagon. When you get hungry between meals or stressed out and crave comfort food, it's common to grab whatever ready-to-eat food is around you. This is especially challenging if you're at work or running errands because the options are more limiting. So, always have snacks nearby.

I bring a snack bag for my kids and I every time we leave the house. You never know when an errand or doctor's appointment might run long. And, my husband packs his office desk drawer with snacks, such as: organic crackers, beef jerky, tortilla chips, and nuts. He also keeps organic cookies on hand, so when there's an office party or birthday celebration, he has something to eat that is decadent but still aligned with his principles.

Joel: You know the old adage about don't shop for groceries on an empty stomach. When you're hungry, you're hungry, and your resistance to junk is pretty low at that point. When your stomach is growling, you just want something, anything. Or when a co-worker brings in that pack of crackers from the vending machine, suddenly you have a craving that drives you crazy.

It's going to happen. Prepare for it by packing some stuff with you. You'd be amazed what you can resist if you have some nibbles accessible. My favorite is jerky - it makes no crumbles and goes in your pocket like an ink pen. It really satiates, doesn't require any refrigeration, and doesn't even require a napkin.

Practical Bite #29: Bring Your Own Solutions

How? Whether you are running errands, attending a social gathering, or traveling, bring your own water and food.

Why?

Joel: This Practical Bite can be socially stigmatizing, so be discreet. You don't want to be THAT person, the one no one wants to be around because all they do is feel guilty around you. Don't walk over to the displayed food and proclaim at megaphone decibels: "Wow, you people eat junk! I can't imagine eating this stuff. I brought my own food so you folks can go ahead and die." That's not the way to win friends and influence people.

Sina: I actually know someone who does that! And yes, it's very off-putting.

Joel: No host wants to have their offering disparaged. No potluck participant wants their contribution disparaged. When Teresa and I go to potlucks, she always brings at least two and often three dishes - more than anyone else. The reason is so I'll have something to eat. She puts it out on the table with all the other dishes, but I make sure I know which ones are hers. Then when I go through the line I concentrate on her stuff.

If I know someone in the group is borderline uncomfortable with industrial fare, I'll ease up to them and softly point out Teresa's dishes. "Oh, thanks. I'll be sure to get them," responds a grateful confidante.

Sina: That's a great idea! The hurdle I run into is cost. Higher quality food, on average, is more expensive. And, bringing three dishes to a party is outside of my budget. But, if you eat beforehand, and bring one dish that your family can eat during the gathering, you'll bring down the cost while blending in socially.

I bring my own solutions wherever I go. This holds true in the literal sense i.e. bring your own water and salad dressing. But it also means to anticipate challenges when outside of your home and come prepared.

For instance, every time I leave the house with my children, I bring filtered water in glass Mason jars and a bag of snack foods. I bet nearly every Mom has experienced a child complaining about being hungry almost as soon as they drive away from the house – even if they just ate a meal! And, it's not uncommon to be out of the house for longer than expected. So, to avoid the possibility of having to buy bottled water, visit a drive through, or grab an unhealthy snack while on the road, I pack water as well as organic snacks that keep well in my bag. My kids favorite "bag snacks" include: trail mix, fruit bars, jerky, dried seaweed, tiger nuts, and dried chickpeas.

Traveling for longer periods of time, such as several days, can be challenging. When my family travels via car, we cook our meals ahead of time and bring them in an ice chest – stored in glass containers. If we are staying in a hotel, I call ahead to see if the room has a mini-fridge. If not, we keep the food cold in the ice chest by refilling it with ice from the hotel. I keep the ice in Ziploc® bags so it doesn't touch the food containers since ice machines are not usually cleaned on a routine basis. Consequently, they can carry pathogens.

In terms of heating the food, some hotels offer a microwave in the room. Others have microwaves you can use in the common dining room. I bring my own toaster oven since I don't use microwaves. It may sound like a lot of work, but preparing our meals in advance allows me to relax during the trip because I know I'm feeding my family healthy food, and I don't have to worry about cooking for several days. It's a win-win!

When traveling via airplane, my family uses a more creative approach. I pack non-perishable foods in our suitcases, such as: beef jerky, nuts, seeds, dried fruit, seaweed, and mixes I've made in advance (See Practical Bite #33). Since, I can't pack enough food to feed our family for the duration of the trip, I search online for restaurants at our destination that are aligned with my principles, such as Organic Krush®. I also call grocery stores in the area to ask if they carry specific products that we eat, including organic produce. If they do, a trip to the grocery store is top priority once we reach our destination. If we are staying with family members or friends, I order non-perishable foods online, such as grain-free tortilla chips and taco shells, and have them delivered to their home.

Again, it may sound like a lot of work, but being prepared allows my family the freedom to travel while protecting our health and standing for our principles. And, if you don't want to cook, there are companies online that deliver organic, pre-cooked meals throughout the United States. As long as you have an address where the food can be sent, you can have meals delivered to you while on vacation.

In terms of parties and social gatherings, as Joel mentioned, they can be challenging because they usually revolve around food. And, when you stand up for your food choices, you are most likely going to stand out. My solution to this dilemma depends on the type of gathering:

- Parties can be tricky because they almost always involve dessert. So, I keep homemade desserts in the freezer that are aligned with our principles. That way, when my children are invited to birthday parties, instead of feeling left out, they can celebrate with the other children while eating a treat they feel good about. Sometimes I call ahead to see what type of dessert the host plans to serve. Then, I make something that looks similar so it blends in.
- If there are snack foods at the gathering, but not a main meal, we avoid temptation by eating a meal right before we go. I also bring snacks for my children because, undoubtedly, when they see other children eating snacks, they will want a snack too. Since kids run around so much, my alternate snacks are not usually noticed.
- If a meal is served, whether it's potluck or provided by the host, we bring our own food. I make it less obvious by bringing each of us a meal in a glass container that is ready to eat and already portioned. That way I'm not attracting attention by taking the extra step of serving each of us food from multiple containers. I simply place each person's food on their plate and then quickly put the glass container back in my bag. Most of the time, nobody even notices.
- If I have a good relationship with the host, I call in advance to let them know they don't need to worry about making food for us. To avoid the host feeling offended, I let them know how excited we are to spend time with them and I explain that we have multiple food sensitivities and it's my responsibility to tend to our individual needs; it's not their responsibility to cater to us. When I take the burden off the host by putting the responsibility on me, the host is almost always relieved.

Maneuvering through social gatherings can be difficult and uncomfortable. I have found that if you come prepared with your own solutions, there is less resistance. However, no matter how much you troubleshoot, there may still be push back. We've been left off the guest list to many gatherings because of our food choices. We've even been uninvited to a holiday celebration with our family! It was devastating at the time, but now I know the push back comes from fear. It's not about me, it's about them. So, let those encounters go. Forgive them for not being the way you wanted them to be, and then release it.

Joel: Sina, if I had the history of near-death health issues you've had, I might be this militant too. But fortunately, I haven't had these so I'm a bit looser in this category. I'm back to the 80/20 rule: eat right 80 percent of the time and that buys you enough health wiggle room to fudge 20 percent of the time. But I know people with incredible sensitivities that if they fudge even a smidgen, they're in pain or even in life-threatening conditions within an hour. I'm grateful beyond words that I don't have any of that; if I did, I'd be a food pit bull like Sina.

Sina: Honestly, if I had not developed a debilitating disease at such a young age, I would not eat the way I do. I ate the standard American diet most of my life with the attitude that I was invincible. After all, I was a competitive athlete; I was strong in my body, mind, and spirit. But when I got sick, everything changed.

I realized that health is a precious gift that most of us take for granted until it's gone. I also realized that I had allowed "sick" to become my "norm." I hadn't noticed it before because I'd look around at my friends and family and everyone was suffering from some type of ailment. So, I chalked it up as being "normal." But, once I was healed, I felt better than I had in decades! So, I continued making changes to my diet and lifestyle. I wanted to see how good I could feel. Could I have more energy than I did as a child? Could I exercise with as much ease as when I was a teenager?

The answer is a resounding yes! I quickly realized that feeling tired, waking up with stiff joints, not recovering as quickly from exercise, and not having the mental clarity I was blessed with in my early 20s does not have to be *my* "normal." So, even though I began eating this way because I was afraid to die, now I *choose* this lifestyle because I want to be the best possible version of me.

I've been on both sides of the health continuum. I know what it's like to nearly die, and I know what it's like to have abundant energy, razor sharp mental clarity, and a love for life that flows from every ounce of your being. I choose health, happiness, and freedom every day of the week and twice on Sundays.

And, while *occasionally* eating toxins in my food is not going to kill me or make me debilitatingly sick again, they prevent me from achieving my best self by placing an unnecessary toxic burden on my body, which ultimately disconnects me from myself and from God. I know I could occasionally consume toxins and go on with my life feeling "fine." But "fine" is no longer good enough. I want extraordinary! Once you've seen and felt what it's like to live your life from a higher state of consciousness – connected with self and God - there's no going back to "normal."

So, I *choose* not to put those chemicals in my body. And, if it wasn't for the disease, I would probably still be chalking up my ailments as "normal." For that, I am deeply grateful.

Joel: Well said. I think the two main points of this tip are these:

1. When you're leaving the sanctity of your own nest, think about your sustenance. What's it going to look like? What's okay to compromise on and what's not okay? The key is to think it through and then plan for it.
2. The second point is that you have many more options, with discretion, than you may think. Buck up; a little weirdness is fine. And don't wear it on your sleeve. Be courageous and realize that if you think, plan, and prepare, you can stay truer to your desires than you might think.

Sina: And remember that going against the grain can be difficult, but the people who are your true friends will understand and support your decision. In fact, now when I bring food to gatherings, most people want to know what I'm eating and they usually ask me for the recipe!

Change can be difficult. Just like you are taking small steps on this journey, allow people the time and space to catch up with you. My in-laws used to be deeply bothered by my food choices. They made negative comments and even referred to me as a "crazy California hippie." But I never pushed my beliefs on them, or acted like that judgmental guest at the dinner table.

Instead, I took responsibility by accepting my diet and lifestyle choices. In other words, I stepped into my power and stopped being apologetic for my choices. I began living my truth, with grace and humility. Amazingly, once I fully embraced my choices, so did they! The negativity and judgment stopped. Just the other day, they asked for my granola recipe! So, give people a chance to meet you where you are. They just may surprise you.

Practical Bite #30: Step Outside The Grocery Store Box

How? Don't limit yourself to your local grocery store. You can often find a wider variety of foods and better deals when you shop online.

Why?

Joel: A mere decade ago I would never have foreseen that I would say this, let alone agree with it, but between then and now, somebody moved my cheese. Are you familiar with the little business book *"Who Moved My Cheese?"* It's about two mice that go through a maze every day to get their cheese. One day they arrive and it's gone. So, they have to figure out a new route to their cheese. It's an allegory, of course, for what happens in business. It mirrors the idea that every ten years or so a business must re-invent itself because its context changes.

Those of you familiar with Michael Pollan's runaway best-seller *Omnivore's Dilemma* know that at that time, I wouldn't ship him a T-bone steak because I didn't believe in shipping. Since that book was written, here is what happened: Uber®, Airbnb®, Amazon Prime®, GrubHub®, Butcher Box®, Wal-Mart® became the world's largest organic vendor, and every large supermarket outfit has drive-up grocery service and surrogate shoppers who pick and pack your groceries for you. In aggregate, all these developments have completely changed the world of retail interface.

The bricks and mortar interface is now more expensive than door-to-door delivery. At the turn of the century (remember Y2K?) that was not the case. Physical aggregation and physical interface were still logically more efficient than cyberspace. But 2020 is not 2000, and today that model inverts. With such amazing technological advancements in the internet of everything, customized distribution with electronic aggregation is now beating out physical facilities.

The other massive change in this technological revolution is internet market access by smaller players. Just 20 years ago, small players couldn't access the electronic shopping cart space because the software was too expensive to either buy or develop in-house. But now numerous templates exist and many ramps allow access to the internet highway. Farms even as small as ours can efficiently offer door-to-door delivery nationwide through these new platforms. It's quite revolutionary.

One additional point to note - sorry, I can't help it. One of my favorite things in all the world is to co-opt something developed for globalization and use it for localization. When our family started Polyface, all of our customer correspondence and marketing went through either snail mail (it was called First Class U.S. Postal Service back then) or telephone calls. Today, we can send out information to all of our customers in a minute, essentially for free. So, while the internet did facilitate global communication, it also made it much easier and cheaper to access neighbors. That's very cool.

Sina: I know that it was difficult to make the decision to begin shipping your products. And, I applaud you for focusing on the positive. You're right, you had to re-invent Polyface or you ran the risk of losing the farm. And, that would be a travesty.

We need our local farms. And, I buy local when possible. But some foods are not available from my local farmers, like organic coconut flour, tigernut flour, and cassava flour. I can find those alternative flours at my local grocery store, but they are expensive. So, my husband found a way to make them more affordable. The exact same products can be purchased online for less money! And, they are delivered to my doorstep. You can't beat that convenience!

It's true that I have received flak from people who are against some of the online retailers like Amazon® and Walmart®. But, that's the beauty of the free market. You don't have to compromise your principles in order to utilize the convenience of buying online. If you don't want to support Amazon® or Walmart® then don't. Find an online retailer that is aligned with your principles.

I purchase food items from Thrive Market®. All of their products are non-GMO, they offer wholesale prices and free shipping, and they use 100% recycled packaging. Plus, with every membership purchased, they give a membership to someone "in need." So, you are helping others while helping yourself. I would rather shop at Thrive Market® than my local supermarket chain because they stand by their principles, which are aligned with mine, and I save money while adding convenience to my life. It's a win-win!

I also buy organic fruits and vegetables from Misfits Market. They ship organic produce directly to your home for up to half the cost of the organic produce in grocery stores. It sounds unbelievable, until you understand their business model.

Misfits Market rescues fresh organic produce that farms and grocery stores can't sell. According to the company, nearly half of the food grown by farmers in the U.S. is never sold; it's wasted. Yet, much of that food is perfectly edible. But consumers don't want to buy produce that isn't "perfect." So, a lot of organic produce never makes it into the supermarkets because they are deemed too big or too small, or abnormal looking, or "ugly" because of small bruises.

Misfits Market sells those unwanted "misfits" to consumers online. In their first year of operation, they already rescued 10 million pounds of misfit produce. That's a cause I can get behind.

Other companies rescue unwated produce as well, such as Imperfect Foods®. In addition, Vital Choice® sells wild-caught fish and frequently offers sales. And, of course, you now have access to the best ecologically-raised meat and poultry because Polyface Farm sells online.

Don't be afraid to step outside of the box we call the grocery store. You may end up lowering your food bill, saving yourself time, adding convenience to your life, finding healthier options and supporting a good cause - all at the same time!

Joel: To close out this Practical Bite, let me give you an example of just how sophisticated the distribution logistics are today. We worked with a fellow several years ago trying to launch a nationwide pastured meat shipping business. He received a lot of pushback for not being local and for an assumed massive carbon footprint per pound delivered. So, he commissioned a carbon footprint study comparing his model to our on-farm store and to a normal supermarket.

The university study concluded he had the smallest footprint of the three venues. Why? Because the average customer who drives out to our farm store does not buy enough at a time. If the average person would buy 100 pounds of product, then our footprint would be smaller, but anything under that, it was cheaper to send it via tractor trailer to a warehouse and then put it on a Fed Ex®, UPS®, or US Postal Service truck - even if the customer lived as close as 40 miles away.

And why was it a smaller carbon footprint than the supermarket? Turns out that all those individual cars waiting to make a left-hand turn burn a mountain of fuel. These distribution empires now have software that takes the days' delivery addresses and automatically creates a route that eliminate left hand turns. That one technological advance saved more than 10 percent of distribution companies' fuel costs, according to industry folks I know.

It's hard for us today to appreciate the finesse of these logistics developments, but they are real and they're here to stay. Then when you add in electric driverless trucks, goodness, things really are changing. Jetsons, here we come. So, the lament heard most of my life that "I can't find an authentic producer around here" no longer holds credibility. You can all get it from Polyface and a host of other super farms around the country. Of course, I love local and would like to never ship again, but somebody moved my cheese. Maybe it'll move back someday.

Practical Bite #31: Stock Up On Sale Items

How? Add a sales fund to your budget. That way, when foods go on sale, you can stock up.

Why?

Sina: This tip sounds simple and you've probably heard it before. But, allow us to show you the power of buying on sale.

The cost of "healthy" food is the number one concern I hear. And, I totally get it. As a homeschooling family, we live on one income. Fortunately, my husband, Donnie, is brilliant when it comes to figuring out how to make "healthy" food more affordable. So, in our family, we divide and conquer: I figure out which foods are optimal for our family to eat, and Donnie figures out how to make those foods less expensive without compromising the quality.

Having a sales budget has tremendously cut down on our food costs. For example, when he was eating grains, Donnie ate a 100% organic breakfast for $0.81 per day. How?

Donnie loved an organic cereal from Cascadian Farms®. Normally, our local Kroger® sells that cereal for $3.29 per box. Sometimes it is on sale at Kroger® for around $2.50 per box. At that price, if you buy 4 boxes, you are getting one for free. But the savings doesn't stop there.

You can save more money by having a sales fund if you look for bulk sales. For instance, every few months, Kroger® offers a bulk sale: If you buy 5 boxes of that organic cereal, the cost is $2.20 per box. Since Donnie keeps a sales fund, when his cereal went on bulk sale, he stocked up with a 6-month supply.

Let's total the cost of one Donnie-sized serving of his cereal (a very large bowl) to see the power of buying on bulk sale:

$0.55 Organic Cereal + $0.26 Organic Milk from Grass-Finished Cows = $0.81 TOTAL

Not only is that organic breakfast less expensive than eating out or grabbing a cup of coffee on the way to work, it's more convenient. Since he didn't have to drive to a fast food joint or coffee shop on the way to work, Donnie could eat an organic breakfast while sitting at the table with his family. It's a win-win!

Joel: Every outfit in the food business has inventory adjustment times. By definition food is perishable, even frozen or dehydrated. It doesn't last forever. Most food businesses try to run a little ahead of expected sales because the one thing customers will never forgive is shortage of product.

And because food is biological, it's not as dependable on the production end as mechanical things. A plumbing factory, for example, can crank out a certain number of 1-inch copper elbows per hour. That's pretty basic as long as the machines function. But in food, you can have drought, flood, bugs, mold, all sorts of issues. This is why farmers always beg for government help: "we're different than all those other businesses."

As a result, feast and famine occur and the final link in the chain is at the retail end. That is where the adjustments must be made. More than likely it's an inventory adjustment and the food company is trying to salvage excess for something rather than giving it away for nothing.

All food businesses have their hot items and their slower items. As a farmer with direct sales, we obviously have to sell a whole critter. We can't just sell steaks. We have to sell the rest of the animal, often called nose to tail. We do the best we can by adjusting our pricing to keep the hot movers (boneless chicken breast) higher priced and the slow movers lower priced. But even in the best of times a year yields some miscalculations and an adjustment is in order. When that happens, we run a sale. I can assure you that most of the time, a sale simply indicates some sort of inventory adjustment.

Or it can indicate a mistake. For example, let's say we take 15 hogs to the abattoir and we need 200 pounds of breakfast sausage but either we or they make a mistake and send it all back as Hot Italian. We might not be able to move all that excess Hot Italian in a timely way. A sale enables us to get our inventory back into equilibrium. You can't imagine how many possible glitches exist in something as unpredictable as growing stuff. Managing inventory is one of the most difficult aspects of our farm; it's far more difficult than raw production. So, jump in; help out a food business trying to get its inventory in balance.

The point is to not automatically assume that because something is on sale it must be defective. Not at all.

If you have a sales budget and storage capacity, including freezer space, you can absolutely buy bulk on sale when it happens and save substantially on your food costs. On our own farm, we've run sales on pork backbone, for example, that are almost immoral. Occasionally we run sales on eggs in the spring, or special pricing on smalls because few people want them. If you ask your farmer for special pricing on slow movers and blemishes, you'd be amazed at the pricing. On our farm, we have a freezer with blemished packages. They might have a tiny tear in a corner or might be misshapen. You can save a pile of money shopping in that freezer.

Sina: I shop in that freezer! We also stock up on meat when Polyface has sales or buy-one get-one free deals. I recently purchased 10 pounds of pork spare ribs because they were on sale for $5 per pound. One time I bought four picnic roasts at 5 pounds each for half off! Like Joel said, we're able to buy large quantities of those sales items because we have a sales fund in our budget and a deep freezer.

Joel: Remember that in order to buy bulk on items that require freezing and refrigeration, you'll need enough of that storage to handle a sudden volume purchase. As you head toward Paradise on our continuum, you'll find your food storage nooks inadequate. I can't imagine anything more truly progressive than to convert your TV room into a large pantry, maybe with a couple of freezers and shelves for canned goods and lots of mouse-proof canisters for dry goods.

One of the biggest impediments to leveraging volume purchase prices is in-home storage. You can get used freezers for less than $100 anywhere. People constantly sell appliances and our experience is that they usually last several years. Maybe not as long as a new one, but certainly worth the money. If you save $100 on one purchase of bulk beef, for example, the freezer is free. Our farm sells what we call a "Larder" of chickens, for example, at nearly $2 off per bird. You have to buy 10 to get that price, but how many families eat 10 chickens a year? Lots. Most eat 50; that's $100 again.

Sina: Donnie found a great deal on our deep freeze during a Black Friday sale. It was $100 brand new. We've more than made up for the cost of the freezer with the money we've saved from buying in bulk and buying food on sale. We also store dried good in our closets.

Joel: The point is that rather than complaining about prices, be proactive and get some storage and a sales fund. That's far more important than a Starbuck's® coffee.

Practical Bite #32: Give Your Family The Freedom To Opt-In

How? Don't force your family to follow the food and lifestyle choices that you have chosen. Instead, create an environment that promotes healthy living while still allowing your family the freedom to opt-in. In other words, don't force them to walk behind you; encourage them to walk beside you. There are many ways to accomplish this goal. We've included some ideas below.

Why?

Joel: My mentor Allan Nation used to say that few things are more unappreciated than unsolicited advice. And if it involves family, the unappreciativeness escalates exponentially. The main idea here is to present an attitude of better rather than an attitude of demonization.

People get really tired of being judged all the time. Instead, happily hum about your changes and infect the family with your happiness rather than your negativity.

Sina: When I began my healing journey, I knew my success would, in part, depend on support from my husband and children. Let's face it, changing your eating habits is challenging enough; you don't want to fight your family. So, I didn't force them to follow a lifestyle I was creating for myself. Instead, I created an environment that fosters healthy living while allowing them the freedom to opt-in.

My children opted-in because I educated them about what's in their food, modeled the lifestyle I wanted them to follow, and allowed them to make their own decisions – even at the young age of 5. For example, I taught them how to read labels so they could decide which foods they wanted to put in their body. Then, I taught them how to create a product comparison, which ended up being a critical tool in their understanding of the chemicals that exist in common foods. For example, for every store-bought dessert they ate, we created a healthier homemade version. Then, we listed the ingredients in our homemade dessert alongside the ingredients in the store-bought version. Next, we researched the associated negative health effects with each ingredient and wrote it down on the paper. Lastly, we read the lists out loud and I asked my children which dessert they wanted to put in their bodies.

Children are very intuitive; after seeing the side-by-side comparisons just one time, they have never eaten store-bought desserts again. So, while it took time to do each of the product comparisons, that approach is much more powerful than simply stating, "Don't eat that dessert because it's not good for you." The product comparisons allowed my children to see the differences between the foods for themselves, and decide if they wanted those chemicals in their bodies. It gave them the freedom to opt-in based on informed consent.

Another approach that is less time consuming is getting your children involved at the grocery store. For example, I showed my children how to look for the Butterfly and the organic label. I turned it into a game by allowing my kids to run up and down the aisles in the grocery store looking for those labels. They loved it! And yes, I sometimes got stares from people who thought my kids were acting out of control. But, looking for the labels gave them something positive to focus on in the store, instead of randomly grabbing items off the shelves, which happened during every grocery store trip before I implemented the Label Game. Most importantly, the Label Game empowered my children by giving them ownership.

Taking ownership allows your children the opportunity to take responsibility for their choices. For example, both of my children began cooking with me before they turned 2 years old. By the time they were 5, I had encouraged them to pick recipes from cookbooks or websites, and guided them as they harnessed their power by learning to cook for themselves.

I struggled for a long time with being able to let go in the kitchen because every time my son, Hunter, would cook with me, he'd make a mess! The floors would be white with a coating of coconut flour while oil and spices were scattered all over the counters. It stressed me out because it was "one more thing on my to-do list" that I had to deal with. But then I realized, the more at ease I became in the kitchen, the more creative Hunter became. It didn't take long before he was creating his own recipes! He turned those recipes into a cookbook at the age of 6, and now – at the age of 10 – he's working on his second cookbook! Kids are amazing. You never know the depth of your child's potential until you let them go and allow them to explore.

Another empowering activity I do with my children is gardening. We started small, with just one plant in a pot that we kept in the kitchen. I bought organic soil and allowed my children to play with the soil and get it all over their hands and body. I got my hands dirty too! Remember, playing in healthy soil adds microbial diversity to your skin, nasal passages and lungs. So, I let go of my concerns. Even when soil was flying through the air and the kids were wiping it on their clothes, I allowed myself to enjoy the laughter of my children as they experienced pure joy building their single-pot garden.

Now, at the ages of 6 and 10, my children build their own outdoor gardens filled with all sorts of fruits and vegetables, such as: pumpkins, squash, watermelons, and cucumbers (my 6-year old calls them "cute-cumbers"). And, they won't let me help! That's probably a smart decision because my children's garden did better than mine this year!

My children also chose to build a bee garden this year. After I taught them that roughly 1/3 of our crops would not exist without bees, they decided to launch a mission to "save the bees" by planting bee-friendly flowers.

All of these strategies took time and effort. But they paid off because now that my children understand the "why," and have chosen this lifestyle for themselves, there is no tension, no conflict, and no arguments. I don't have to tell them to eat their vegetables at the dinner table, or remind them not to eat the samples handed out at the grocery store. And, it's deeply rewarding to see my children stand for their principles and fight for something they believe in.

It's also important to meet yourself where you are. You don't have to build an entire vegetable or bee garden with your children. Start with just one plant, in one pot – like we did. You don't have to do formal product comparisons. Start with playing the Label Game. And, then build on it by teaching them how to find and read the ingredient label. Then, pick one ingredient on the package and show them how to look up any adverse health effects. Take it one step at a time because opting-in doesn't happen overnight; it's a journey. So, give your children the space and time they need to figure out *their* principles and decide how *they* want to stand for them.

Now, let's talk about spouses.

Joel: Get it in their mouth. Authentic food tastes good and makes you feel good. Nothing beats "try this, just for fun." Who doesn't respond to some food teasing? Sounds sexy to me.

Sina: I guess everyone is different. In in my experience, it's best not to force your spouse to eat a certain way. It's funny because Donnie, my husband, used to eat the exact opposite of my kids and me. He bought the cheapest foods because he thought he was "getting a deal," and he'd eat nearly any processed food. For breakfast, he used to eat donuts and chocolate milk. He never ate vegetables, and the only fruit he would eat is green apples.

My friends would routinely make comments such as, "I can't believe you let him eat that." I always thought that was a fascinating comment because it's not my right to force him to eat the way I think he should eat. Each of us has the right to eat what we want. So, I don't force my beliefs onto others. Besides, like you said, nobody likes to be told what to do – not kids, not adults, and certainly not spouses.

So, I have never told Donnie what to eat. In fact, I did the exact opposite; I made no comments at all. Meal times were difficult because he would eat something completely different from my children and me. And, of course, my children wanted to "eat what Daddy's eating" because they are boys who want to be like their father and the processed food is addicting. Initially, I responded by telling my kids that Daddy is an adult and he can choose what he wants to eat, but we aren't eating that food because it's not healthy. That didn't go over well! They just kept asking for "Daddy's food."

Immediately, a divide formed in our family and there was tension each time we sat down to eat. Then, one day, Hunter said, "Why can't I choose what I eat?" That's when it hit me: If I don't give him the responsibility of making his own food choices now, while he's still under my supervision, he's going to move out one day and rebel – likely by eating the foods that "Daddy eats." Or, he was going to start sneaking food, like I used to do as a child. So, that's when I started teaching my children about what's in their food and giving them the choice to opt-in.

Meanwhile, my husband was hearing me teach my children about how the chemicals in our food are not safety tested by the FDA, and how GMOs are "presumed" to be GRAS, and how rBGH can contribute to prostate cancer. So, he began making small changes all by himself. For instance, instead of conventional milk, he started buying organic milk. Instead of Pop Tarts®, he started buying the organic version. I was thrilled! Yet, I said nothing.

Then, Donnie saw my miraculous recovery from the autoimmune disease, largely through changing my diet. Over those several months, he made more changes to his diet. He switched to organic cereal and bread. Again, I said nothing.

Later, as my children learned more about what was in their food, they asked their father to stop eating those chemicals. I remember one day when we sat down to eat as a family, Hunter looked at his Dad and said, "I don't want you to eat that food anymore because I don't want you to die." Donnie didn't say anything, but I could tell it hit him hard. He continued to make small changes. Again, I said nothing.

The tipping point came when Donnie edited my first book. He realized that the government is not actually making sure our food is safe. And, that nobody knows if the 10,000 chemical additives in our processed foods are safe. And, then he looked around and noticed that everyone around him seemed to be sick, or have at least one family member who was sick. Even his friends were sick, and they were in their 30's! That's when he made the connection between the sick food supply and all of the sick people. Again, I said nothing.

It took about a year of baby steps, but now, Donnie eats all organic foods, no grains, and no dairy! He's even spoken at one of my events on how to make healthy food more affordable. That's remarkable considering where he started! But, importantly, he made those choices on his own by educating himself and seeing how my health and the health of our children has improved through dietary changes. By not hounding him to change or dictating what he "should" eat, Donnie had the space to figure out what he thought about the food and decide what he wanted to do about it. He opted-in.

Again, people might surprise you, if you give them a chance.

Practical Bite #33: Create Convenience

How? Keep the convenience of prepared mixes in your life while standing for your principles and adding trust to your food supply by making your own dry mixes in batches. This method can be used for any type of home-made mix, including: pancakes, waffles, biscuits, cakes, cookies, tortilla shells, and bread. Here's a recipe for grain-free, dairy-free, egg-free, soy-free, sugar-free pancakes that are high in fiber. Shockingly, they taste good!

Grain-Free, Dairy-Free, Egg-Free, Soy-Free, Sugar-Free Pancakes

Dry Ingredients:

- 2-½ cups garbanzo bean flour
- ½ cup arrowroot powder
- 1-½ cups tiger nut flour
- 1 Tablespoon coconut flour
- 1 teaspoon Real Salt®
- 2 teaspoons baking soda

Wet Ingredients:

- 3 cups filtered water
- 3 Tablespoons coconut vinegar
- ¾ cups avocado oil
- Additional avocado oil for cooking pancakes on skillet

Instructions:

1. Line up 12 dry glass jars that are 64-ounces each (or use 24 dry glass jars that are 32-ounces each).
2. Add dry ingredients to all 12 jars, one ingredient at a time. (If using 32-ounce jars, add the garbanzo bean flour to one jar and the remaining ingredients to the second jar).
3. Place lids on each jar, label the jars, and store in pantry. Mixes will last as long as the expiration date listed on the individual dry ingredients.
4. When ready to make one batch of pancakes, add wet ingredients to the bottom of a blender. Next, add one 64-ounce jar of dry ingredients (add 2 jars if using 32-ounce jars; 1 jar of garbanzo bean flour and 1 jar of the remaining dry ingredients). Blend on high for several minutes, scraping down the sides to ensure all of the dry ingredients are thoroughly mixed. (If pancakes taste gritty, blend longer.)
5. Cover the bottom of a skillet with avocado oil. Heat pan so it's very hot (The hotter the pan, the crispier the outside of the pancake. So, if you like soft pancakes then keep the pan on medium heat). Pan is ready when drops of water sizzle and pop. Pour ½ cup batter onto pan. Let cook until the pancake is easy to flip, roughly 3 minutes per side. For a soft center and crunchy exterior, cook on one side and then fold onto itself (like folding an omelet) and cook for an additional 3 minutes.
6. Eat with fresh fruit or maple syrup.

***Side note:** Some alternative flours can be finicky about ambient temperature. Consequently, more flour may be needed if the pancakes are too thin and more water may be needed if they are too thick. Play around with the recipe until you reach your desired consistency.*

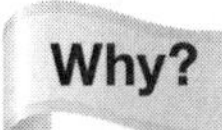

Why?

Joel: My bride of 40 years, Teresa, is a wizard in the kitchen. She majored in Home Economics in college and then taught a semester of high school while one of the Home Ec. teachers was out on maternity leave. We were high school sweethearts so we kind of went through college together too. I remember some of her projects involved kitchen efficiency and the single most important aspect was "do like things together." That was axiomatic in culinary training.

In other words, don't flit around the kitchen; do all the knife work at once. Then do all the stirring at once. But for the big picture, this includes preparing things at once. If you have a prepared mix time, you can do several types of mixes at once. In full transparency, she doesn't buy or prepare mixes beforehand. Everything is scratch but she's so efficient in the kitchen, somehow, she seems to get it all done fast.

Here's my story as to why you don't want to buy mixes. Many years ago, when we were just beginning to produce lots of eggs, we would take them once a week to an egg farm that had cleaning, candling, weighing, and boxing equipment. I ducked under the candling hood one day and asked the lady operating it what she did with the cracks.

Egg candling simply means you shine a bright light through the egg and you can see the yolk, air sack, blood spots (if any exist) and spot the most hairline crack. The eggs were on a conveyor that went over a bright light. Everything was under a canvas hood like a dark room to help see what the bright light illuminated.

Now realize that these eggs had just come through the washer that was full of manure and chlorine. Eggshells are porous, and of course cracked eggshells are even more porous. Occasionally an egg would still have a fleck of manure on it even after coming through the washing gauntlet. When she spotted a cracked one, she'd pick it up and put it in a carton beside her. To my question "what do you do with those eggs?" she answered "we take them over to an extraction company. They dump the eggs in a giant cylinder and press everything through a mesh screen that keeps the shells on one side and squeezes the liquid through to the other. That's what goes in prepared mixes in the grocery store."

In case you missed the picture, remember that nobody cracked these eggs and put their insides in the press. The whole eggs went in there - manure, chlorine, insides and outsides.

The whole thing gets mashed and the screens separate the liquid from the solids. After that, I've always told people "if you buy cake mixes in the store, make sure you have to add eggs." But, of course, the eggs are just one questionable thing.

Making your own mixes is fun and if you do several at a time, you can enjoy the future convenience but you won't be eating chicken manure.

Sina: One of the most challenging areas of my diet is not having the convenience of store-bought mixes, such as cake mixes or pancake mix. I rarely find a processed food that I'm willing to eat, let alone a mix that is aligned with my principles. So, my family decided to make our own mixes in order to add convenience back into our lives.

I used to make a recipe only when I needed it. So, if my kids wanted pancakes for breakfast, I'd get out all of the ingredients and make one batch of pancakes. That got old very quickly! It's time consuming and daunting when you are cooking from scratch every day. So, we came up with a better method that saves time and energy.

We prepare dry mixes ahead of time and store them in glass jars. Instead of making just one mix when we want to eat pancakes, we make 12 mixes. We simply line up 12 jars and add one dry ingredient to each jar at a time. For instance, we add tiger nut flour to each jar and then we add coconut flour to each jar and then baking soda, etcetera until every ingredient has been added to every jar.

This simple method saves an enormous amount of time and energy. For example, imagine how much time it takes to bring all of the ingredients out to make one batch of pancakes, find the recipe, bring out all of the measuring utensils and the bowl, make the batter, and then put all of the ingredients away and clean the measuring utensils. It takes me roughly 7 minutes to do the prep and clean up for one batch of pancakes. By making 12 jars of pancake mix at one time, I only have to get the ingredients out once and clean up once. Consequently, I save 77 minutes!

Plus, the assembly line approach saves even more time because each time you add the same ingredient to the 12 jars, you get faster. It doesn't take as long to add a ¼ cup of flour to jar 12 compared to jar 1. That means, each successive jar takes less time to make than the first jar. Consequently, we use this method for all sorts of home-made mixes, including: pancakes, waffles, biscuits, tortilla shells, and bread rolls.

The key is to pick a time to make the mixes that's convenient for you. Instead of trying to make them in the morning while trying to get the kids ready for school and get yourself to work on time, wait until it's convenient. Maybe that's while listening to a podcast or watching a television show. My husband makes his biscuit mixes while watching football. He once told me, "I might as well do something with my hands while watching football." That works for me! One less thing I have to do in the kitchen! Another option is to get your children or grandchildren involved. I pay my children to prepare the mixes. They earn 25 cents per jar, which encourages involvement in their food supply, helps them practice fractions, promotes team work, and fosters their entrepreneurial spirit. And, it reduces my time in the kitchen!

Making mixes in batches is time well spent: you add back the convenience of mixes while standing for your principles and increasing your trust in your food supply. Win-win-win!

Joel: Moving your participation this far into the food system is not only good for your health, it's good for your spirit. Snuggling into the comfort of something you've sourced and prepared yields emotional satiation like few things. Think of how you feel when you pull off any project that you developed, shepherded, and saw to fruition, including the fulfillment on the faces of others involved with the project. That whole experience is incredibly affirming. Whenever you participate in your provenance at this level, it offers the same kind of emotional high, but this time it's from your family. That's even better.

Practical Bite #34: Sprout & Grind Your Grains

How? If you choose to eat grains, pick an organic, ancient, sprouted grain and grind it using an in-kitchen mill, either electric powered or hand cranked.

Why?

Joel: We don't do this in our house but we know plenty of people who do. A simple hand-operated grinder lets you enjoy the freshest flour imaginable.

Once you have your mill, you'll want to experiment with all sorts of minor grains like spelt, amaranth, quinoa. For more common grains, you'll want to find old varieties that are now more available than they were just a couple of decades ago. The market for heritage type grains is expanding, as well as the production. That's a good thing and you'll enjoy trying some of these extremely old genetics.

Sina: I don't grind grains either because I don't eat them. However, if I did, I would consume organic, sprouted, ancient grains.

Ancient grains are generally defined as grains that are largely unchanged over the past several hundred years. Examples include: einkorn, emmer/farro, Khorasan or durum wheat (Kamut®), sorghum, teff, millet, quinoa, amaranth, and spelt.

When eating grains, choose organic. Organic means the grains are not allowed to be sprayed with most pesticides or herbicides, or grown using sewage sludge or most synthetic fertilizers. And they cannot be grown from genetically modified (GM) seeds.

While GM wheat is not currently on the market in the United States, there is a growing movement to get GM wheat on your dinner plate. In fact, several GM wheat varieties have already been created in the laboratory and field trials have occurred in the United States. In addition, rogue GM wheat has been found in Washington, Oregon, and Montana. Interestingly, the USDA could not figure out where the GM wheat in Oregon came from, so it closed the investigation in 2014. Therefore, the safest bet is to buy organic.

In addition, glyphosate is sometimes sprayed on conventional grains as a pre-harvest desiccant. Spraying the crop with glyphosate stresses or kills the plant, which accelerates drying and speeds up the ripening of the grains. While this method gets the crop to market sooner, it also means there is more glyphosate residue on the grain by the time it reaches market compared to only using glyphosate during the growing process. So, choose organic because glyphosate is sometimes used to desiccate grains, including: wheat, oats, rye, buckwheat, corn and millet. (It's also sometimes used on beans, lentils, peas, flax, sugar beets, canola and potatoes).

Once you have chosen your organic grain, sprout it. Spouting grains increases their digestibility, as well as the availability of some nutrients and bioactive compounds. For instance, studies have shown higher levels of antioxidants, including vitamin C and tocopherols, in wheat following sprouting.

There are many websites that teach how to sprout grains. Here's a basic recipe to get you started:

Sprouted Grains

Ingredients:

1 pound whole grains
1 tablespoon vinegar

Instructions:

1. Place grains into a large glass mixing bowl. Add warm water until covered roughly 2-inches. Stir in vinegar. Cover bowl and set it on the counter for 18-24 hours.
2. Drain and rinse well. Pour grains into a fine-mesh sieve and rinse well with water, stirring grains with your hands.
3. Twice a day for 2-3 days, rinse and stir the grains until a tiny sprout emerges at the end of the grains.
4. Transfer grains to dehydrator trays and dehydrate for 12-18 hours.
5. Once the grains are firm and dry, grind into flour using a grain grinder.

Since neither Joel nor I mill our own grains, I reached out to Sue Becker, from The Bread Beckers®, to provide additional insight on this subject. Here's a glimpse into our conversation:

Sina: Sue, I've heard you say that "real bread" cannot be found in the grocery store. Can you elaborate?

Sue: "Real Bread" is made from whole grain flour that has had none of the bran and germ stripped away and is milled just before making the bread so that all of the vital nutrients are still viable.

In the late 1800s, the huge steel rolling mills came on the American scene. These mills crush the wheat into flour. The flour is then sent through screens that sift all of the nutrient rich bran and germ away, leaving only the protein and starch portions of the grain, known as the endosperm or more commonly, white flour. These steel rolling mills virtually replaced the local stone mills, and for the first time in history white flour and white bread became the bread for the rich and poor alike.

Today, these rolling mills are used by all large commercial flour mills and all flour is milled this way, even what is labeled whole grain. To make whole grain flour, they simply recombine some of the bran and germ back into the white flour according to a legal government standard.

To be labeled "whole grain", the bread you find in the grocery store shelves must list this whole grain flour as its first ingredient. However, these whole grain loaves may also contain chemical preservatives, dough conditioners, multiple sweeteners, and added ingredients such as pure gluten (the extracted protein of white flour). The addition of such large amounts of gluten greatly diminish the fiber to flour ratio and upset the naturally occurring balance of these components. These chemically laden loaves are no comparison to "real bread" made from "real" freshly milled flour with all its nutrition still intact.

Sina: The bottom line is, you can't trust the "whole grain" label in the grocery store, correct?

Sue: Some misleading marketing verbiage will say things like "made from whole grains." Well, white flour is made from whole grains. Or labels state "wheat bread" but caramel coloring to turn it light brown are added. The customer reads "wheat" bread, sees the brown color and thinks whole wheat or whole grain. Yet, read the ingredients and you'll see enriched white flour! Or, the label states multi grain and while the bread is made using different whole grains for the flour, the bran and germ are stripped away. In other words, it's really white flour.

Sina: Just like any other food in the grocery store, it's critical to read beyond the label when purchasing breads and other grain products.

It's equally important to find a reputable source of grains. For example, grains are susceptible to mold. And mold produces mycotoxins, which can lead to chronic inflammation in your body and subsequent disease, including cancer. According to the World Health Organization, whole grains "are regularly contaminated with aflatoxins [a type of mold]."

Mold can grow on grains either before or after harvest, but most of the mold is believed to stem from how grains are stored in warm, damp and humid conditions. And, it's important to find grains without mold because, according to the FDA, "When the grain is processed into final products like flour or feed, the visible mold may be removed, but the majority of toxins are not and can still cause poisoning."

So, how can someone find grains that do not contain mold?

Sue: Know your source and where the grain is grown. Warm, humid climates are the most susceptible to the problem of molds and mycotoxins. More rainfall during a growing season makes for more moisture in the grain. Then the warm weather during storage can compound the problem by contributing to conditions suitable for mold. But technology and improved ventilated storage conditions have greatly reduced the susceptibility, even in these areas.

Colder, dryer climates, such as Montana, have very little problem with mold and mycotoxins. The cold growing season and storage (200 days below freezing) are optimal for producing dry grains and cold storage, conditions not as susceptible to mold.

When there is an unusually wet growing season (which is rare), the grain elevator in Montana that we use takes extra precautions to ensure the grain is dry, and has their wheat tested by a federally approved laboratory to detect mold or mycotoxins. As mentioned above, their growing conditions and storage make it less likely to have a problem. It is our opinion, that Montana grows the best bread making wheat.

Sina: Do you cook with all types of grains, or do you elevate some grains over others?

Sue: I like to use a variety of grains, usually based on the end product I want to enjoy. For example, if I want corn bread or southern grits, I will, of course, choose corn. If I want a soft muffin or biscuit, I will choose soft wheat, spelt or maybe even buckwheat or sorghum. If I want to make a yeast leavened or sour dough bread, I will choose a hard wheat, spelt or rye. I mostly use organic grains, as I have them readily available. I have not used sprouted grains.

Sina: If someone wants to mill their own grains, how do they find a good, reliable mill that is affordable?

Sue: Well, of course, I am biased here and would say they can find a "good mill" at Bread Beckers® in Woodstock, GA or online at www.BreadBeckers.com as well as nutritional and cooking support. We have many articles, as well as video classes, on milling and baking bread.

After 28 years of milling all my flour and making all the bread for our large family (9 children), and 27 years in the grain mill business, we highly recommend the Wonder Mill® by Grote Molen. It is fast, clean, durable, easy to use and requires no cleaning. It uses stainless steel milling heads so there is no oil residue on the milling heads like there is in stone mills. The capacity is 12 cups of flour in one (fast) milling and the flour falls directly into a closed flour cannister. The speed and closed container are very important features. I do not like the dust created when the milled flour falls into an open container. The Wonder Mill® generates very little friction to the grain so very little heat to the flour and mills 1 pound of flour (about 3 cups) in less than 30 seconds.

The flour from the Wonder Mill® is beautifully fine and produces very soft breads, cakes, cookies, muffins or pancakes. Everything your family will love to consume. The cost of the Wonder Mill® is very affordable – much less than other mills on the market.

It is also very durable. I have had mine for 26 years, used nearly daily, and have never had it repaired. Our ministry in Haiti has used two Wonder Mills®, daily for three years now to mill flour to make bread for 600-800 children every day. They have never been repaired!

I do not recommend grain mill attachments that some mixers offer to mill flour. They are very slow, produce coarse flour, fall into an open container (producing a lot of dust) and can cause extra strain and heat to the motor of the mixer.

Some people choose to start with a blender but usually end up getting a designated grain mill. The flour from even a high-powered blender might be a good starting place but generally the flour is somewhat coarse and will therefore produce a denser bread. Start here with caution as the denser bread might just turn your family off to the idea of freshly milled whole grain bread.

Sina: Do you recommend milling the grains right before use to preserve the nutrient content and reduce oxidation or rancidity?

Sue: Yes. Once the grain is milled and the flour is exposed to the air, oxidation begins to break down and destroy many of the nutrients. So, having a mill in home, and milling the grain into flour just when you are ready to use it is ideal.

With the right mill (such as the Wonder Mill®) this step is about as easy as taking a flour canister out of your cabinet. The mill does all the work for you. Simply, turn it on, pour the dry grain or bean into the hopper, and in just 1-2 minutes you have nutritious freshly milled flour.

Sina: If someone wants to use freshly milled grain in an existing recipe, what is the conversion factor?

Sue: It is super easy to convert any recipe calling for white flour to freshly milled whole grain flour. For most yeast bread recipes, the conversion will basically be 1:1 using hard red or hard white wheat. You will want to use a hard wheat as this has the higher protein content for the necessary gluten formation to enable a good rise from yeasted breads.

For pastries, such as cakes, cookies, biscuits or pie dough, you will want to use soft wheat for a mild flavor or spelt, emmer or einkorn if you want a slightly nuttier flavor. The general rule of thumb when converting a white flour recipe to one of these freshly milled pastry flours is to use about ¼ cup more freshly milled flour for every cup of white flour called for in the recipe. For example: if a cookie recipe calls for 2 cups of all-purpose white flour, you will use 2 ½ cups soft wheat, spelt, emmer or einkorn flour.

I use freshly milled flour for ALL of my baking. In 28 years, I've not found any recipe that I could not make with freshly milled flour. And the good news, my family likes the freshly milled flour version better. And the icing on the cake – it's nutritious as well as delicious.

Sina: Will you share one of your favorite recipes as a jumping off point for our readers?

Sue: Certainly! Start simple, get some basic recipes that your family enjoys and choose the grain accordingly. Wheat is the king of bread making for a reason. It works well in most every bread application, whether yeasted or a quick rise using baking powder.

When I first started milling my flour and making all the bread for our family, I had 5 young children that I homeschooled. So, this change had to be easy.

I started with our 4 family favorite breads – basic sandwich bread or rolls, muffins, pancakes and a coffee cake that we loved. These basic recipes can be found in our small Recipe Collection (AKA the *Bread Beckers® Recipe Collection*) or my *The Essential Home Ground Flour Book*. Below is the recipe for the basic bread:

Basic Yeast Bread Dough (Makes 2 – 1 lb. loaves)

This is a great basic recipe for any bread baker and can be a "go to" dough for dinner rolls, buns, cinnamon rolls, doughnuts, pizza dough and more. Using only a few ingredients, the dough is easy to make and is very forgiving whether too much or too little flour is added. This recipe uses no milk or butter and the egg is optional, as is the gluten. Perfectly sized recipe for a 2 lb. (1 kg) automatic bread maker.

Ingredients:

- 1-½ cups hot water
- 1/3 cup oil
- 1/3 cup honey
- 2 teaspoons salt
- 1 Tablespoon rice bran extract (optional)
- 1 teaspoon gluten (optional)
- 1 egg (optional)
- 4-4 ½ cups hard wheat flour
- 1 Tablespoon yeast

Instructions:

1. In a large mixing bowl or bowl of stand mixer, combine hot water, oil, honey and salt, egg, if using and rice bran and gluten if using.
2. Add ½ of the flour and mix until a thick batter forms. While continuing to mix, add the yeast and the remaining flour to form a soft dough. Knead for 5-10 minutes until smooth and elastic. Let rise – shape into loaves as desired. Let rise in a warm place until doubled in size.
3. While loaves rise, preheat oven to 350°.
4. Bake risen loaves for about 30 minutes until the internal temperature is 180-190 degrees.

**To use an automatic bread maker for kneading the dough, place the ingredients in the bread machine pan in the order listed.*

**I do not typically use either the rice bran extract or the gluten. So, these ingredients really are optional. But some people prefer the softer texture and slightly better rise that these ingredients give.*

SECTION 3:

Meet Real Food

CHAPTER 5

Shift From High Quality Processed Food To Whole Food

You've swapped low quality processed foods for higher quality processed foods. That's great! I bet you've already realized that those higher quality processed foods, while still a step in the right direction, contain weaknesses, such as: nutrient loss, fortification with synthetic chemicals, lack of a healthy microbiome, and misleading labels. The next category will help you fill those holes.

Moving along the road map, the next category is whole foods, which includes foods that are sourced from the ground or the animal. These foods contain no additives, and have undergone minimal or no processing. Examples include: fruits and vegetables in their native state, eggs, and whole pieces of meat – think of a chicken breast with the bone and skin still attached.

By switching from higher quality processed foods to whole foods, you achieve huge health gains while still receiving the convenience of buying food from the grocery store. For example, whole foods contain minimal or no preservatives, artificial or natural flavoring or coloring, GRAS chemicals, artificial sweeteners, or synthetic fortification. And, they do not undergo the significant loss in nutrients that occurs with heavily processed foods. Thus, choosing whole foods instead of processed foods increases your health by reducing the toxic burden on your body and nourishing your microbiome.

Choosing organic whole foods lowers your toxic burden even further. Organic means the produce is not allowed to contain GMOs, be sprayed with most pesticides or herbicides, or grown using sewage sludge or most synthetic fertilizers. And it cannot be irradiated. Organically-raised animals are not allowed to be given hormones, antibiotics, or fed GMOs. Consequently, organic whole foods generally contain a healthier microbiome than their conventional counterparts, as well as higher levels of micronutrients, which your body needs to be healthy and thrive.

Whole foods also contain functional molecules, or health-promoting compounds, such as carotenoids, anthocyanins, isoflavones, and other phytochemicals. Plants produce health-promoting compounds in response to various stressors, such as changes in the environment or pathogen/herbivore attack. Those functional molecules help protect the plant against disease. When you eat those functional molecules, they also help protect you against disease, including inflammatory diseases.

In addition, both plants and humans produce microRNAs, which are short segments of RNA that can regulate gene expression. Recent studies have revealed that when you eat whole foods, you consume microRNAs. Those microRNAs can enter your blood and tissues and regulate your gene expression. In other words, the plants you eat are literally turning your genes on and off.

We are learning that microRNAs are involved in the regulation of many biological processes, including: insulin secretion, cholesterol metabolism, aging, immune responses, cell death (apoptosis), as well as the growth and development of nerve cells, cardiac cells and skeletal muscle cells. In fact, a study published in the medical journal *Current Eye Research* in 2012 reported that curcumin (found in turmeric) increased the level of a microRNA that suppressed tumor growth. In other words, the microRNA exhibited anticancer effects.
We don't fully understand the mechanism. However, we know that when a plant is under

stress, it can make certain microRNAs that turn on stress-responsive genes, which increases its chance of survival by making it more resilient. For example, there are microRNAs that enhance tolerance to heavy metal exposure, nutrient deficiencies, and oxidative stress. When you eat those plants, you are eating some of those microRNAs, along with the health-promoting compounds produced from their regulatory response. Therefore, you are benefiting from the plant's adaptive response to the environment. That means, if you want to be healthy, the type of food (i.e. whole foods) and the quality of food (i.e. organic) is just as important, and possibly more important, than your DNA.

Whole foods also offer more trust in your food supply because, compared with processed foods, there is less processing, therefore, less opportunity to add chemicals. And, since there is less of a supply chain (i.e. fewer companies handle the food), there is less reliance on labels.

Eating whole foods also helps you reclaim freedoms you have lost. For instance, by choosing whole foods, particularly organic whole foods, you opt out of the centralized food system that the government has created – the system that is making you sick. By speaking with your dollars, you send a message to the government and food industry, which shifts the market. If you want to change your food supply, speaking with your dollars is the loudest voice you have. And, choosing whole, organic foods over processed foods screams freedom.

Practical Bite #35: Count Quality, Not Calories

How? Stop counting calories and start eating organic whole foods.

Why?

Joel: We humans have a limitless capacity to make simple things complex. Something as simple as eating is now surrounded with a bookshelf full of diets, calorie counters, and laboratory manipulation. A few people have always been fat. Remember "The Fat Lady" in Old Maid®? Growing up, I knew one fat woman and one really fat man. But just one of each. Today, everybody knows several.

Those trim and fit people in our old ancestral black and white photos did not get that way by counting calories. To be sure, many of them worked hard, which burned up a lot of energy. But they didn't fixate on calories. They just ate whole foods because Duncan Hines® hadn't been invented yet. Or Hot Pockets®.

Sina: I used to count calories when I wanted to lose weight. I had a small notebook where I'd write down everything that I ate, along with a running total of the calories I consumed. If I reached my caloric limit for the day, I'd stop eating. Or, I'd exercise to burn more calories so I could eat more. I believed that if I burned more calories than I consumed, I would lose weight. That sounds logical, but it's actually not true.

Our culture is fixated on calories, as though counting calories is the magic solution to weight loss and health. We have watches and phone apps that count calories for us, and weight loss programs designed entirely around caloric intake. And, remember the Nutrition Facts Label that is included on every food package sold in America? It's focused on calories too! Look at the label. Calories are the first item listed, in bold. And, now there are even calories listed on menus.

Yep, that's your tax dollars at work. With 2/3 of Americans either overweight or obese, the government decided to step in and "save us" from ourselves by requiring all chain restaurants with 20 or more locations to post calorie contents on their menus. The government thought that if you knew how many calories were in your cheeseburger, you would opt for the salad instead. Seriously? Do we really need the government to tell us there are more calories in a cheeseburger than a salad?

Clearly, I'm not a fan of the government trying to change our behavior. But what bothers me the most about this government mandated caloric rule is that the emphasis is placed on the calorie and not the quality. It assumes "a calorie is a calorie," which is what I was taught in graduate school. But, that's not true. Not all calories are created equal.

If you ate 500 calories of soda and 500 calories of broccoli, would they have the same effect on your body? Of course not! They are calorically the same, but they are not the same nutritionally. And, your body instinctively knows that truth. Let's break this down a little further so we can dispel the calorie myth once and for all.

Do you know how calories are determined?

Joel: A calorie is a unit of energy - the amount of energy to raise the temperature of a gram of water one degree Centigrade. Today, it's often expressed in physics as 4.1868 joules. It's energy. Obviously, though, a calorie of gasoline energy will not do in my body what a calorie of pork chop will do. And a calorie of pork chop is not all that comes with a bite; it includes a lot of other stuff. Ditto for carrots or eggs. Calorie is such a tiny portion of the measure of a food item it's practically unimportant. Which is Sina's whole point.

Sina: Exactly! And the method used to determine a calorie is flawed. Specifically, a food is placed in a machine, called a bomb calorimeter. It's burned until there's nothing left but ash. The amount of heat given off during the burning process is measured as calories. Yep, that's actually how calories are determined.

Well, people complained that it was not an accurate system, so a second system was developed in the late 1800s. It still relies on measurements from the bomb calorimeter, but it indirectly estimates calories by utilizing a calculation that uses an estimate on top of another estimate on top of a third estimate. Essentially, scientists estimated the grams of protein, carbohydrate and fat in a given food and then subtracted the number of calories they thought were lost through poop, urine, and heat. Using this method, it was determined that fat releases 9 calories per grams while protein and carbohydrate both release 4 calories per gram. Those values probably sound familiar because they are still used today.

Can you see some glaring flaws with this method?

Joel: I'm thinking. Let's see, could it be that our bodies, as well as food, are not just calories but are interacting with enzymes, bacteria, minerals and all sorts of things? Perhaps I'm not just a test tube? Help me out here, Sina.

Sina: You are on the right track. This laboratory experiment uses a closed system, which means the food is not affected by the environment (i.e. only heat is released). So, if you take our example of soda versus broccoli, it is true that in a laboratory setting, using a closed system, both of those foods would release the same amount of energy because they both contain 500 calories of heat energy.

But our bodies are not closed systems and our gastrointestinal tracts are not bomb calorimeters. We are complex systems that interact with our environment.

For example, burning food in a bomb calorimeter boils down to just one reaction: oxygen combines with a carbon source (i.e. food) and breaks it down into carbon dioxide, heat energy, and whatever carbon bits are left over (i.e. ash). In contrast, digestion in your body requires a whole bunch of chemical reactions. Those chemical reactions require an enzyme in order to work properly, and most enzymes require at least one cofactor, such as a vitamin or mineral. That means, your ability to efficiently digest food depends on many factors, such as:

- Stress level
- Nutrient deficiency status
- Ability to make enough acid and digestive enzymes
- Composition of your microflora
- Timing of your previous meal
- How the food was prepared i.e. if it's cooked and pureed versus raw
- How the different foods in your current meal interact with each other
- How many times you chew each bite, etcetera.

In other words, unlike a bomb calorimeter, the efficiency of your digestive system changes based on your environment and your individual state of being. So, you may be able to harness 300 calories from a meal one day and then only harness 230 calories from that same meal the following week. Hence, you cannot compare calories obtained by burning food in a machine with calories obtained by digesting food in your body. It's like comparing apples to oranges.

Besides, food is not just calories. Food is information; with every bite of food, you send instructions to your body that can either create health or create disease.

Let's continue with our soda versus broccoli example. When you drink the soda, it's essentially pure sugar. There are no fiber, vitamins, minerals, or phytonutrients to help your body process the calories. Consequently, your gut readily absorbs the glucose sugar in the soda, which spikes your blood sugar. Insulin is released by your pancreas to deal with the large sugar load, which results in a high blood insulin level. High insulin increases inflammation, raises triglycerides and lowers HDL (the "good" cholesterol), raises blood pressure, and increases storage of belly fat.

If that wasn't bad enough, you still feel hungry because insulin blocks leptin, which is a hormone released by the brain that tells your body you are full. So, you may in fact be full, but your body thinks you are hungry, which causes you to over-eat. And, now you are craving more sugar because your pleasure-based reward center was triggered. So, you become addicted to sugar and nothing tastes good unless it's super sweet.

Let's compare that to 500 calories from broccoli. Like soda, broccoli is a carbohydrate. However, broccoli is relatively high in fiber and low in sugar, which means it is more slowly digested. When foods are slowly digested, they do not cause a spike in blood sugar or insulin. Consequently, you do not end up with inflammation, increased triglycerides, or fat stored around your belly. In contrast, the broccoli fills your stomach, which sends a signal to your brain that you are full. Soda does not do that. Also, the pleasure-based reward center is not triggered when you eat broccoli, which means you don't become obsessed with seeking out and devouring highly refined sugar. You also get a dose of phytonutrients, which increase your ability to detoxify, and vitamin C, which helps protect you from cancer and other inflammatory diseases. And, broccoli contains glucosinolates and sulphorophanes, which can help balance your sex hormones and reduce your risk of developing cancer.

I can go on, but I think you get the point: You can eat two different foods that have the same number of calories and end up with very different biological responses in your body.

One food can heal you while the other foods can make you sick – even though you consumed the same number of calories. So, I no longer count calories. It's a waste of time.

Joel: Whew! This is why I wanted to write this book with Sina. I like hitching my wagon to this horse because it's going to truth places. Now I'm thinking the problem with us humans is that we take the complex and make it simple, which is opposite what I said before. Okay, so we mess up everything; how about that?

This might be a good place to offer a couple of stories from the farmyard. They might not fit perfectly, but I think they are in the ballpark. The first involves how grass changes potency in a drought. When we have a herd of cows grazing along in a pasture, depending on time of season and rainfall, two identical-looking blades of grass can have huge differences in nutrient satiation.

In a drought the grass concentrates minerals. In a wet time, the grass contains way more water. It's the same grass and it's green. But the cows need 150 pounds of the wet grass to meet their daily nutritional requirements and they only need 100 pounds of the drought-stressed grass. You know wine makers love drought in their vineyards because it makes the grapes explode with sugar by concentrating minerals.

Now for one more story. If you recall from Practical Bite #9, many years ago, we suddenly had a problem in our broiler chickens. At about one week old, some would develop malformed feet that crippled them and soon they'd die of starvation because they couldn't walk to feed and water. I looked through my poultry books and found the culprit: curled toe paralysis. What caused it? Riboflavin deficiency.

The symptoms developed from friction in the nerve sheath. The friction set up a staph infection creating the paralysis. The orthodox cure, of course, was antibiotics. That's what the industry used. Being a lunatic farmer, I grabbed my nutrition books to find foods high in riboflavin. Greens and organ meats.

Suddenly I realized why it stopped when I put the birds out on pasture. As soon as they started eating the green grass, they got enough riboflavin and the problem stopped. But could I prevent it in the first place? I isolated the ones with the paralysis and fed them beef liver. Now remember, these were birds with a staph infection. It was like a miracle. In about

48 hours, these birds that literally pulled themselves around with their wings - it was really pitiful - were up and walking around. Their staph infection went away not with antibiotics, but with nutrition.

Here's the point. Neither the grass difference for the cows nor the diet difference for the chicks indicated a difference in calories. Calories did not change. It was nutritional density. That's what changed. If you really want to change your life, change your nutrition and forget about calories; we're far more complicated than a laboratory burn test and some assumption darts thrown on the table.

Sina: And, if you still want to count calories then keep this in mind: Not only is the method for calculating calories inaccurate, many peer-reviewed scientific studies have concluded that calorie labels themselves are inaccurate. In fact, it's common for the calorie content to be under-estimated. For instance, in 1993, a study published in the *Journal of the American Medical Association* concluded that, of the items tested, the calories listed on the food package were off by 85% in locally prepared foods and 25% in regionally sold foods. The authors concluded, "These findings suggest that food labels may be inadequate sources of caloric monitoring. Health care professionals should consider the accuracy of caloric labeling when advising patients to use food labels to help monitor their caloric intake."

More recently, a 2010 study published in the *Journal of the American Dietetic Association* concluded that some restaurant foods contained up to 200% more calories than what was listed on the menu. And, in 2014, a study revealed that common snack foods also contained more calories than what the label stated, but were still within the FDAs allowable limit. So, how much wiggle room does the FDA allow when it comes to telling you how many calories are in your food?

The label can be off by 20% and still be in compliance! So, if a cheeseburger actually contains 300 calories, it can be listed as only containing 240 calories. That's a big difference for someone who is basing their daily food intake on calories!

Joel: One of the privileges I've had in my life is getting acquainted with numerous gurus in the wellness field. Sina is one, but many others are out there. My favorite question whenever I meet a new one is "if you could get your clients to make one change in their life, what would it be?"

Normally the answer is some permutation of eating whole foods. It might be drinking soda or eating industrially-prepared processed foods. But in the end, it boils down to eating as close to whole as possible.

Sina: I agree. There are so many different diets on the market because nobody really knows what you should eat. There are a lot of opinions and a lot of disagreements. Even dietitians and nutritionists can't agree on what you should eat. However, eating more whole foods is the *one* thing that nearly every single person in the health field would agree on.

Eating whole foods comes with a lot of advantages. For instance, I'm often asked how I control my weight if I don't count calories. It's actually a simple answer; I eat whole foods. In fact, a study published in 2019 in the scientific journal *Cell Metabolism* connected processed foods with weight gain. Specifically, study subjects stayed at a research clinic for twenty-eight days, which allowed researchers to control their diet. Half of the group was fed processed foods for two weeks (such as sugary cereal, packaged muffins and sandwiches) and then switched to unprocessed food for the following two weeks (such as yogurt with fruit and stir fry over rice), while the other half did the reverse order. Subjects were allowed to eat as much as they desired. On average, when consuming processed foods, subjects ate roughly 500 more calories each day compared to the unprocessed diet. Consequently, subjects gained roughly two pounds in two weeks on the processed diet and lost roughly two pounds on the unprocessed diet, on average.

When you switch from a processed food diet to a whole food diet, you don't have to worry about counting calories because when you eat whole foods, your body self-regulates; it works the way it was designed to work. You stop over-eating because you are no longer blocking the hormonal signal that tells your body you are full. You stop craving sugar because you are no longer triggering the pleasure-based reward center in your brain that drives you to seek out and devour the sweetest foods. You stop storing belly fat because you are no longer spiking your insulin levels. And, you feel more emotionally stable because you are no longer on the roller coaster of sugar highs followed by that inevitable afternoon crash.

There is a caveat. Eating whole foods does not mean you get a free pass to eat fruit all day. Yes, fruit is a wonderfully nutritious whole food. But it still contains sugar. So, I eat it in moderation.

Joel: When Sina and I say whole foods, we're also not advocating a raw food diet or that you can't do anything with food. We're saying that coming into your kitchen, you want food with no ingredient list except that food.

Teresa makes our own granola for a breakfast cereal. I'm not a big grain eater, but every once in a while, a bowl of hearty granola is great - on a morning when she wants to sleep in. She's made this stuff for decades by buying whole components, mixing them together, and roasting them on a cookie sheet in the oven.

It makes the house smell like a bakery when she does it, but it's all basic ingredients like crimped oats, coconut flakes - all things that have no ingredient list. She puts it in a big one-gallon Tupperware® canister and I can enjoy it whenever I want. The only ingredients are: Crimped Oats; Coconut; Honey. Then you cook, bake, mix and whatever else you want to do with it.

Sina: Excellent point, Joel. Eating whole foods can be as simple as a salad with guacamole, sweet potato stuffed with veggies, vegetable soup, grilled chicken with steamed vegetables, or an apple with nut butter. It doesn't have to be complicated.

Do yourself a favor and stop counting calories. Stop picking your foods based on an inaccurate food label that perpetuates the myth that all calories are created equal. It's simply not true. So, don't base your food choices on a concept that you now know is wrong. Let the stress of calorie counting release from your mind and body.

Instead, eat whole foods - the foods God intended you to eat. Your body recognizes whole foods. It knows how to digest and metabolize them. And, whole foods contain the micronutrients that you need in the form that God intended you to eat. But, remember to choose organic!

Organic means the produce is not allowed to contain GMOs, be sprayed with most pesticides or herbicides, or grown using sewage sludge or most synthetic fertilizers. And it cannot be irradiated.

If you're not ready to switch to an all-organic diet, that's okay! Flip the page to find out how to make a slow transition while getting the most health benefits for your dollar.

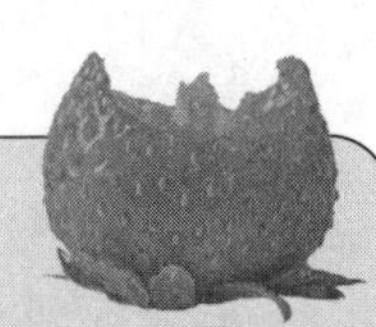

CHEW ON THIS

Check out this quote from David Baer, a research physiologist at the U.S. Department of Agriculture's Human Nutrition Research Center in Beltsville, Md. He's referring to listing calories on the food label:

"If we're going to put the information out there on the food label, it would be nice that it's accurate."

Practical Bite #36: Avoid The Dirty Dozen®; Choose The Clean Fifteen®

How? If you want to decrease your pesticide load but can only afford to buy organic fruits and vegetables when it matters the most, choose organic when they appear on the Dirty Dozen® list and choose conventional when they appear on the Clean Fifteen® list. The lists can be found at www.EWG.org.

Why?

Sina: When I switched from conventional to organic produce, I didn't change everything at once. It took time to adjust to the higher cost, so I took baby steps. I began by choosing organic versions of the produce that were most contaminated with pesticides. To help with that prioritization, I utilized the Dirty Dozen® and Clean Fifteen®.

Each year, the Environmental Working Group (EWG) releases an annual report of the dirtiest and cleanest produce. The Dirty Dozen® is a list of the 12 fruits and vegetables containing the most pesticide residues. The Clean Fifteen® is a list of the 15 fruits and vegetables containing the least amount of pesticide residues. Here are the lists from 2019:

DIRTY DOZEN™	CLEAN FIFTEEN™
Strawberries	Avocados
Spinach	Sweet Corn
Kale	Pineapples
Nectarines	Sweet Peas Frozen
Apples	Onions
Grapes	Papayas
Peaches	Eggplants
Cherries	Asparagus
Pears	Kiwis
Tomatoes	Cabbages
Celery	Cauliflower
Potatoes	Cantaloupes
	Broccoli
	Mushrooms
	Honeydew Melons

The EWG creates these lists by analyzing data from the U.S. Department of Agriculture and the U.S. Food and Drug Administration. Each year, those government agencies test some of our produce for the presence of certain pesticides and their residues. (Glyphosate is not included in the analysis.) The EWG analyzes those test results and provides an assessment for consumers - for free. For example, in 2018, they analyzed test results from more than 38,800 samples of 47 types of conventional produce. Some of their key findings included:

- A total of 230 different pesticides and pesticide break down products were detected.
- Most pesticide residues remained on the produce even after they were washed. Sometimes, pesticide residues remained even after the produce was peeled.
- 22 different pesticides or pesticide residues were found on one strawberry sample.
- Nearly 70% of non-organic samples contained at least 1 pesticide.
- 40% of all non-organic spinach samples contained DDT, which is a neurotoxic insecticide that is banned in the U.S.

Every year I share these results with my children, which helps strengthen their resolve. At the age of 5, I taught them the difference between organic and conventional. Then, I let them choose which version they wanted to eat. Both of my children chose organic, without hesitation. Even at that young age, they instinctively knew that eating chemicals was not good. In fact, they won't even eat the yummy foods at birthday parties unless it's organic. And, it's funny because when my children aren't getting along and they want to poke fun at each other, they will yell, "Oh yeah, well you eat conventional food!" My work is done.

Joel: That's hilarious!

Folks, if you're going to pick apples, some are within reach and others are higher up. Pick the easy fruit first is an old saying that developed when people still had personal knowledge about picking fruit. It makes no sense to climb up a precarious ladder and risk falling when down below you bushels of fruit await picking. You can never pick the whole tree at once; you have to start somewhere, so it may as well be the mostest the quickest.

Different fruits and vegetables have different susceptibilities to bugs, fungus, molds or whatever malady is out there. Some are simply harder to grow than others. Over the years, chemical protocols for the most fragile have been much higher than the ones less fragile.

Some conventional produce sees quite limited chemical application so switching to organic may not save you a lot of chemical exposure. But other produce is literally drenched in multiple applications. I know farmers who grow sweet corn, for example, who spray it every single week to make sure nobody ever sees a worm in an ear. That's what I call bathed in chemicals. It makes sense to start switching there for maximum protection.

You might wonder how today's produce in America can still contain DDT. It's been banned for decades, so why is it still showing up on our food? The answer may surprise you as much as it did me.

Believe it or not, a chemical company can manufacture a product in which DDT is a component, but since it's only part of the whole formula, DDT is neither listed on the label nor identified in any way as the product. This is more of that sleight of hand that the regulator/corporate fraternity contrives when they have their problem-solving sessions.

When the final compound breaks down, it breaks down into its constituent parts. Compounds do break down over time, but each has a different breakdown anatomy. For example, when chemical companies say "breaks down in the soil" they are partially true. The number one catalyst for detoxifying anything is organic matter. Organic matter is primarily carbon. Ever heard of carbon filters on water? Or chelation therapy? That's almost Roto-Rooter® carbon pumped through your veins.

Carbon loves to attach to things, including toxins. That's why compost piles are such detox wonders. Even the conventional poultry industry now recognizes that composting mortalities (chickens that die) is as good or better than incineration. On our farm, we compost everything that will decompose because it's the safest, easiest, best way to dispose of dead things. I've instructed my family many times that when I leave this earthly abode, I want them to throw my body in the compost pile; at least then it can help feed worms and grow stuff. It makes a great place for disposing wayward bureaucrats, too.

The point is that when the industry says "breaks down in soil" the question is what kind of soil? You can pour almost anything on high carbon soil and it'll break down into less toxic material. But most farmers are not using carbon-rich soil. The 5-10 percent organic matter soils that the Europeans found when they landed here have been gradually reduced to

1 percent or even less in some cases. On our farm, in half a century, we've taken the soils from 1 percent to a bit more than 8 percent with steady composting and good grazing management.

So how do we still have DDT showing up on our plates? Because if it's simply one of the ingredients, it's okay. The final product is not DDT and that makes it okay. But in the breakdown, however long that takes, the ingredients return to their pre-combination as part of the breakdown process. And the less organic matter in the soil, the slower the breakdown. That's what we need to understand.

Sina: If you haven't already switched to organic produce, pick the low hanging fruit first. Buy organic when produce appears on the Dirty Dozen® list and buy conventional when produce appears on the Clean Fifteen® list.

Practical Bite #37: Buy A Slow Cooker Or A Pressure Cooker

How? Go to a store that sells kitchenware, like Target® or Walmart®, and purchase either a slow cooker or a pressure cooker. Even easier, order one on-line.

Why?

Joel: Teresa and I are such fans of the slow cooker or crock pot that we give them for wedding gifts. These things can make your marriage go stratospheric because nobody needs to know anything about cooking to make fantastic meals. And it's so easy nobody is tired from kitchen prepping, leaving more time to enjoy marriage, you know. And more energy. Enough. Technically, slow cookers and crock pots are not the same thing, but they're pretty close and I'm not going to parse out the difference here.

Whenever someone asks me how to cook meat, especially, I ask them if they have a slow cooker. If our country is lacking one thing in the culinary space, it's kitchens with slow cookers. People, this is the most important utensil in the kitchen. Perhaps it's stigmatized by the word "slow" and people assume it means cooking is slow. Yes, cooking is slow, but that doesn't mean the meal is slow. In fact, we think this is the fastest way in the world to fix a meal. Before leaving for work in the morning, throw everything in. Frozen meat, some veggies like onions, carrots, potatoes. Any time after 4 p.m., dinner is ready.

If you get tied up and don't get home until 6 p.m., it's ready. If you really get tied up and don't get home until 8, it's still ready. It's not burned. It's not dry. It just sits there all day at 40 watts of power bubbling and filling the house with meal prep perfume and it's ready any time you want to eat. If you use a pretty slow cooker, you just move it to the table and it becomes the serving dish. It's nearly foolproof. Meat is always succulent and tender.

We think it's the fastest, easiest, most convenient way to fix a dinner. I see these sidebars about the 45-minute meal, or the 30-minute meal. Let me tell you, the crock pot offers a gourmet 10-minute meal. You just throw it in and leave; the machine does all the work.

Sina: When I started cooking all of our meals from scratch and trying to eat more whole foods, I was quickly overwhelmed and tired. It's a lot of work! But then, I started using a slow cooker and the process became so much easier. I was able to create an entire meal simply by throwing ingredients into the pot and walking away. And, cleanup was simple because it's just one pot.

One of my favorite kitchen strategies is to load my slow cooker with healing whole foods in the morning so that when dinner time rolls around, I can relax with my family instead of scrambling to find something "healthy" for us to eat. I also use the slow cooker to prepare batches of meals. For instance, I'll cook a stew, soup, or meat dish and then store it in small glass containers in the freezer. That way, I don't have to cook multiple times each day because I have ready-to-eat frozen meals already prepared. And, if I'm working late or I get sick with a cold or I just don't feel like cooking, I don't feel stressed about making dinner because I can simply re-heat one of my frozen homecooked meals.

I have an Instant Pot®, which serves as both a slow cooker and a pressure cooker. I use the pressure cooker function from time to time because it cooks my food so much faster than the slow cooker function. However, there's debate regarding whether or not food should be cooked in pressure cookers. The concern is that the high pressure may destroy some of the nutrients or beneficial elements contained within the food. So, I use it sparingly, but the pressure cooker was essential in my healing journey.

I couldn't digest any form of meat for years. I tried eating red meat, chicken, turkey, pork, fish and seafood, but nothing worked. Eating a single fork-full resulted in painful bloating and cramping. It was a huge problem because I also couldn't eat grains, beans, or legumes. Consequently, I was becoming deficient in protein. So, I began using the pressure cooker because, compared with the slow cooker, the high temperature forces more of the protein and connective tissue to break down, which means the meat is pre-digested to a greater extent. The strategy worked! I was able to eat small portions of meat and, therefore, quickly reverse the protein deficiency.

So, pressure cooking can be a useful tool if someone has difficulty digesting and absorbing nutrients. I still use the pressure cooker when I'm in a hurry because it cooks so much faster than the slow cooker. But, when time allows, I opt for the slow cooker. Regardless, using a slow cooker or pressure cooker is a huge timesaver. It's my favorite kitchen tool!

Practical Bite #38: Use Your Slow Cooker Or Pressure Cooker

How? Here's a quick and easy recipe to get you started:

Chuck Roast with Veggies

Ingredients:

4-pound chuck roast
2 onions, chopped
3 carrots, chopped
3 potatoes, peeled and cubed
2 celery stalks, chopped
1 cup water or beef broth
4 teaspoons onion granules
4 teaspoons garlic granules
2 teaspoons Real Salt®

Instructions:

Add water (or broth) to the bottom of the slow cooker. In a small bowl, combine seasonings. Rub seasoning mixture on all sides of the roast. Place roast in cooker and add vegetables. Place cover on slow cooker and cook on low for 8-10 hours. Enjoy!

Why?

Sina: Now that you have a slow cooker or pressure cooker, use it.

I laugh because when I first learned about the Instant Pot®, I told my husband I had to have it "right now." I was convinced that it would help me heal. So, I became relentless in my pursuit, like a bulldog. My husband finally said okay, with the caveat that I had to "actually use it." So, I promised to use it "all the time" and then rushed to order it online. I got the Instant Pot® in 2 days, and then it sat in the box in my pantry for nearly 6 months.

It wasn't that I didn't want to use it; I didn't know how to use it. And, at that point, I was so tired that it felt like one more daunting task added to my to-do list. But then, I got tired of listening to my husband make subtle comments about how I said I "needed it" and "promised" to use it. So, I took it out of the box, realized how easy it was to use, and never looked back.

Joel: This is such a great story, Sina, because it shows how intimidating new routines can be. This isn't the difference between your 10-year-old car and the 2-year-old car you just bought. When you sit in them, they both have a steering wheel, probably in about the same place, a gas pedal, ditto, and a brake, ditto. They're fairly similar.

But when you start cooking in an Instant Pot®, it's really different than using a frying pan on the stove or a roasting pan in the oven. It's a really different gizmo, and different gizmos are intimidating. Here we have someone as dogged and creative as Sina, and she can't bring herself to look at this new kitchen gadget for 6 months. It's like an imposter on my comfort zone. Yes, folks, we both get it.

On our farm, we have a zero-turn mower. Those of you who operate these things will laugh at me. It doesn't have a steering wheel. I'm scared to drive it. Yes, I've driven it a little, but it scares me to death. I'm afraid I'm going to run it into the swimming pool or through the flower bed. And that would not make Mama happy; we all know the end of that: when Mama ain't happy, ain't nobody happy. So fortunately, I have a couple of people, including my grandchildren, who run that thing like a pro. Glad I don't have to learn.

So, I get it. I get the new thing. But this isn't a lawn mower. It's not a Caribbean Cruise. It's your life, your health, your happiness, your integrity. Take it out of the box. Play with it. You'll be a pro in no time and, like Sina, will laugh at yourself that it intimidated you for so long. Goodness, you'd think it was a snake in that box.

Practical Bite #39: Don't Trust The "Gluten-free" Label

How? When you see a processed food labeled as certified "gluten-free," flip it over and read the ingredient list. If it contains any of the following ingredients, leave it on the grocery store shelf: wheat, barley, rye, oats, sorghum, millet, teff, triticale, spelt, durum, einkorn, emmer, corn, rice (except wild rice), groat, graham, amaranth, buckwheat, or quinoa.

And, look out for "hidden" sources of gluten. Food additives and GRAS chemicals are commonly derived from corn or wheat. Examples of ingredients that may contain gluten are: citric acid, MSG, natural or artificial flavors, natural or artificial colors, vegetable protein and gums, maltodextrin, and modified food starch.

Instead of trusting the "gluten-free" label, choose whole foods that are naturally gluten-free, such as: fruits, meat from 100% grass-finished cows, wild-caught fish, wild rice, and vegetables.

Why?

Sina: When I say "gluten," which foods come to mind?

Joel: I always think bread, crackers - anything baked with grains. I guess I'm like most people?

Sina: Yes, most people think that only wheat, barley, and rye contain gluten. That's because of the FDA. They decide what is considered gluten-free. But their definition is based on outdated information from World War II.

During the 1944 "Winter of Starvation," a pediatrician in the Netherlands observed improvements in his patients' symptoms during a wheat shortage. Consequently, he began testing other foods on his patients, including rye. These foods were staples in that country, at that time, so he naturally characterized gluten-containing foods based on what the people were readily eating.

Today, we know there is not just one gluten protein. There are hundreds of gluten proteins, which means there must be more that we haven't discovered yet. We also know that gluten isn't just in wheat, barley, and rye. Gluten is in *all* grains, including corn and rice. But the

FDA does not acknowledge this current information. Instead, they base the "gluten-free" food label on outdated and inaccurate information, which puts some of us directly in harm's way.

Remember when I said that corn surrounds you on all sides in the grocery store? That means gluten surrounds you on all sides in the grocery store. And, what are most certified "gluten-free" processed foods made of? Corn and rice!

That's concerning because we know that people who react to the gluten in wheat (alpha-gliadin) may also react to the entire family of gluten proteins – including the gluten in corn and rice. I did. That's one of the main reasons why I couldn't heal my gut for such a long time. I was eating "certified gluten-free" foods thinking I was helping myself heal. But I was actually misled by that label because those foods still contained gluten, in the form of rice and corn, and I reacted to them. Every time I ate those foods, my body mounted an immune response. That protective response created inflammation throughout my body, which contributed to the rapid progression of the autoimmune disease.

The bottom line is: the current food labeling laws do not support a true gluten-free lifestyle. They add to the confusion because they support a *traditional* gluten-free diet, which is a gliadin-free diet (i.e. gliadin is the type of gluten found in wheat, barley and rye). The current food labeling laws do not support a *true* gluten-free diet, which removes all forms of gluten.

Once I learned about the "gluten-free" labeling farce, I had a very difficult time letting go of my anger. I trusted that label. And, why wouldn't I? People with celiac disease and gluten sensitivity are told by doctors, dietitians, and nutritionists that those "certified gluten-free" foods are "safe" to eat. But that label kept me sick!

For a long time, I was angry with the FDA, food companies, and "experts" who were recommending those products. But then, I realized it's my responsibility to know what I'm eating. I knew that blindly trusting a label would come with consequences. But I didn't realize the consequence would be life-threatening. Trusting that label greatly contributed to my slow, agonizing decline in health. Once I made that connection, I decided to take responsibility for every bite of food that entered my mouth.

So, I began researching deeper into this area. You'll never guess what I found out!

Joel: I'm not sure I want to know!

Sina: Yes, this was the most upsetting part for me. The fact that corn and rice contain gluten, and the fact that they can make some people sick, is not new information. We have known **since the late 1970s** that gluten in corn can affect people with celiac disease and irritable bowel disease! A study published in *Clinical Experimental Immunology* in 1979 reported that people with Crohn's disease, ulcerative colitis and celiac disease had elevated antibodies when they ate corn. The authors concluded that the increase in antibodies suggested "increased mucosal permeability," which is another name for leaky gut!

Here's the kicker: The corn that was used in that experiment was the same corn used in the manufacture of Corn Flakes®. The authors of the study stated, "We are grateful to Kelloggs Ltd for suppling samples of the maize used in the manufacture of cornflakes." Yet, if you look at a box of Corn Flakes® on the grocery store shelf, it still carries the label "gluten-free."

Just to be clear, the maker of Corn Flakes® is not doing anything illegal. Technically, they are following the FDA labeling guidelines. The root of the problem is people, like me, who have blindly trusted this label. It's our responsibility to know what we put in our bodies. We must look beyond the labels in order to find the truth so that we can give informed consent.

Joel: We're certainly building the case for personal responsibility and freeing ourselves from dependency on government-approved labels. As this Practical Bite unfolds, Sina, I can feel people getting despondent and depressed, like "where do I turn?" Fortunately, you love research - you have an earned PhD for crying out loud - and you know the chemistry, the language. But the average person doesn't have that platform.

So, when you try to make it easier to absorb, to actually respond, you end up opting out of the supermarket. I know it sounds crazy, but this whole issue is what drives Paleo, Keto and other themes based on prehistoric norms. Rather than sifting through all the modern stuff, just skip the whole modern deal and build your own historically normal provenance. That begs the question: did anyone 200 years ago eat crackers?

That's a simple question, but it speaks to this issue because it helps us understand how profoundly abnormal modern western eating really is. I wrote a book about this called *Folks,*

This Ain't Normal. I'd love to see an anthropologist take the modern supermarket and compare the percentages of its contents to a larder from 200 years ago. People ate grain but it was very little. People ate apples but it was a lot more. That sort of thing. I think most of us cannot imagine how different our daily intake looks today compared to our forebears.

So, what's the safest thing to do? When I come to a chapter like this, I want to curl up in a fetal position and not face the world. It's that frustrating and discouraging. The sheer effort to vet things; it's maddening. So, what's the easiest thing to do?

For me, and Sina may disagree, it's just to opt out. I don't care if I have another slice of bread or a cracker the rest of my life. Really; I'm not kidding. Historically people did well on extremely simple diets. This is one of the things Dr. Weston A. Price found when he searched the world for cultures with many centenarians. Most had fairly simple diets. Milk, meat, eggs, nuts, some vegetables, and few grains, usually fermented in some way. You can live on a lot worse than this. I think I could live on eggs for a long time. I know people who have done milk fasts, where for weeks they only drink whole raw milk.

I'm not advocating craziness here; all I'm suggesting is that we don't have to be addicted to grain-based diets. And realize that all fake meat is grain based. That should give us all pause.

Sina: I agree that opting out is the safest option. Instead of trusting the "gluten-free" label, choose whole foods that are naturally gluten-free, such as: wild rice, fruits, meat from 100% grass-finished cows, wild-caught fish, and vegetables.

Let me add, there is a lot we don't know about gluten. For example, do gluten sensitive individuals *always* react to the glutens contained in corn and rice? Not necessarily. Research indicates that at least 50% of people will develop gastrointestinal inflammation and antibodies to corn, but we don't know the exact number yet. It's probably much higher than 50% because these populations can develop a decreased ability to make antibodies, and that's one of the main markers used to determine if there's a reaction to gluten.

My clients *always* do better when removing all sources of gluten from their diet, including all grains, as well as foods that contain gluten-mimicking compounds, such as: quinoa, buckwheat, amaranth, and dairy. The ones who don't remove all sources of gluten, usually don't make a full recovery. We see this pattern in the scientific literature as well.

Many studies have shown that the majority of the time, a traditional gluten-free diet (no wheat, barley, or rye) fails to fully heal the gut lining in celiac or gluten sensitive people. For instance, in 2009, an article published in *Alimentary Pharmacology & Therapeutics* concluded that after 16 months on a traditional gluten-free diet, only 8% of people healed their gut lining, 65% had persistent inflammation, 26% had no change, and 1% got worse. The authors concluded that, "Complete normalization of duodenal lesions is exceptionally rare in adult celiac patients despite adherence to [a traditional gluten-free diet]." In other words, the certified "gluten-free" foods are not helping people heal their gut and may actually be preventing them from healing.

But there is good news! As awareness increases, some scientific studies are calling for a re-evaluation of the use of corn and rice in "gluten-free" products. So, maybe we'll see a change in the market soon. But, for now, our grocery stores are filled with corn and rice. "Gluten-free" foods are still recommended by well-intentioned medical doctors and dietitians. And, the FDA has not announced any plans to revise their definition of "gluten-free."

But you can be the solution! Now that you know the truth behind the "gluten-free" label, harness your power:

- Share this information with friends and family so we can help others while also moving the market together.
- If you have tried the traditional gluten-free diet and still can't heal yourself, check your ingredient labels for gluten-containing compounds. It may be one of the triggers preventing you from achieving a full recovery.
- Instead of trusting the "gluten-free" label, choose whole foods that are naturally gluten-free, such as: wild rice, fruits, meat from 100% grass-finished cows, wild-caught fish, and vegetables.
- For a list of processed foods that I eat, visit www.HandsOffMyFood.com. But please keep in mind that unless you grow the food yourself or know your farmer, there's always a chance that your processed food could contain gluten. For instance, it's common for manufacturers to change ingredients or ingredient sources, to unknowingly mislabel products, or recall a product due to cross contamination. There's no guarantee when you put your trust in the label.

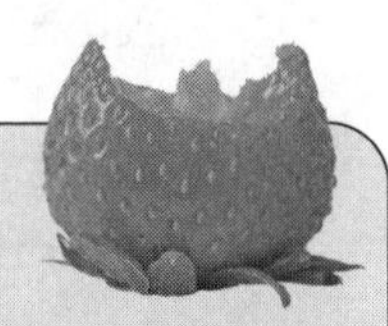

CHEW ON THIS

People who follow a traditional gluten-free diet are more susceptible to arsenic poisoning, largely from consuming rice. Even though rice contains a form of gluten, it is widely used to make "gluten-free" processed foods, such as: cakes, muffins, brownies, pudding, pie, cereal, and pizza. And, rice is susceptible to arsenic contamination (See Practical Bite #48).

It's common to rely heavily on "gluten-free" processed foods when someone decides to "go gluten-free." Since most Americans consume at least 75% of their calories from processed foods, it's logical that you'd simply swap out your gluten-filled processed foods for "gluten-free" processed foods, which contain rice. Therefore, it's not uncommon for people eating a traditional gluten-free diet to have higher levels of arsenic in their body. In fact, a study published in *Epidemiology* in 2017 reported that people eating a traditional gluten-free diet had 50% higher levels of arsenic in their urine compared with people eating a non-gluten-free diet.

If you choose to be gluten-free, you can reduce your chance of developing arsenic poisoning by consuming a *true* gluten-free diet, which does not contain any rice except wild rice. Wild rice is naturally gluten-free, but be sure to soak it first!

Practical Bite #40: Peel Your Apples

How? If you buy apples from your grocery store, look at the ingredient list for the wax that most likely coats the apple. If you are okay eating those ingredients then eat the apple. If not then remove the skin of the apple, or buy direct from a local farmer you trust.

Why?

Sina: If you don't want to eat wax, you most likely need to peel your apples! That's right, apples can be coated with wax. In fact, many fruits and vegetables are commonly waxed, including: apples, plums, peaches, tomatoes, peppers, cucumbers, and squash. Even organic produce can be waxed. Why are your fruits and vegetables waxed?

By the time your produce ends up in your local grocery store, it has gone on an adventure. Most of the time, your produce is grown in distant places, including: Mexico, Turkey, and even China! Since they travel an average of 1500 miles to reach you, the fruits and vegetables are often picked unripe, coated with wax, and then some are gas-ripened before arriving at your grocery store. The wax coating helps maintain freshness, inhibit growth of mold, and prevents bruising while on that long journey.

Aside from the fact that eating wax is not appetizing, the wax can contain corn derivatives. So, if you are trying to avoid gluten, peel your apples. The wax can also contain preservatives, fungicides, and plasticizers. But those chemicals must be safe for you to eat, right?

Maybe and maybe not. The FDA is in charge of regulating wax on your produce. Not surprisingly, the chemicals in the wax are commonly GRAS. So, you take a risk every time you eat wax-coated produce.

It can be tricky figuring out if your produce is coated with wax. According to the FDA Compliance Policy Guide for Safety and Labeling of Waxed Fruits and Vegetables, if produce is waxed, it must be clearly labeled. Specifically, when in package form, the label has to state that wax was applied. If the produce was received in bulk containers at the grocery store, it is the responsibility of the store "to display the food to prospective purchasers either with the labeling of the bulk container plainly in view or with a counter card bearing the required information."

In my experience, the ingredient list for the wax is challenging to find. I rarely find it on labels or packaging. Instead, I have to hunt for it by asking the produce manager for the ingredient list. If the manager does not have it, I ask for the name of the supplier of the specific fruit or vegetable I want to eat. Then, I call the supplier and ask for the ingredient list for the wax. Sometimes they are forthcoming and sometimes not. But it gets even trickier.

Sometimes the supplier is both a farmer and a distributor. In that case, either the farmer or the distributor could have applied wax to the produce. So, you have to call both! That's a lot of work, especially when you are hunting down wax ingredients for multiple fruits and vegetables. So, what do you do?

Unfortunately, you can't effectively wash off the wax by rinsing your produce under water. By definition, wax is not water soluble. There are products you can buy to remove the wax, but you won't remove all of the chemicals. In fact, nobody knows how much of the chemicals are absorbed into the produce. So, peeling your produce is a better strategy to reduce your exposure to the wax and accompanying chemicals.

But the peel is rich in fiber and other healing nutrients, including antioxidants. So, if you want to avoid the chemicals and the wax while still receiving the nutritive benefits provided by the skin, you can grow your own or find a local farmer you trust. With local purchases, since the produce doesn't travel far, it's not usually waxed.

But here's the catch: Even though their produce may only be on the truck for 24 hours or less, some local farmers who sell produce in grocery stores are using wax. Apparently, in order for local farmers to compete with bigger suppliers, the produce has to look just like the produce from big suppliers, which are often waxed. So, when purchasing from local farmers in the grocery store, you still need to make sure the produce was not waxed.

Fortunately, local farmers who sell directly to consumers – such as through Community Supported Agriculture (CSA) and farmers markets – do not usually wax their produce.

Joel: That's right, Sina, and ditto for nearly all vegetables. First, local producers who sell through the artisan market generally subscribe to a more natural approach to life, and that includes not waxing their vegetables. Second, conscientious local growers take better care of their vegetables because the eyes-to-plant ratio is more than it is in a large commercial outfit.

I was in Colorado on a large organic produce farm while they were picking zucchini squash.

A group of about six workers walked behind a gigantic processing machine that was pulled by a tractor. This processing machine had conveyors on it and it straddled the squash rows. The workers picked the zucchinis, tossed them into a hopper which fed a conveyer that brought them to a long sorting deck. Under a canopy, other workers sorted the incoming squash into various bins. The whole apparatus was probably 25 or 30 feet wide. When all the bins were filled, a fork lift put them on a trailer so they could be transported to a wash and pack facility. I hope by now you're thinking: "Wow, that's a lot of bumping and thumping." You'd be right to think that.

All that hard handling created blemishes which reduce eye appeal and actually open up the vegetable for deterioration. Kind of like skinning your knee opens your body up for infection. The point is that waxing has both cosmetic and shelf stabilization benefits. But your local produce grower doesn't have this kind of equipment, this kind of acreage, and these kinds of workers. At a smaller scale, more care occurs throughout the process, from planting to harvest. By patronizing that more careful grower, you not only vote for a different kind of production model, you also invest in a healthier alternative.

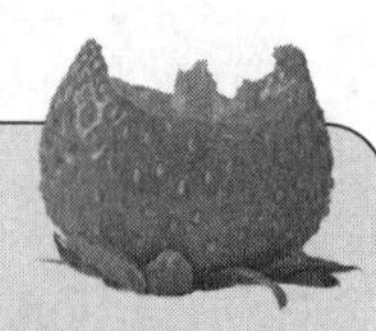

CHEW ON THIS

Wouldn't it be nice if new varieties of produce were chosen for nutritional content and taste? Most commercial varieties are not. They are chosen for ship ability. Think about it. If the winner of the variety contest is the one that can best handle jittering in the back of a tractor trailer for 2,000 miles, what's the criteria for selection? Cardboard. That's what ships without damage. You can ship cardboard from here to the moon and it's still cardboard. So, tomatoes taste and feel like cardboard. Apples feel like cardboard mush. If you want pop-in-your-mouth flavor and juice, along with super nutrition, you want to eat varieties that won't ship well.

Practical Bite #41: Cook A Whole Chicken

How? Here's a simple recipe to get you started:

Cook A Whole Chicken

Instructions:

1. Place a whole frozen chicken (roughly 5 pounds) in your slow cooker or pressure cooker.
2. Add 4 cups filtered water.
3. Directly on top of the chicken, sprinkle 2 teaspoons Real Salt®, 1 Tablespoon granulated garlic, 1 Tablespoon granulated onions, 1 teaspoon basil, 1 teaspoon sage, and 1 teaspoon oregano.
4. Coarsely chop 1 onion, 3 celery sticks, and 3 carrots. Add to the cooker.
5. Pressure cook on high for 8 minutes per pound of chicken, or slow cook on high for 4-5 hours or low for 8 hours. (If you plan to cook the chicken on low heat, it's recommended you first cook it on high heat for one hour before you switch to low heat to ensure the chicken is at the correct temperature for food safety purposes.)
6. When the chicken is done, the meat will fall from the bones and you'll have a broth in the bottom of the cooker. Remove the chicken from the cooker, and shred. Drizzle some of the broth on top of the chicken to moisten. Alternatively, if you want the chicken to have golden brown skin then transfer the whole chicken to a baking dish and broil in the oven for 4-5 minutes or until the skin turns brown and crispy.
7. Drink the broth as is or turn it into a nutrient dense bone broth by placing the bones back in the cooker along with one coarsely chopped onion, 3 cut-up celery sticks, 3 cut-up carrots, 2 teaspoons Real Salt®, 2 teaspoons vinegar, and just enough water to cover the bones. Cook on high pressure for 90 minutes or slow cook for 24-72 hours. Strain the bone broth through a cheesecloth. Store in the refrigerator for up to one week, or freeze for one year.

Why?

Joel: A few years ago, we had a problem with our checking account so Teresa went in to get it straightened out. One of the bank gals spent a couple of hours with her and finally figured it all out. The bank didn't charge us for it - probably because we're such a huge customer.

To express our gratitude, though, the next time she went to the bank, Teresa brought a care package. She put in a couple pounds of sausage, ground beef, a couple of steaks, two dozen eggs, and a young broiler chicken. The next day the bank lady called: "thank you for all that wonderful food, but what do I do with a whole chicken? I've never had one before."

Now folks, this lady was a grandma. She was a product of the 1960s, not the 1990s. The desperate state of our domestic culinary arts is epic. So, don't be scared of a whole chicken. You can even check on it throughout the day; don't worry, it won't run away. It'll still be in there cooking when you check on it.

Sina: Cooking with a whole chicken is a lost art. My parents used to cook a whole turkey on Thanksgiving, but the rest of the year we ate boneless, skinless chicken breasts when we could afford it. Consequently, I grew up not knowing how to cook a whole chicken.

When I got sick, I learned about the healing power of bone broth. It can help heal leaky gut syndrome by assisting in the repair of the lining of the gastrointestinal tract and supporting the growth of good bacteria in the gut. Thus, it also supports the immune system and helps lower inflammation. That means, bone broth can help you heal from food sensitivities and inflammatory diseases. Bone broth can also help improve digestion, decrease bloating and gas, promote healthy bowel movements, reduce joint pain, increase bone strength, provide stronger immunity against common colds, and promote healthy, youthful skin, nails, and hair.

In order to make broth, you need bones. Hence, the need to learn how to cook a whole chicken. The bones, skin, and connective tissues (such as ligaments and tendons) are packed with beneficial nutrients, including: collagen, gelatin, amino acids, antioxidants, and trace minerals like potassium and calcium. Think about all of the nutrients we throw away each time we don't utilize the bones, skin, and connective tissues. Those parts of the chicken are invaluable for our health. We're throwing away the best parts!

It's fascinating because while we readily discard the best parts, ancient cultures from around the world consumed them for thousands of years in various forms – including broth. Yet, most people I know don't consume broth nor do they know how to make it. This is another example of how we've lost touch with the power of food as we've become separated from our food supply.

Fortunately, we are slowly realizing the power of broth as more people are becoming chronically sick. In fact, broth has become a staple in many modern healing protocols, such as the GAPS diet (Gut and Psychology Syndrome Diet). There's even a bone broth fast that is used as a tool to help reverse disease, digestive disorders, food sensitivities, fatigue, pain, and brain fog.

Joel: Right now, in 2020, and I expect this to hold for a long, long time, you can buy a genuine 5-star pastured whole Polyface chicken for less per pound than industrial fecal boneless skinless breast at Wal-Mart®. Every person who buys regular brand-name boneless skinless breast from a supermarket would be financially ahead and certainly nutritionally ahead to buy a whole chicken from a local authentic pastured food-crafter.

"But I don't know what to do with the rest of the chicken," some people lament. Well, pull it off the bones and make a casserole. Melt the bones in your slow cooker and make bone broth, like Sina admonished. Few things pack the punch of real pastured chicken broth; it's like the elixir of the gods. And I'm not saying that to sell chickens; well, maybe I am. But around the bones, in the bones, and in that dark meat lurks tremendous nutrition your microbiome is begging for; satiate it.

Sina: I buy my whole chickens from Polyface, but if you're not ready to step onto the farm, you can still save money by purchasing a whole chicken in the grocery store, compared with buying individual chicken parts. For instance, a whole organic chicken at my local grocery store is currently $2.99 per pound while boneless chicken breasts are $5.99 per pound. And, if you want the breasts air chilled, it will cost you $7.99 per pound. Even organic chicken thighs are more expensive than a whole organic chicken, at $3.99 per pound.

When I used to buy boneless, skinless chicken breasts, the price per pound was more than a whole chicken but I thought I was getting a bargain because I didn't have to deal with the bones and skin. Who eats bones and skin? Now I know that I was paying more and missing out on the benefits of bone broth, collagen, and the many other nutrients contained in those chicken parts.

So, buying the whole chicken is a win-win: you save money while utilizing the full spectrum of nutrients that a chicken has to offer.

Practical Bite #42: Cook One Meal Using Whole Foods

How? Cooking with whole foods can be intimidating. Start with easy recipes and work your way up to more complex meals. Here are a few recipes to get you started (adjust the quantities in each recipe based on your needs):

Egg Muffins

Instructions:

Heat oven to 350°F. Line 5 strips of uncured bacon in a large glass casserole dish, making sure the individual strips do not overlap. Cook for roughly 20-25 minutes or until reaches desired doneness, turning once. Break or cut into small pieces. Set aside.

Sauté ½ cup diced onions in avocado oil or grass-finished butter over medium heat until tender. Add roughly 2 cups diced vegetables to the pan, such as: mushrooms, bell peppers, or spinach. Sprinkle with Real Salt®. Cook until tender then set aside.

Wisk together 12 eggs in a bowl. Set aside. Grease muffin tin with oil or butter. Pour beaten eggs into muffin tins, filling ¼ of the way.

Next, add cooked vegetables and bacon to each muffin tin. Evenly distribute the remaining beaten eggs into the tins. Bake for 18- 20 minutes.

Let cool then remove from tins. To re-heat egg muffins, cut a slit on top of the muffin and place a pat of grass-fed butter into the cut then warm in toaster oven.

Muffins keep for 5 days in the refrigerator or a month in the freezer.

Chicken Salad

Instructions:

Cook a whole chicken as outlined in Practical Bite #41. Shred the chicken from the bone.

Chop lettuce, tomato, cilantro, carrots, celery, bell peppers, jicama, and any other vegetable you desire. Place shredded chicken on top of salad. Add sliced avocado.

For a quick dressing, drizzle avocado oil over salad, squeeze a lemon wedge on top (or add a splash of vinegar), and lightly sprinkle with Real Salt®.

For a more flavorful dressing, add the following ingredients into a glass container and shake until combined (adjust salt as needed):

1 cup avocado oil or extra-virgin olive oil
1 Tablespoons coconut vinegar
4 Tablespoons water
1 teaspoon freshly squeezed lemon
4 teaspoons Italian seasoning
1 teaspoon salt
1 teaspoon honey or maple syrup (optional)

Chicken and Broccoli

Instructions:

Cook a whole chicken as outlined in Practical Bite #41. Or, place bone-in chicken thighs on a glass pan, drizzle avocado oil on top and bake on middle rack at 350°F for 50 minutes or 425°F for 35 minutes. Bake until there is no pink at the bone and juices run clear.

To steam broccoli, add water to a pot and place the steamer inside the pot. Cover with lid. When water is hot and steamy, add the broccoli florets into the steamer basket. Cover with lid and cook for 5-6 minutes. If you overcook the broccoli, it will lose its vibrant green color.

Place broccoli and chicken on plate. Generously drizzle avocado oil on top of chicken and broccoli, and sprinkle with Real Salt®. Garnish the plate with chopped watermelon.

Sautéed Greens

Instructions:

Heat avocado oil or grass-finished butter in pan on medium heat. Chop an onion and greens of your choice, such as: kale, spinach, swiss chard, or collards. Add a handful of onion to pan, if desired, along with the stems of the greens. Sauté until onion softens.

Then, add the leaves of the greens. Stir gently until the greens begin to wilt, roughly 3-5 minutes. Just before removing from heat, add freshly minced garlic and Real Salt®.

If desired, add a squeeze of lemon juice, using fresh lemons. If the change in color of the greens bothers you, blanching and shocking the heartier greens before sautéing can help maintain their color.

Naked Burger with Yucca (or Sweet Potato) Fries:

Instructions:

Make a quick and easy meal by purchasing a bag of yucca fries or sweet potato fries (read the ingredient label to make sure nothing is added, except possibly non-iodized salt).

Cook fries based on the recipe on the bag. While the fries are baking, heat avocado or coconut oil in a large pan over medium heat.

Shape hamburger meat into the desired number of patties. Cook in pan until patties reach desired doneness. Serve patties on a bed of lettuce with tomato slices, avocado slices, pickles or sauerkraut, and sprinkle with Real Salt®. Yucca fries are delicious dipped in guacamole.

To quickly make guacamole: mash one avocado in a bowl with a fork. Squeeze half a lime into bowl. Add ¼ teaspoon Real Salt®, ¼ teaspoon granulated onion, and a minced clove of raw garlic. Mix together.

Chicken Fajita Bowl

Instructions:

The morning before you want to eat this meal, soak wild rice as outlined in Practical Bite #48 and marinade the chicken as follows: add 1/4 cup avocado oil or olive oil, 2 teaspoons granulated onion, 2 teaspoons granulated garlic, 2 teaspoons Real Salt®, and 2 Tablespoons ground cumin to a glass container and mix together.

For spicy chicken, add ½ teaspoon chili powder to the marinade.

Place two chicken breasts in the container and coat with the marinade. Seal and refrigerate overnight.

The next day, cook rice as outlined in Practical Bite #48. Then, add avocado oil or coconut oil to bottom of sauté pan. Once hot, add thinly sliced onions along with red, green, and yellow bell peppers. Sauté until the peppers are soft and then remove to a plate.

Add about a tablespoon of oil to the pan. Then, place the marinated chicken meat in the pan and cook for 5-7 minutes until no longer pink inside. Serve over rice with guacamole and tomatoes.

Why?

Joel: You have to crawl before you walk. Doing something is far better than doing nothing. Even if the something is the wrong thing. Even if the something doesn't turn out very well. If your whole foods are sourced correctly, you'll be surprised how forgiving they'll be on the tongue.

I had a lady in the farm store the other day who had her 6-year-old son with her. He was a tiny, anemic-looking child. His mother said he was finicky and simply wouldn't eat. She bought a couple dozen eggs, noting over her shoulder as she left "he doesn't like eggs." Two days later she called on the phone.

"My son is eating six eggs at a sitting!" she said excitedly. It wasn't because she was a good cook. It was because the eggs changed. In our home, we use a crock pot or slow cooker all the time. You can put well-sourced grass-finished beef in there and it'll be wonderful without any salt, pepper or other seasonings. Cooking doesn't have to be intimidating if you use great provenance and simplicity.

Sina: I agree, cooking with whole foods doesn't have to be complicated. It can be as easy as steaming vegetables and grilling a piece of meat, or making a salad with home-made dressing. But, when I started cooking whole foods, I felt very insecure because I was taught how to cook using primarily processed foods. So, using whole foods to make a meal felt unfamiliar. Hence, I followed recipes to the letter! Then, one day all of that changed.

I decided to make mashed parsnips using a recipe from a well-known chef. I followed the recipe exactly. When the parsnips were ready, I was so excited to take that first bite! I called my kids into the kitchen to try my newest food adventure. They bounced into the room shouting, "Me first! I want to try it first!" I handed each of them a spoon full of my parsnip masterpiece, which they quickly shoved into their mouths. Almost immediately, their smiles turned into a look of utter disgust. I said, "It can't taste that bad." So, I put a spoonful in my mouth and, almost immediately, I made the same yuck face. My parsnip masterpiece was awful! Even my dogs wouldn't eat it! All five of my dogs left the mashed parsnips untouched in their bowls.

That experience shattered my fear of cooking with whole foods because I realized that I don't have to be "perfect," and not every dish I create is going to taste good. And, that's okay. Afterall, if a famous chef published a dish that inspired the yuck face, surely there's room for everyone to grow.

So, now I view cooking with whole foods as an adventure; an experiment where sometimes I'll fail and sometimes, I'll hit a home run. Of course, following recipes from well-known chefs will undoubtedly lead to more home runs. But I find joy, and a sense of accomplishment from creating my own recipes. And, now I'm comfortable in the kitchen so I don't even measure ingredients most of the time. My kids say that watching me cook is like watching a cooking show because I'll smell the spice to decide which flavor to add and then I'll just throw some in the pot. Or, I'll create a new cookie recipe by asking my body which ingredient combinations sound good. It's a lot of fun, and it's freeing to step outside of the recipe box and let your imagination run wild! Although, it does get me into trouble when I'm trying to write down recipes to share.

Joel: Mastery requires repetition. We all know wizards in the kitchen. You don't have to be one, but I guarantee you that you'll become one if you spend any time there.

Again, we tend to be successful on the things we put our attention on. If you really put effort into something, chances are you'll do better at it than the thing you neglect. Rather than feeling inadequate in the kitchen, make up your mind to do one thing in there. Just one. It's okay if it's not perfect. Don't burden yourself with too difficult a goal up front. Commit to one thing; don't worry about the second thing.

In our house, Teresa does virtually all of the cooking. Whenever I do a media interview and people ask me if I cook, I smile and respond: "I've only cooked twice in my life. Two times for about 9 months." Women get it right away. Men it takes a little longer. Yes, Teresa's two pregnancies were not the most enjoyable times of her life.

You know what I did? It was barbaric, but it worked. I simply put equal portions of canned tomatoes (from our garden), canned squash (from our garden), and canned green beans (from our garden) in a pot and heated them up. Then I sprinkled cheese over the top - or dumped cheese, if you know what I mean - and it was wonderful. In the morning I threw a piece of meat in the crock pot and it was ready for supper. So, I'd put my mishmash, the crock pot meat, and then applesauce (from apples we purchased and made our own applesauce), plus some pickled beets or pickles on a plate, and call my bride to supper.

That was the default supper anytime she was not feeling well. Sometimes that's what I ate for days on end. But it's good stuff; it's fine. And I knew the routine was temporary. I love eggs. Breakfast is my favorite meal of the day and the one I feel most comfortable doing. I do a 60-second omelet that's to die for. If you throw in some cheese, diced onions, diced peppers, and diced tomatoes, oh my, it's heaven. Who can't eat that a couple of times a day? Meals don't have to be complicated.

By the way, if you've noticed, a common theme of my cooking is cheese. I figure you can put enough cheese on a cow pie and make it delicious. Some extra cheese can cover up a multitude of sins. So, use liberally.

Sina: I'll add one caution: I never use nonstick pans or nonstick utensils because they are the most prominent source of the man-made chemical PTFE (polytetrafluoroethylene); the brand name is Teflon®.

PTFE belongs to a family of compounds called PFAS (per- and polyfluoroalkyl substances), which are known as "forever chemicals" because some of them accumulate in the environment and body. According to the EPA, "exposure to PFAS can lead to adverse health outcomes in humans." Examples include: tumors, reproductive and development issues, liver and kidney issues and immunological effects in animals. Among humans, exposure can lead to cancer, thyroid hormone disruption, low infant birth weight, and increased cholesterol.

The two most well known PFAS chemicals include:

1. PFOA – formerly used by DuPont® to make Teflon®
2. PFOS – formerly used to make 3M's Scotchgard®

Both of those chemicals were banned in the United States after serious health issues became known. So, a new generation of PFAS chemicals were created to replace them. Would you cook your food on pans that were made using the new generation of chemicals?

I choose not to. Instead I use stainless steel pots and pans. Cast iron is also a good option. In terms of cooking in the oven, I use clay pots, glassware and cookie sheets that are not coated with nonstick material.

Practical Bite #43: Save Time & Money By Batching & Storing

How? To save time and money while adding convenience into your life, prepare large batches of food and store them in single serving glass jars. Here's an easy meal to get you started. It's called Salad in a Jar:

Salad in a Jar

Instructions:

1. Decide how many jars of salad you want to make. If you want to eat one salad each day of the week then use 7 jars, such as Mason jars. Arrange the jars in a line on the counter.
2. Chop all of your preferred salad ingredients. Don't add avocado or any items that might brown until you are ready to eat the salad. To save time, use a food processor to grate carrots. Then, switch the blade and use the food processor to slice cucumbers, celery, beets, and anything else that can be prepared without having to get out the knife and chop it by hand. If you have kids or grandkids, line up the ingredients on a cutting board, like large mountains, to make it fun for them to create their own salad jars.
3. Begin making your salads by adding salad dressing to the bottom of each glass jar.
4. Next, add the ingredients that you don't mind exposing to the salad dressing (such as celery, peppers, tomatoes, carrots, cucumbers and beets). This first layer will protect the other layers from getting soggy.
5. Then, add the ingredients you don't want swimming in the dressing, but are still okay if they get wet (such as mushrooms, beans, lentils, corn, peas and broccoli).
6. Delicate ingredients, like cheese and hard-boiled eggs, are added next.
7. Then, add rice, couscous, pasta or quinoa (Omit if grain-free, except for wild rice and grain-free pasta).
8. Add lettuce as the last vegetable.
9. Top with nuts, seeds, croutons, or any other items that you don't want exposed to moisture. (For a grain-free crouton recipe, visit www.HandsOffMyFood.com)
10. Place lids on all 7 jars. Refrigerate; making sure the jars remain up-right so the dressing does not touch the lettuce. The shelf-life will depend on the ingredients you selected. Typically, lettuce lasts 7 days without browning. Just prior to eating, add avocado and freshly grated ginger and turmeric.

Why?

Joel: A few years back once-a-month cooking was the rage. Do you remember that? The whole point was to take one day a month (or two) and do all the cooking for the month; all the meal prep. It was developed by a busy home school mom who had to create time in her life. By compressing all the cooking into one or two days a month, the total time spent in the kitchen dropped substantially. That may be extreme, but today's technology of freezing and refrigerating makes such a notion possible when it wouldn't have been a scant century ago.

One of the most intriguing things to me, in this domestic culinary space, is that at the very time in history when we've never enjoyed so many labor-saving techno-gadgets, we've never been more reluctant to prepare our own food. As food prepared outside the home escalates north of 50 percent these days, our techno-glitzy kitchens sit idle, and that's a shame. Never in history has cooking been more efficient.

Never before has from-scratch cooking been easier. And yet here we are buying highly processed foods and going out to eat routinely. Right when we got liberated from the drudgery of the wood fire and wooden water bucket, we decided to abandon the heart of the home. This may go down as the greatest cultural contradiction in history. You can't go beyond labels without ending up in your kitchen. On the beyond label journey, at some point you will find yourself parked in the kitchen. Embrace it. Rest in it. Love it. Hug your fridge.

Sina: I admit it; I'm a fridge hugger! I love creating healthy meals in my kitchen, as long as I'm not stressed. My biggest stressor is feeling like I don't have enough time. And, that's why I batch cook.

Hands down, batching food has been my biggest time saver in the kitchen. For instance, every time you want to make a salad for lunch, think about how long it takes to get all of the ingredients out of the refrigerator, get out the cutting board and knife, chop up each item, get out a bowl to hold the salad, clean the cutting board and the knife, and put away any leftover ingredients. The time adds up quickly.

Now imagine if you made 7 salads at the same time – one salad for each day of the week. You only have to take the ingredients out of the fridge once, get the cutting board and knife out once, and clean the cutting board and knife once. You do chop up more of each ingredient, but that doesn't take much additional time since you're already chopping. Overall, you save time because you only do the prep work and clean up once, but you get 7 meals!

It takes me roughly 30 minutes to make 7 Salads in a Jar. I think it's pretty amazing that you can make your lunch for the entire week in just 30 minutes! Plus, the salads store well and are portable. I simply grab one and take it on-the-go. As long as it stays up-right, the lettuce remains crisp.

The key is to make the salads when you are not stressed or rushed. Don't wait until you are rushing out the door for work or you're really hungry. Make the salads when it's convenient for you. Maybe it's while streaming a podcast or watching a show on television. I make Salads in a Jar as soon as I return home from the grocery store, which saves even more time because the groceries are already out on the counter. One week, I made the mistake of putting away the groceries before I made the salads. I was tired and thought, "I'll get to it later." The week passed and I never got around to making those salads. As a result, I lost my free time that week! So, now I plan ahead by making sure I have enough time and energy to make the salads as soon as I get home from the store.

Salads were the first meal I batched, but practically any meal can be prepared in large batches and stored in glass jars or containers. It's a great way to save time in the kitchen and add the convenience of ready-to-eat frozen meals back into your life. Here are some of my favorites:

- ❖ I make large batches of soups, stews and broths and store them in single-serving jars in the freezer.
- ❖ I also cook 2 pounds of ground beef at one time. I use half of the meat that week and freeze the other half to be used later. That way, if I want to make pasta sauce, for example, it takes less time because the meat is already cooked. I just add it to the sauce.
- ❖ Likewise, when mushrooms are on sale, I sauté large batches and freeze them in small glass containers to be used later in sauces or a frittata.
- ❖ Instead of cooking one package of bacon, I cook 4 at a time in the oven using multiple glass pans. I slightly undercook the bacon and store half of it in the freezer. When

I'm ready to eat it, I finish cooking the bacon in the toaster oven by heating for a few minutes at 350°F.

- ❖ When cooking spaghetti squash or yams, I cook twice the amount I need for dinner and store half in the freezer. To save more time, I prepare the yams before storing them. For instance, if I want to eat mashed yams for dinner, I cook a large batch of yams in the oven, then I puree all of them in the food processor with coconut milk and cinnamon. I store half in jars in the freezer for ready-to-eat meals.
- ❖ When organic vegetables are on sale, I buy large quantities and batch cook them to add to my ready-to-eat frozen meal collection. Some vegetables freeze better than others. I don't freeze broccoli or spinach, for example. But green beans and brussels sprouts freeze exceptionally well.

Some less obvious examples of foods you can batch and store in the refrigerator in single serving jars include: no bake oatmeal, yogurt parfaits, bacon and eggs, and burrito bowls. Again, if you make 7 jars at one time, you have breakfast or lunch already made for the entire week! You can even batch guacamole. I started storing batches of guacamole in jars to save money. When avocados are on sale, I purchase a bunch and create large batches of guacamole, which I store in the freezer in glass jars. Because of the method I use, only a small amount of browning occurs, which mixes right into the guacamole once defrosted. For the recipe, visit www.HandsOffMyFood.com

Joel: One of Teresa's favorite time savers is pre-cooked chicken. We use stewing hens for this process. These are laying hens who have come to the end of their productive life. Although they are tough, they have orange fat and a taste that's out of this world. All gourmet chefs prefer them for making stock.

Using a large roaster pan, we can fit about 8-12 of these old stewing hens. At 350 degrees for 4 hours, the meat literally falls off the bones. We let it sit for an hour to cool down and then pick it all off. We pour the inch and a half of golden broth off and freeze that in quart containers. With a pair of scissors, she cuts up all that chicken into chunks and puts it in quart freezer containers (about 2 pounds per). This procedure gives us a whole inventory of precooked, pre-chunked chicken ready for a casserole at a moment's notice.

It's a life saver when you have 30 minutes to fix supper. Or when unexpected guests show up. You can put on a real feast in just a few minutes because you batched a cooked chicken inventory beforehand. Talk about freedom.

Sina: I love that idea! I'm going to incorporate pre-cooked chickens into my kitchen plan. Thanks Joel!

One last tidbit to close out this Practical Bite. When re-heating left overs, I encourage people to use something other than a microwave. I re-heat food using the oven, or a toaster oven, or on the stove using stainless steel pans. We got rid of our microwave a few years ago when I realized that I was spending a lot of time and money on procuring and cooking the highest quality foods and then I radiated them in the microwave!

Research suggests that microwaving your food may actually change the structure of some of the compounds, including: amino acids, fatty acids, vitamins and phytonutrients. In fact, some studies have reported that when food is microwaved, it can result in a reduction in vitamins, antioxidants, and phenolic compounds, as well as inactivation of some healing components. So, don't work against your goal by microwaving your left overs. It takes a little longer to re-heat food using a toaster oven, but it's worth it!

Practical Bite #44: Eat A Daily Helping Of Microbes From Ferments

How? Buy unpasteurized fermented foods from reputable sources or make your own. Almost any fruit or vegetable can be fermented. Here's a recipe for sauerkraut to get you started:

Sauerkraut

Ingredients:

1 large head of shredded cabbage
2 Tablespoons Real Salt® or Himalayan Salt

Instructions:

1. In a large glass bowl, mix cabbage with salt. Let sit for 10 minutes.
2. Next, massage the cabbage for about 10 minutes to release the juices.
3. Then, pack the mixture into a large glass container (such as a wide mouth mason jar). Make sure all of the cabbage is submerged at least 1-inch below the liquid to prevent spoilage. Add filtered water to cover, if needed. You can also tuck an extra cabbage leaf on top to make sure all of the cabbage is submerged. Cover container tightly with lid.
4. Place in a cool location on a plate for 3 days. Check every day to make sure cabbage is completely submerged in liquid.
5. After 3 days, store in refrigerator. You can eat it after 3 days, but it improves with age. Store in airtight container in the refrigerator for up to 6 months.

Why?

Sina: I used to think of microbes as "bad." Hence, I tried to get rid of them in my house and on my body. I used antimicrobial soaps, antimicrobial hand sanitizers, antimicrobial house hold cleaners to "disinfect" my home from microbes that could be lurking on the door knobs or bathroom counters, and I used antimicrobial sprays to kill the microbes that could be floating in the air. And, when I caught a cold, I dutifully took the antibiotics that are handed out like candy in many doctor's offices. In a nut shell, I believed what the medical establishment and media have been pedaling for decades – microbes are "bad" and must be killed or they can make you sick.

Society is currently fighting a war on microbes. And we're losing – quite badly, I might add. Remember superbugs? They are microbes that are resistant to most antibiotics, which means if you get an infection from a superbug, antibiotics most likely can't help you. I had MRSA, so I know first-hand how serious superbugs can be. It took two rounds of very potent antibiotics to beat the MRSA down to a level where I could function, and it still came back. So, I understand the fear around superbugs. But the media and medical establishment use that fear to push antibiotics and antimicrobials. Case in point: you can find antimicrobial hand sanitizer receptacles at the entry of most hospitals, doctor's offices, and grocery stores. And, almost every Mom I know carries a small bottle of antimicrobial hand sanitizer in her purse. Again, I understand the fear. But, let's stop for a moment and asked ourselves, "Why do we have superbugs?"

We created superbugs! They are a result of us trying to kill off microbes. In an attempt to sterilize our offices, homes, food, and bodies, we have liberally used antimicrobials. Each time you use an antimicrobial, it places an environmental pressure on the microbes and they adapt accordingly. In other words, they get stronger. As they get stronger, they become resistant to the current antibiotics. So, scientists have to create new, stronger antibiotics. And, then the microbes adapt to those new antibiotics and become even stronger – hence the term "super bugs." It's a vicious cycle we have created. And, scientist say that if we continue down the current path, in the end, the microbes will likely win. So, what can you do about it?

Don't be lulled into fear mongering. Microbes have gotten a bad rap, but these misunderstood tiny miracles are essential for your life and longevity. Remember, you are more microbe than human. So, when you kill them off, you are killing off pieces of yourself. Consequently, you are more susceptible to developing an inflammatory or chronic disease. Simply stated: You would die without your microbes.

While it's true that pathogenic microbes can make you sick, most microbes do not. Again, it comes back to balance. I don't like to use the terms "good" and "bad" microbes because all microbes serve a purpose and are not "bad" unless they are not kept in check. But, for simplicity, dysbiosis is commonly explained by stating there are "good" bacteria and "bad" bacteria and when you don't have enough of the "good" guys, the "bad" guys can increase to a level that promotes disease. If you recall, that's what happened to my son when he developed symptoms of autism, and that's also why I developed MRSA.

Fortunately, I no longer have MRSA. But, it's not because I took antibiotics. I don't have MRSA because my body fought it off after I gave it the microbes it needed to rebalance my microbiome. Initially I used probiotic supplementation, which was a fantastic way to jump start my efforts toward rebalancing my gut. But I got caught in the common probiotic trap – I relied on probiotics long-term instead of transitioning to better food and lifestyle choices.

You simply cannot develop a healthy, balanced, *diverse* microbiome by relying on probiotic supplements. They provide a very large quantity of only a handful of microbes. Relative to the number of microbes naturally present on and in our bodies, probiotic supplements create a sort of monoculture, thereby decreasing your diversity. So, even though those microbes are considered "good," too much of a good thing can be bad.

In fact, you can actually develop small intestinal bacterial overgrowth (SIBO) from having too many "good" bacteria – such as an overgrowth of *Lactobacillus* or *Bifidobacterium* species. And, since most probiotics currently on the market contain large quantities of *Lactobacillus* or *Bifidobacterium* species, you can end up with too many of those "good" microbes, making your condition worse. Thus, while I initially relied on probiotics, I transitioned to fermented foods.

Compared to probiotic supplementation, fermented foods provide a *diverse* array of "good" microbes while also providing B vitamins, enzymes, and organic acids, which can stimulate the growth of "good" bacteria. Plus, there are many types of fermented foods to choose from, such as: sauerkrauts, vinegars, kombucha, yogurt, kefir, tempeh, natto, wine, beer, cured meats and sourdough bread. Cultures have consumed fermented foods for longer than we've been practicing agriculture and it's actually easy to do. Let's take sauerkraut, for example. Sauerkraut is fermented cabbage. Essentially, microbes (such as yeast and bacteria) that are naturally present on the cabbage, your hands, and in the air digest the sugars in the cabbage. It's a win-win because the sugar content of the food decreases while the beneficial bacterial count increases.

Fermented foods are relatively simple to make and can offer huge benefits to your health. They can improve digestion, help mitigate infections, including *H. pylori*, and help manage inflammatory diseases such as arthritis, cancer, and diabetes. Studies have also shown that fermented foods can decrease anxiety.

You can save money by making your own fermented foods, but there are good store-bought options available when you just can't find the time. Remember to always read the ingredient label because sugar may be added. Also, sometimes the beneficial bacteria have been killed off or inactivated through processes like pasteurization, baking, or filtering. So, I buy raw sources from reputable companies when I don't have any homemade ferments available.

On a side note, some people cannot tolerate fermented foods. For example, people who have SIBO, Candida overgrowth, or histamine intolerance may experience worsening symptoms when consuming fermented foods. When I started eating fermented foods during my healing journey, even one teaspoon resulted in GI discomfort, including gas and bloating. So, I consumed a soil-based probiotic supplement until my body was ready to transition to ferments.

Joel: Believe it or not, refrigeration is a fairly modern invention. In our myopic tendency, we assume that the way things are is the way they've always been. A healthy reminder that we live in aberrant times with indoor plumbing, supermarkets, and refrigeration keeps us appreciative of food history. That humans have lived a lot longer — a lot longer — without refrigeration than with it may sound peculiarly unprogressive or even cultishly nostalgic, but our modern blip in historical terms should be kept in perspective to protect us from unwise directions. The refrigerated and frozen aisles in the supermarket may indicate a newfound access to abundance and food security, but they also represent an unprecedented change in the way we preserve and store food.

That change, in turn, dramatically changes what enters our mouths, our stomachs, and our digestive tracts. Connecting the history to today is the link that illustrates the magnitude of our changes. I'm convinced, especially after spending lots of time with millennials, that not 3 percent ever sit and meditate about how profoundly different the material entering their mouth is from the material entering the mouth of great-great-grandma in 1850. The average person today, for some strange reason, thinks frozen pizza, squeezable cheese, and clam shells of refrigerated micro-greens from 2,000 miles away was commonly ingested in 1850. It was not.

While great-great-grandma was much more prone to die in childbirth, or die from infections caused by burns (those hoop skirts were a terror with open hearth cooking) or to get any number of infectious diseases from lack of sanitation, she did not die from cancer, heart disease, Type 2 diabetes or all the other modern chronic non-infectious mortality causes. At least she was healthy right up until she caught on fire cooking supper.

So, if you didn't have a freezer or refrigerator, how would you preserve things so you had something to eat during the winter? Hmmmm? Home canning did not come into vogue until after 1900. Just stop and think for a minute. If I came over and took away your freezer and refrigerator AND your supermarket, what would you eat in January? Where would you find it? This is where the larder comes in. You'd find it in your larder. The larder contained cured and dried meats, dried herbs, vegetables, and grains (both beans and grains for flour). The root cellar held out as long as possible with storage vegetables like root crops. I didn't mention one big one on purpose: fermented foods.

Fermentation enables food to be preserved without refrigeration and freezing, at ambient temperature. That is why fermented foods abound in every culture from the beginning of recorded history. If there's one food preservation technique ubiquitous in longevity and region, it's fermentation. Wine preserved grape nutrition during the off season. The American Whiskey Rebellion we all read about in high school history class was all about western Pennsylvania apple growers shipping brandy to Philadelphia as a way to preserve their apple crop before refrigerated warehousing. And as a way to ship it. A two-week bouncy ox cart ride was hard on apples, but bottles of brandy nestled in straw offered apple nutrition to far-flung urban centers.

Why do I belabor the historical nature of fermentation? Because if for no other reason than food security, stocking your home with fermented goodies is a way to take panic off your emotional table when the power goes out or the blizzard comes. Or the Chinese. The point is that fermented food, from dairy to cucumbers, have formed a foundation for domestic food security a lot longer than the Costco® warehouse. When you bet on a football team, you want to bet on the one with the winning record. In the case of food, the longest winning record goes to fermentation, not the local supermarket. This dependency on non-refrigerated storage actually developed a healthy gut flora and fauna. Antiseptic cryovac packages of veggies shipped from the other side of the world not only create a large carbon footprint, but also lack nutrition compared to proximate compost-grown produce preserved with fermentation.

Whether you do the fermentation or get your ferments from a friend or trusted commercial source, realize that those jars hearken back to an era when people by and large were immune to cancer. What a shame that right at the time we freed ourselves from hoop skirts and the threats of the fireplace, we embraced a new threat: microbiome sterility. While I'm pleased to recommend not burning to death, I'm also pleased to recommend fermented food and beverages to flood our internal microbes with cousins.

Practical Bite #45: Add One Prebiotic Each Week

How? Each time you shop for food, choose one prebiotic. Take it home and eat it, preferably raw. Examples of prebiotics include: jicama, onion, garlic, asparagus, chicory root, leeks, celery, dandelion greens, under-ripe bananas, Jerusalem artichoke, and tiger nuts. Here are some easy ways to add prebiotics into your daily diet:

- ❖ Add raw garlic to your salad, hummus, guacamole, or broth.
- ❖ Add chopped dandelion greens to your salad.
- ❖ Add an un-ripe banana to your smoothie or eat the banana with a scoop of tiger nut butter.
- ❖ Add tiger nuts to your trail mix.
- ❖ Chop up jicama into French fry-shaped sticks. Eat them plain or on a salad.
- ❖ Spread tiger nut butter on celery sticks and you'll eat two prebiotics in one meal.
- ❖ Add onions when grilling vegetables or as a topping on your burger.

Why?

Joel: Every living thing needs a food source. Whether it's a cow, you, or the microbes in your intestines, life eats. Feeding good fiber into your system provides lots of feedstock and surface area for colonizing microbes. Think of your gut as a big long potluck dinner table. All the people going through are the microbes and they're taking a little of this, a little of that. Would you be disappointed if you went to a potluck and only one dish was on the table? I would.

From the list above, notice how many things tend to be identified with spring. In a garden and yard situation, onions, asparagus, leeks, and dandelions all scream spring. Why would nature offer all these things in the spring? Because over the winter we've been eating a lot of stored food that generally has less fiber in it.

Sina: Currently, there is a lot of attention in our culture directed toward getting probiotics into our diet, which is good. But we forget that probiotics need to be fed in order to be healthy and to multiply. Probiotics eat prebiotics, which are a type of non-digestible fiber. Like other high-fiber foods, prebiotics remain undigested as they pass through the upper part of the gastrointestinal tract. Once they reach the colon, they are fermented by gut microflora. In other words, as they move through your gastrointestinal tract, they provide food for your beneficial bacteria.

Prebiotics are a powerful tool to have in your toolbox because they can positively affect everything about your health. For starters, prebiotics help maintain a balance and diversity of intestinal bacteria, particularly increasing the number of beneficial bacteria, such as *Lactobacilli* and *Bifidobacteria*. And, you don't have to eat prebiotics for weeks or months before they have an effect. In as little as 24 hours after eating a prebiotic, your intestines will already contain more beneficial bacteria!

That means, in just 24 hours, you can begin to lower your overall inflammation, and decrease your overall disease risk. In fact, studies have shown that consumption of prebiotics can:

- ❖ Lower your risk of cardiovascular disease
- ❖ Improve digestion
- ❖ Lower your stress response
- ❖ Help regulate hormonal balance and stabilize mood
- ❖ Enhance immune function
- ❖ Lower your risk of obesity
- ❖ Aid in weight loss
- ❖ Lower your likelihood of autoimmune reactions
- ❖ Protect bone health

So, be kind to yourself by adding one prebiotic to your grocery list each week. You can make it fun by turning it into a game, like we did. Each week while at the grocery store, my children run around the produce section hunting for prebiotics. They each choose one, take it home, and prepare it for the family to eat. It sounds simple, but that game gives them ownership of their food choices, which motivates them to eat prebiotics.

Joel: Who doesn't like celery? With peanut butter? Dandelions often grow in lawns; don't spray them. Eat them. What we often call weeds are more often than not nature's Rx. Asparagus is one of the easiest things to grow around your home. It's a perennial so it doesn't need to be planted but once in your lifetime. It comes up every spring; you don't have to do anything to make it come up. Probably one of my most favorite spring traditions is hunting asparagus and eating it raw, right in the garden. The stalks we have here in our garden, unlike the ones in the store, are literally nearly an inch in diameter. Those fat stalks are sweet as sugar and tender as peas. Yum.

Sina: Start simple. Each week, pick one prebiotic and eat it. When possible, consume it raw. You'll save time and your beneficial microbes will love you for it! The next week, change it up; pick a different prebiotic and eat it. Rotating your prebiotic foods will help increase the diversity of your microbiome. Like Joel said, don't bring just one dish to the potluck; make your microbes happy by bringing an array of dishes they can choose from!

Practical Bite #46: Spice It Up!

How? Utilize herbs and spices to add flavor to your food while boosting your microbial diversity, resilience, and overall health and well-being. Here are some easy ways to incorporate more herbs and spices into your diet:

- ❖ Add fresh, raw cilantro, ginger and turmeric to salad by chopping up the leaves and stems of the cilantro and using a potato peeler to add small slices of turmeric and ginger root.
- ❖ Add a clove of raw, pressed garlic to guacamole or bone broth just before serving.
- ❖ Toss a handful of fresh mint into a smoothie.
- ❖ Make pesto using basil and a squeeze of lemon.
- ❖ When cooking ground beef, add cumin, a pinch of ground red pepper flakes and, Real Salt®.
- ❖ Create mint tea by gently simmering a handful of mint in water for 20 minutes, covered with a lid. Turn the heat off and let it rest for 10 minutes.

Why?

Sina: I think we can all agree that our nation is getting sicker. Look around and you'll see kids with all sorts of food allergies and developmental issues, while adults are being diagnosed with autoimmune diseases and cancers in their 30's. Clearly, part of the reason we are sicker is because of the food we are eating. But, that's only part of the equation. We are also getting sicker because of what we are *not* eating.

When nutritionists and dietitians give dietary recommendations, the focus is usually on the macronutrients. They tell you how much carbohydrate, fat, and protein you should eat and even the type you should eat, such as skinless chicken breasts instead of a fatty steak. Sometimes they will throw in a line about the importance of taking a multivitamin and mineral supplement or an omega-3 capsule. But, you most likely won't hear a nutritionist or a dietitian talk about getting enough herbs and spices in your daily diet. We simply aren't taught the value of God's medicine in school.

But, did you know that herbs have been consumed for thousands of years by cultures all over the world? Even the Bible talks about the healing properties of herbs and essential oils.

And, our ancestors ate herbs regularly. They ate plants largely for their nutritional (energy) value. But they also ate herbs alongside those plants as daily medicine.

It's interesting because until approximately 100 years ago, herbs were not only a main part of our diet, they were our main remedy for all health issues. In fact, roughly 80% of the world still uses herbs and other natural medicines as their first line of defense against disease. And, several countries are currently fighting for herbals and other natural remedies to be the first medicines used to treat illnesses in hospitals. Yet, in America, medicinal plants freely grow in our backyards, but we kill them with Roundup® and other herbicides because we view them as unwanted "weeds." That's how far removed we are from our natural food supply.

Herbs and spices are essential for our health and wellness. They offer a wide array of health benefits, such as: reducing inflammation, decreasing stress, increasing energy, improving immune function, enhancing mental ability, and detoxifying the body. For example, eating garlic can decrease your risk of cardiovascular events and slow the progression of atherosclerosis. Cinnamon not only tastes delicious; it can help normalize blood sugar levels in people with type 2 diabetes by improving their ability to respond to insulin. Clove can decrease inflammation and may also trigger cell death of colon cancer cells. Turmeric can decrease pain and improve memory, while ginger can reduce nausea, as well as pain and swelling related to conditions such as osteoarthritis and rheumatoid arthritis.

Studies have also shown that eating herbs and spices can help balance your microbiome by increasing your beneficial bacteria while decreasing potentially harmful bacteria. They can also change the concentration of metabolites produced from those bacteria, such as short-chain fatty acids, bile acids, and lipopolysaccharides (LPS), which are correlated with metabolic diseases like type 2 diabetes and obesity. Trimethylamine-N-oxide (TMAO), which is linked with cardiovascular disease risk, has been reported to decrease following consumption of specific herbs. The list of benefits goes on and on, but I think you get the point.

Joel: It's as important to eat more of the positive as it is to eat less of the negative. Lots of times when we talk about eating properly, the discussion slides toward what we should NOT eat. I get it; we're hard wired on the negative side. We love to complain more than construct. But actually, much of the change in our modern American diet needs to be in the realm of adding, not subtracting. Adding bits and pieces of superior food, like herbs.

We hope that you leave this book feeling freed to embrace lots of good stuff in your life rather than feeling food imprisoned. Herbs are one of those liberating things that can free us up from a host of maladies and spice (literally) up our lives.

Sina: Spicing up your food is another motivator for eating at home. When my husband decided to stop eating out and start cooking at home, he initially felt deprived. He missed the flavors of his favorite fast foods – the hot and spicy sauce from Buffalo Wild Wings® and the tangy, sweet flavor of Chipotle® rice. So, I suggested we reproduce the recipes at home, using fresh, organic, whole ingredients. He was skeptical at first, but after trying my version of Chipotle® rice and calculating how much money we saved by making the rice at home, he was hooked! So, you don't have to miss out on your favorite flavors just because you cook at home. You can replicate any recipe. And, by adding more flavors through herbs and spices, you are feeding your body healing compounds on a daily basis. It's a win-win!

Because our culture is so far removed from the concept of eating a daily dose of God's medicine, it can be difficult to grasp what it looks like. Don't make it harder than it needs to be. It can be as simple as adding cilantro to your taco, or ginger to your salad, or brewing a cup of mint tea. And, it doesn't have to cost money!

Herbs grow freely in my backyard year-round because I don't spray with chemicals, which means I have access to free food all year! Last week, my children and I made a salad by foraging in our yard. We harvested a few leaves of lettuce from our garden, and then went on a scavenger hunt. We picked plantain leaves, chickweed, and dandelion leaves. Then, we topped off the salad with violets and dandelion flowers.

It's funny because I never thought about eating from my backyard until, one day, I brought home lettuce from the grocery store and my husband jokingly asked, "Why do you spend money on lettuce leaves when you can just eat the leaves off the trees in our yard for free?"

He was completely joking, but it sparked my curiosity: Why did I elevate one type of plant over another? In that moment, I realized I was limiting myself to what the grocery store thought I should eat. Just like we tend to limit ourselves to what the nutritionists and dietitians think we should eat.

Don't let them box you in. God has provided you with a treasure trove of free food and medicine. It's all around you. All you have to do is stop standing in its way. Stop spraying it down with chemicals or ripping it up from the earth and throwing it away under the guise that it's just a "weed." Leave it alone and let it provide for you. Let it heal your body, mind, and spirit.

Joel: While some toxic things do exist, like pokeweed, for example, most of those wild plants out there are edible and highly nutritious. Plenty of plant identification sites exist on the internet to aid you in your herb journey.

Sina: And, if you don't want to forage for your herbs and spices, buy them fresh at the grocery store and make sure to choose organic. For a real treat, grind your own spices. My favorites spices to grind are: cinnamon, cumin, nutmeg, and black pepper.

Compared with pre-ground spices, freshly ground spices usually contain more flavor as well as higher levels of healing compounds, including: essential oils, antioxidants, and anti-inflammatory compounds. However, freshly ground spices deteriorate just like pre-ground spices. So, I buy as many spices as possible in the whole form and grind them just before adding them to a recipe. You can grind them using a mortar and pestle, or a spice grinder or coffee grinder.

Grinding your own spices also increases trust in your food supply. For example, pre-ground spices can contain additives, which don't have to be disclosed on the label. Some spices contain rice, flour, or corn starch fillers, which means they contain gluten. There have also been reports of low-cost imitation products being sold as a pure spice. Even potentially carcinogenic industrial dyes that are banned for human consumption have reportedly been added to products to make the spice appear fresher.

In fact, consumer concern regarding adulteration of spices was so high that it forced the FDA to conduct a "risk profile on pathogens and filth in spice." According to the report:

> "Microbial pathogens that have been found in spices include *Salmonella, Bacillus spp.(including Bacillus cereus), Clostridiumperfringens, Cronobacter spp., Shigella,* and *Staphylococcusaureus.* Filth adulterants found in spices include insects (live and dead

> whole insects and insect parts), excrement (animal, bird, and insect), hair (human, rodent, bat, cow, sheep, dog, cat and others), and other materials (decomposed parts, bird barbs, bird barbules, bird feathers, stones, twigs, staples, wood slivers, plastic, synthetic fibers, and rubber bands)."

Again, grind your own spices whenever possible.

I also grind chia seeds, which are not technically a spice but they contain healthy fats that can deteriorate quickly, becoming rancid. If you ingest rancid fats, it can result in inflammation. Therefore, chia and flax seeds are additional ingredients that are worth taking the time to grind just prior to adding to a recipe.

Grinding your own spices only takes a few minutes and it adds wonderful flavors, beneficial healing compounds, and trust to your meal. Just try it. I bet you'll be hooked too!

Practical Bite #47: Breathe In Microbial Diversity

How? Visit as many different "healthy" ecosystems as possible, and take deep breaths. Get out of your house or office and go for a walk in the park, drive to the mountains and hike, sit on the sand at the beach and take deep breaths as you watch the waves crash on the shore, visit your local farmer, read a book under a tree with your shoes off (as long as the grass isn't sprayed with pesticides), or finally go on that camping trip your kids have been begging to do for months. Get back into nature and just breathe.

Why?

Joel: Inhale. Go ahead. I give you permission. Inhale deeply. What does it feel like? Sterile? Stuffy? Metallic? Just like we have different ecologies on the land, we have different ecologies in the air. The air is full of stuff. You know that stream of sunshine coming through the window? Notice all the dust in that light?

That's in air all around us, but we don't see it. I like to think that the Peanuts® comic strip with Pigpen with the swirling dust cloud around his head is actually more normal than abnormal. That is actually the way the air looks through an electron microscope. It's not empty space; it's teaming with both living and nonliving particles.

We can walk in and out of different air ecosystems simply by changing location. Perhaps the worst air in the world is in long flight jets. That cabin air gets cycled and cycled and cycled. Big buildings are a close second, regardless of what kind of air filters they have.

The most intoxicating air? The good stuff? That's out in the pasture or in the woods. The earth's air filters are leaves. As a gentle reminder, grass blades are leaves too. Just like we need different foods, we also need different air. Well, maybe I don't since I'm out here on the farm all the time. But if you live in an urban setting, getting to a highly vegetated setting can bring all sorts of healing to your body via air with different stuff in it.

Sina: We previously mentioned that microbial diversity is required for optimal health, abundant energy, and true happiness. Diversity is so important, that I consider microbes to be an essential nutrient. Just like vitamins, minerals, and water are known to be essential for life, so are microbes. Consequently, I make sure my family gets a daily dose of "healthy" microbes.

And, I vary the source so we create resiliency through building a *diverse* ecosystem in and on our bodies.

One of the most effective ways to increase microbial diversity is to breathe in the air from different "healthy" environments. Get out in nature and breathe in the microbial diversity from as many different ecosystems as you can. Stay there for a few hours, if possible. You'll not only repopulate your microbiome, you'll improve your mental health and recharge your battery.

You may not have time to travel to distant places, and that's okay. Find your local park or botanical garden. Even easier, walk down the street and you'll be surrounded by microbes that are different than the ones you normally encounter while at home or the office. There's always some place you can visit that will offer different and "healthy" microbes for you to breathe. Obviously avoid ecosystems you consider to be polluted, like subways or places near freeways. But don't make it harder than it is; just start by finding some place in nature that is close to your house and breathe.

Joel: Few things energize me in the summer like lying down in the pasture before dark. Sometimes I go to the woods and just lie down for a while. All those spores from mushrooms, the pollen from tulip poplars and the dust stirred by squirrels scampering adds to the microbial diversity on my insides. Spending time in an outside that's beautiful is a great way to populate your insides with beauty. And by the way, I can't help but make a shameless plug here for visiting your farm. What better compliment could you add to your food than to breathe in air from the place where it was produced? You've heard of companion planting in the garden (some plants like others). How about companion inhaling with your farmer and your food?

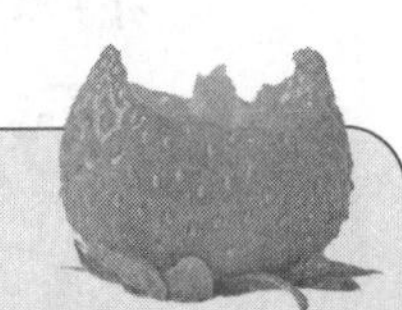

CHEW ON THIS

While you're out in nature, breathing in microbial diversity, give yourself an energy boost by walking on the grass with bare feet – as long as the grass is not sprayed with chemicals. This is called "grounding" or "earthing."

Since you are energy, you carry charges in the form of electrons. You can become deficient in electrons for many reasons, including stress, which can contribute to disease and unwellness. Fortunately, the Earth's surface contains almost a limitless supply of free or mobile electrons. You can absorb those free electrons through direct contact with the Earth.

It's theorized that those electrons can help prevent and reverse disease, as well as promote overall wellness. For instance, a study published in the *Journal of Environmental Public Health* in 2012 suggested that grounding can promote physiological changes and increased well-being, including better sleep and a reduction in pain. One proposed mechanism is the neutralization of reactive oxygen species, which would reduce acute and chronic inflammation.

So, go grab some electrons! It's easy to do and will help you feel energized. Simply shuffle your feet slowly over the grass so that your feet remain in contact with the grass the entire time. Better yet, while you are grounding, say 10 things you are grateful for – out loud. You might be amazed that something so easy can profoundly boost your energy and your mood.

Practical Bite #48: Say No To Arsenic In Rice

How? Limit your intake of processed foods that contain rice or rice derivatives. On the ingredient label, look for the word "rice" in a variety of forms, such as: rice vinegar, rice bran, rice germ, rice starch, rice syrup, or rice protein. When preparing rice, you can remove as much as 85% of the arsenic by following this protocol:

1. Place rice in a metal strainer and rinse under water for at least one minute.
2. Transfer rice to a large glass bowl and add 6 times as much water as rice. For example, if you are soaking 1 cup of rice then add 6 cups of water.
3. Soak for 24-48 hours, rinsing occasionally by pouring out as much water as possible and then re-filling the bowl with water.
4. After 24-48 hours, place the rice back into the metal strainer and rinse under water for at least one minute.
5. Cook the rice in a stainless-steel pot in 6 times as much water as rice. Again, if you are cooking 1 cup of rice then add 6 cups of water.
6. When desired texture is achieved, remove from heat and place the rice back into the metal strainer and rinse under water for at least one minute. If rice is too wet then squeeze out some water by pressing down on rice with a spoon.

Why?

Joel: But Sina, are you serious? You mean I have to think about what I'm going to eat 48 hours in advance? Really? Don't you realize that more than 50 percent of Americans have no clue what they're going to eat for dinner even as late as 4 p.m.? This doesn't sound very convenient. Of course, I'm partly joking with my poking, but it's a real conundrum, isn't it? When you get right down to it, food planning is the real bugaboo, isn't it?

Sina: Absolutely! I never used to plan my meals. In fact, food was an afterthought – something I squeezed into my busy schedule, often between meetings or while driving in the car. So, I totally get it. But I'm asking you to do something that is inconvenient because we are learning that arsenic poisoning is more common than previously thought. And, with a little planning, it's avoidable.

When I was debilitatingly sick a few years ago, I had arsenic poisoning and it was awful. I experienced chronic fatigue, muscle weakness and cognitive deficits. Have you heard of brain fog? Some days the brain fog was so bad that when reading a children's book to my 5-year old son, I could not follow the story line! It felt like I wasn't myself – like my mind slowed down to a crawl and I was trapped in a single moment while life continued to march forward all around me. To rid my body of the excess arsenic, I underwent several rounds of "natural" chelation, which was also very fatiguing. How did I even get arsenic poisoning? From eating rice!

Rice can contain inorganic arsenic, which is a heavy metal that can be toxic to your body. It doesn't matter if the rice is white, brown, wild or organic; all types are susceptible to arsenic contamination. In fact, brown rice commonly contains more inorganic arsenic than white rice.

You may not think you eat a lot of rice. But, since rice is subsidized by the government, it can be found in a plethora of processed foods, including: crackers, cereals, granola bars, cookies, energy bars, breads and baby foods.

That's a potential problem because consuming inorganic arsenic can lead to disease. Even the FDA acknowledges it's a health concern: "Consumption of inorganic arsenic has been associated with cancer, skin lesions, cardiovascular disease and diabetes in humans." The CDC classified it as a carcinogen, and the International Agency for Research on Cancer declared inorganic arsenic to be a category 1 carcinogen – that means it is known to cause cancer. If all of these agencies know it can cause disease then why is arsenic in our rice?

Arsenic is naturally present in the soil. There are many forms of arsenic, but we generally separate them into two broad categories: inorganic and organic. The current health concern is centered on inorganic arsenic, which is thought to be the more toxic form. The reason there's too much inorganic arsenic in some farming areas is partly because it was sprayed on crops for decades. It was actually used as a pesticide. And, even though it was largely banned in the 1980s (certified pesticide applicators are still allowed to use arsenic compounds), inorganic arsenic is still present in undesired quantities in some farming areas because it can remain in the soil for decades.

Rice is particularly susceptible to higher levels of arsenic because it is the only major cereal crop that is grown under flooded conditions - the rice sits in water. And, arsenic is water-soluble, which means it would rather leave the soil and float around in the water. So, the rice gets exposed to the arsenic and sucks it up. It just so happens that rice is exceptionally good at absorbing arsenic and holding onto it. Consequently, arsenic is showing up in all types of rice, as well as processed foods containing rice derivatives.

Joel: Orchards were such a heavy user of arsenic-laden pesticides that old orchard sites are still considered the most arsenic-toxic properties in rural America. Part of the property search often includes whether or not it contained an orchard during the 1940s-1960s and if so, a soil sample is in order.

On farms, arsenic has been used not only in pesticides, but also in animal feeds as an appetite enhancer. It is now prohibited in chicken feed, where it was primarily used, but I've seen enough noncompliance in the industry that I've become dubious about anything that is prohibited.

Sina: The good news is that you can reduce your chance of getting arsenic poisoning by reducing your intake of processed foods containing rice derivatives, and by soaking your rice.

The soaking protocol might sound time-consuming, but it's actually a time-saver. Yes, you have to plan ahead, but soaking the rice allows it to sprout, which results in less cooking time. So, for me, the protocol is a win-win. There is one catch: some nutrients, such as folate and thiamin, can be lost when you rinse and soak rice. For me, the lost nutrients are not a priority. My priority is to remove the arsenic. I make up for lost nutrients by adding leafy greens, grass-finished beef and other nutrient-dense foods to my diet.

What's really cool is that while consumers can protect themselves from arsenic poisoning, farmers can actually help correct this health problem that we are currently facing, right Joel?

Joel: Yes. The antidote to soil toxins, regardless of origin, is organic matter (OM). That's the decaying material in the soil and all the soil life, from earthworms to actinomycetes. It's linked to soil carbon and is a measure of all the living components (as opposed to nonliving like water, air, and mineral) in the soil. Think of OM like a sponge or buffering agent. I sometimes call it the soil's Alka Seltzer®. It absorbs and neutralizes toxicity. As a side note, whenever you hear a chemical company say "our poison (of course, they don't use that word, but that's what it is) breaks down in the soil" they are telling a half truth. The ability of soil to break down toxins, including eggs laid by pest insects, is directly tied to its OM content.

As a general rule, the higher the organic matter, the more protective and functional the soil. Do you know the quickest way to destroy organic matter? Tillage. All that stirring and hyper-oxygenation is like throwing gas on a fire; it literally burns out the organic matter. That's why grass-finished beef is the ultimate land healing tool; those cows don't require any tillage for grains. Of course, in mainstream agriculture, a lot of grain is fed to herbivores, but that's not nature's template. If the soil has a toxin, then, adding carbon like wood chips or leaves, adding compost, and even stopping the stirring (tillage) all ameliorate the problem over time.

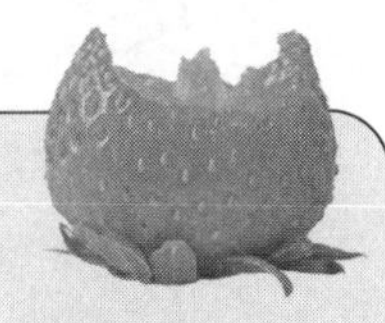

CHEW ON THIS

The FDA acknowledges that babies are highly susceptible to arsenic poisoning because rice intake is roughly three times greater for infants than adults, in relation to body weight. They also acknowledge that exposure to inorganic arsenic during infancy and early childhood can have neurotoxic effects. So, what's the FDA doing about it?

The FDA proposed a limit on the amount of inorganic arsenic allowed in infant rice cereal; however, it's merely a suggested limit. Companies do not have to adhere to the FDA recommendation. Across the top of the FDA document that contains the suggested arsenic limit, it states, "Contains Nonbinding Recommendations."

Clearly, the FDA is not going to swoop in and save us from arsenic. But you don't need the FDA to provide a solution. Be your own solution! Read your ingredient labels and soak your rice.

Practical Bite #49: Listen To Your Body

How? Instead of adhering to a specific diet or following dietary advice from "experts," listen to your body. Nobody knows your body better than you. As long as you can differentiate between what your body needs and what your mind craves, you are the best dietitian or nutritionist that money can buy.

You already listen to your body to some extent. For instance, you've probably experienced a sugar high followed by the inevitable sugar crash. You may have felt tired, unmotivated, cranky, and had a bad craving for more sugar. That sugar crash is your body's way of telling you to "knock it off." Or, perhaps you have experienced heart burn after eating spicy food. When that happens, it's common to reach for antacids. But your body is not telling you that it needs an antacid. It's telling you it doesn't want to eat that spicy food. If you've ever craved a greasy cheeseburger, perhaps your body wanted the fat or the iron or the protein. Maybe you've felt bloated after eating foods that your body didn't want, or you felt sluggish or got a headache or brain fog. These are all ways your body is communicating with you to tell you what it needs. Your body is always talking to you. But, most of us have forgotten how to listen.

Here are a few easy ways to start listening to your body:

1. The next time you crave sugar, pause and ask your body if it really wants sugar or if it's tired. Close your eyes, take three deep belly breaths, and then say these words out loud, "Body, are you tired?" Allow yourself to sit in the silence and wait for the answer. Listen with an open mind, and your body will respond. If the answer is that your body is tired, resist eating the sugar and instead take a nap or sit quietly for 5-minutes, with your eyes closed and muscles relaxed, to recharge your battery.
2. Likewise, if you need caffeine to make it through your day then ask your body if you are doing too much. Say these words out loud, "Body, do I need caffeine because I'm doing too much?" If the answer is yes then evaluate yourschedule. Consider removing items from your "to do list" or building in rest periods throughout the day. Even adding 5-minutes of rest or meditation canturn your day around.

3. Many of us eat to reward ourselves, or we eat when we're sad or bored, or because the clock says it's time to eat. In our modern world where food is abundant, eating only when you are hungry has become a skill. Next time you want to eat, check in with your body first. You may actually be tired, thirsty, or eating based on addiction or emotion. Close your eyes, take three deep belly breaths, and ask, "Body, am I hungry?" If your body responds that it needs food then eat. However, if your body shows you emotions like boredom, anger, anxiety, or fear then consider refraining from eating. Instead, recognize that when your motivation to eat stems from addiction or emotion, it is common to crave unhealthy foods in that moment. So, pause, breathe through it, acknowledge the emotion, and give your body the opportunity to tell you what it needs on an emotional level.

Why?

Sina: For decades, I struggled with my cholesterol. Even though I cycled 100-miles a week, hiked on the weekends, lifted weights, and wasn't overweight, my HDL was consistently below 35 mg/dL and my triglycerides were close to 300 mg/dL. So, the doctor sent me to a dietitian. At that time, I was in graduate school earning my doctoral degree in Nutrition, but I went to the dietitian anyway because I was scared. I believed the medical doctor when he told me I was at risk for early-onset heart disease and may need medication – in my late 20's. So, I diligently followed the dietitian's advice.

I cut the fat out of my diet and ate a lot more carbohydrates. It was horrible. Each time I wanted to eat, I had to count the grams of fat, specifically saturated fat, on the Nutrition Facts Label. Consequently, I stopped eating eggs, butter, and red meat. I replaced my 2% milk with non-fat milk and bought low-fat cheese. And, I consumed oatmeal for breakfast every day, which tasted horrible without the added butter and brown sugar. I even ordered my pizza meatless, with half the cheese!

I followed that protocol for over a year. And, when my blood values came back, they were worse! My total cholesterol increased by 90 points, my HDL dropped below 30 mg/dL, and my triglycerides jumped to over 300 mg/dL for the first time in my life.

Both the dietitian and the doctor could not explain my results. Since I had a food journal, which proved that I diligently followed the diet, they both said my "bad" cholesterol values were genetic. Consequently, there was "nothing" I could do to improve them except take medication.

I never took the medication. But I lived in that space of fear for over a decade, thinking I was doomed to get heart disease and eventually die from a heart attack. After all, both of my parents and my Grandparents have heart disease, so I figured it must run in the family – like the doctor said.

Then, one day, I learned that your genes do not dictate your health. Thanks to a little discovery called epigenetics, we know that you are not doomed by your genes. You can actually turn them on and off with your food and lifestyle choices, as well as your thoughts. In other words, just because your Mom and Dad have high cholesterol doesn't mean you will have high cholesterol. And, just because your Grandparents had diabetes doesn't mean you will develop diabetes. You can change your disease outcome based on *your* choices.

So, I chose not to buy into the limiting beliefs of the doctor and the dietitian. Instead, I started listening to my body. Since low-fat wasn't working, I switched to a higher fat diet that included lots of saturated fat from good sources, such as: coconut oil, raw milk, and beef and butter from grass-finished cows. And, I started drinking bone broth, including the fat! I remember the first time I cooked bone broth in my crockpot. When it was ready to eat, I opened the lid and saw a thick layer of melted fat sitting on the top. I nearly gagged! I didn't know how I was going to force myself to drink the fat, but I wanted to be healed, so I scooped a ladleful of broth into a coffee mug and gulped it down. And then, the strangest thing happened – my body wanted more! It loved the fat! So, I drank a mug-full with every meal that day. I felt fabulous! I had so much energy, and I didn't experience my usual 3 o'clock energy crash. Needless to say, I was hooked!

I've been eating a relatively high-fat diet for roughly 5 years, and my lab values are better than ever! My HDL is 75 mg/dL and my triglycerides are 49 mg/dL! Not to mention, my energy is through the roof!

I was surprised at how high my HDL climbed because I exercise much less than I used to -

before I had kids. When my HDL was below 35 mg/dL, I was exercising intensely at least 5 days a week for at least an hour a day. Now, my HDL value is fantastic and I do considerably less intense forms of exercise, including: walking, yoga, Pilates, gardening, housekeeping, and meditation. In fact, most of my exercise comes from trying to keep up with my kids!

I'm not saying you shouldn't do intense exercise. My minor was Exercise Physiology, so I am biased toward the value of physical activity. But I find it fascinating that exercise did not improve my HDL; removing carbohydrates and adding saturated fat did. I would never have figured that out if I had continued listening to the doctor and dietitian instead of listening to my own body.

Joel: What an incredible story. You are one of the few who stepped off the treadmill. That would be the treadmill of orthodox-think. Isn't it interesting that most people know, deep down, that there's something rotten in Denmark - politicians, bureaucrats, and corporate executives? Who trusts these folks? We have a collective disdain for what is generally known as "the system," or the "powers that be," but then we worship their minions in the system and follow their advice like good little boys and girls. Why? What you did, stepping off that orthodoxy treadmill, is well-nigh impossible unless you're highly unusual. I'd say you qualify for that, Sina.

But we grow up disempowered to think we can make decisions. We went to school where inquisitiveness was subject to a bell. We took tests that arbitrated what was worth learning. We followed a course of study that a test said we might like or a guidance counselor thought would suit us. I could go on in this vein, but you get the point. At no time in human history has a culture been more dispossessed of personal authority and autonomy. We have coaches for everything. Investments. Resumes. Wellness. You name it, someone is a coach for it.

I think it follows complexity. You can't work on your car anymore. You can't work on your computer. You can't even work on your kitchen blender. We've gradually been reduced to dependents psychologically, and that disempowerment extends right over into health and food.

We don't trust ourselves to know anything, so we don't listen to our own bodies. I know some things make me feel bloated and others make me feel super. Some make me wake up and others put me to sleep. Some makes me constipated and some makes elimination gentle and easy. Awareness is doable. It's my body, my life.

Sina: What you said about growing up feeling "disempowered" deeply resonates with me. Beginning at a very young age, we are taught that we should listen to "experts" instead of listening to ourselves. And, since everyone else is following those "experts," it's very difficult to not be a sheep.

It took a long time for me to stop out-sourcing my problems to "experts" and to start listening to my body because I didn't trust myself. I bet hardly any of us *truly* trust ourselves. And, it's partly because of our culture. As you said, we are trained to find answers outside of ourselves. Consequently, if we get a cold, we see a doctor. If we have high cholesterol, we see a dietitian. If we have pain in our back, we see a chiropractor. If our foot hurts, we see a podiatrist, and so forth. We have trained ourselves to become dependent on other people and, in the process, we have become disconnected with ourselves.

Think of all the time you spend seeking diet advice. Some of us know all of the latest diet trends, we ask friends what they eat, we buy cookbooks that sit on our bookshelves collecting dust, we read blogs hoping to gain insight into the "secret" of how to be healthy, and we buy books – like this one – hoping that an "expert" will reveal the magic formula that we've been desperately seeking. I know because I used to do the same thing.

But, have you tried asking your body what it wants to eat? And then *really* listening for the answer? If you want to know which foods are right for your body, stop searching for the answer externally and start listening to yourself.

When I was sick with an autoimmune disease, a friend offered me great advice: "The answer doesn't lie in your checkbook. The answer is inside of you. Stop paying people for *their* answer and start listening to *your* light within."

She's right. The answers are within you. When you receive answers from other people, their bias comes along for the ride. This book is full of bias. That's why, early on, we encouraged you to pick and choose the Practical Bites that resonate with you. Because only *you* know what's right for *your* body. Once you start seeking answers from within, and you check in with yourself on a daily basis, you begin to reconnect with yourself. Over time, trust is rebuilt and as you become whole again, you become freer, healthier, and more joyful.

It took some time for me to understand how to put that truth into practice. My leap of faith occurred that pivotal day when I made the decision to do the complete opposite of what the doctor and dietitian recommended. It's funny because I agree with Joel that what I did those many years ago was "unusual." I certainly received a lot of pushback from friends and family. My Dad thought I was "killing" myself. But, now there's a stockpile of scientific evidence supporting my unorthodox decision – that *some* of us can benefit from eating more healthy fats, including saturated fat. Maybe you're one of those people?

If you listen to your body, it will tell you if it wants more fat. If you listen to the medical establishment, nutrition field, and the government, you will continue to reinforce the limiting belief that fat is "bad." Those organizations can't get behind the numerous studies that have shown that some people thrive on a higher fat diet. Why? Partly because it means reversing course and admitting that the dietary advice they have been selling us for over 50 years is wrong. Can you imagine the backlash that would occur if people found out that the advice we've been following from the government and trusted institutions, like the American Heart Association (AHA), has actually *caused* disease?

Joel: Well, lots of us are waking up to it, and hopefully when a million people read this book, those numbers will increase. Sina, I want to make sure people don't think we're just crackpot conspiracists. But we do agree that groupthink does not exist just because credentialed experts enter the room. You think kindergarteners are peer dependent? Try going to a medical conference or an agriculture expo. You've never seen such peer dependency and groupthink.

Sina: I think it's so common because our brains are hardwired to "fall in line," like good little sheep. It's an evolutionary adaptation designed to give you the best probability of survival. For instance, let's pretend you are gathering berries with your buddies and suddenly one of them starts running in the opposite direction. Your brain tells your body to follow him because he is most likely running from a predator, like a lion. So, you start running too. You don't even really know why you are running, but your instinct tells you to run. In that situation, being a sheep is beneficial.

But we are no longer prey; we're not trying to avoid being lunch for a hungry lion. We have the luxury of listening to our bodies and forging our own path. Yet, it's difficult to go against the grain because we are still hardwired to go with the masses.

Fortunately, you can break your dependency by developing a trusting relationship with yourself. When you trust yourself, you are able to more effectively exercise discernment. Consequently, when you receive advice or hear about the latest diet craze, you can check in with yourself and allow your body's innate intelligence to tell you if that dietary approach is appropriate for you. In that way, you become your own "expert."

Joel: So, it all comes down to trust. Of course, we all need expert opinion from time to time, but goodness, don't be afraid to go with your gut. And choose experts who adhere to your philosophy of life. Why go to an expert who thinks life is mechanical, or who pushes drugs for everything? Think!

Perhaps the biggest decision anyone has to make is who they're going to trust.

Sina: Absolutely. Because the consequences of that decision are enormous. So, before you freely give your trust to "experts," know their motive. Everyone has a motive. Even the government and trusted health organizations, like the AHA, have motives. To find their motive, you can usually follow the money.

For instance, today everyone knows it's bad to eat man-made trans fat – the type of fat that can be found in Crisco©. It raises LDL cholesterol and lowers HDL cholesterol. But, did you know that in the 1900s, the AHA actually advised Americans to eat Crisco© if they wanted to avoid heart disease? The medical director of the AHA posed on camera with a bottle of Crisco©. Why?

I can't say for sure, but it might have something to do with the $17 million (in today's money) that Procter & Gamble® gave to the AHA. Procter & Gamble®, of course, was the maker of Crisco©. And, before receiving that money, the AHA was a small group with practically no money and very little influence. Oh, how money can change people.

You can also follow the money to understand why we have certain harmful food policies in America. It's sad but, the FDA is notorious for its revolving door. For instance, we previously mentioned Michael Taylor. He was the attorney who crafted the FDA's policy that unleashed GMOs into our food supply with no long-term testing and no oversight. He repeatedly moved back and forth between working for the FDA and working for Monsanto. Dr. Margaret Miller helped get rBGH approved by increasing the allowable level of antibiotic residues in milk after rBGH failed to meet the requirement. She studied rBGH while working for Monsanto and then joined the FDA where she became the Branch Chief of the division that evaluated her own research. Dr. Susan Sechen also helped get rBGH approved. She conducted studies on Monsanto's rBGH drug while in graduate school and then was hired by the FDA to review her own studies! She even published articles supporting Monsanto's rBGH drug while she was an FDA employee. The list goes on and on at the FDA.

And, I would be remiss if I didn't mention the motive behind the government's Dietary Guidelines. Those recommendations are largely determined by the food and drug industry. A group of 11-15 "experts" on the Dietary Guidelines Advisory Committee make recommendations for what Americans should eat. Their recommendations become the Dietary Guidelines. In 2015, the *British Medical Journal* revealed that the Committee relies on systematic reviews from groups like the AHA and the American College of Cardiology, "which are heavily supported by food and drug companies." In other words, when you consent to the Dietary Guidelines like a good little sheep, you are following the advice of people who are pushing the processed foods and pharmaceuticals that are actually making us sicker.

Speaking of pharmaceuticals, did you know that Big Pharma funds nutrition "experts", research studies, professional conferences, and student events on college campuses?

Joel: Yes, just like Big Ag funds farm research. Years ago, I finally heard stupid advice from a PhD animal scientist once too often. He did a weekly radio show and talked about pinkeye in cattle. He advised the orthodox antibiotic injection in the conjunctiva of the eye. It's hard to administer to a cow (she's big and doesn't cotton too much to me pulling her eyelid down so I can poke a syringe in there). We had years of success by just feeding a good quality dehydrated seaweed – kelp - to our cows. Neighbors had blind animals running around and we just never had a problem.

So, I called the professor and invited him to the farm. He stopped by and I showed him our program, our cows, and explained how organic iodine in the kelp kept the infection at bay. He was diplomatically polite and even curious - even intrigued. He said he'd love to run some trials on it and I assured him I'd be glad to collaborate with him on the trials. When I pressed him a few months later about doing the research, he simply and matter-of-factly responded: "I'll do it as soon as you give me seed money to do the research."

You'd think these publicly funded scientists would be able to do research they thought was important. No; they do research that gets industry seed money. And since I didn't have $10,000 of seed money, the research never happened, and many years later, he was still dispensing drug advice for a condition easily rectified with good nutrition. Cow care is not different than people care.

Sina: That's the main reason I left academia; I didn't want to be at the mercy of funding agencies. They don't reward thinking outside of the box. Instead, they give money to researchers who are willing to stay inside the orthodox cage and play their game, by their rules. I think it's pretty obvious by now that I'm a rule breaker. In fact, I may not even be on the game board! But that's the mentality you need if you want to get off the treadmill.

Look, I'm not suggesting you never see a medical doctor again or that you stop reading nutrition articles. Everyone needs guidance. And, seeking opinions can help broaden your knowledge and perspective. So, by all means, continue to educate yourself, continue to seek advice, and continue to see your medical doctor. But, don't follow the advice just because you've been taught to be a sheep or because everyone else is doing it. Nobody can tell you exactly what your body needs. "Experts" can make generalized recommendations. And, the really good "experts" can run tests to narrow down your body's needs. But, there's no one size fits all approach to eating. And, nobody has that magical eating plan you've been searching for – except for you.

As previously mentioned, your body's dietary needs change based on many variables, including: the seasons, stress level, activity level, hydration status, nutrient deficiency status, etcetera. If you lock yourself into one type of diet, such as Paleo, Keto, or High-Carb, you become more focused on adhering to that diet than listening to your body. In essence, you become a slave to the confinements and limiting beliefs of that dietary protocol. You also run the risk of losing variety in your diet, which is critical for disease prevention and reversal (See Practical Bite #50)

Just like our ancestors did not count calories, they did not calculate percentages of macronutrients (i.e. protein, carbohydrate, and fat). Your body is more unique than a cookie-cutter diet. It's also more resilient! Your body was not designed to be confined to a strict ratio of macronutrients. It was designed to handle adversity, including differences in macronutrient content due to seasonal changes and availability, as well as times of scarcity due to lack of food. Remember, a little stress on the body can be good.

Once you can effectively communicate with your body, you will most likely discover that your needs change with every meal. You'll likely have an over-arching preference for a certain macronutrient composition – such as more fats or more carbohydrates or more protein. But, on a meal-by-meal basis, your specific needs will change based on your current state of being.

For instance, as previously mentioned, my body almost always wants higher fat meals. The amount of fat I eat is not high enough to be considered the Keto diet, but it's higher than most Americans eat, and it certainly contains more fat than the high-carbohydrate diet promoted by the government. My diet would also not be considered Paleo because, when it comes to protein, sometimes my body wants a small amount of meat, and sometimes it doesn't want any. Usually it loves bone broths, but I can go for days without eating meat and my body is happy.

Since I listen to my body and change my diet accordingly, I don't fit into any of the man-made dietary boxes. I used to live inside that box. And, every time I went off a diet, I would feel bad about myself, as though I "cheated" or I "failed." Now I live outside of that box. I choose to harness my power by remaining open to new information, but ultimately listening to my own body.

So, I encourage you not to fall into the trap of picking someone else's dietary protocol and rigidly adhering to it. And, I encourage you to stop trusting Big Brother or the AHA or any other "expert" who tells you they know what you should eat. Instead, start trusting yourself. You already know everything you need to know about how to be healthy, happy, and free. You just have to tap into the light inside of you.

Joel: So, trust yourself to make decisions for your own body. Listen to your gut. Rely on yourself whenever possible. But, none of us can know everything, so we have to choose our advisors. Choose wisely, Indiana Jones.

Practical Bite #50: Cycle Your Foods

How? Cycling means you temporarily remove entire food groups from your diet for a given period of time. After that time period, you bring that food group back and you remove a different one. For example, all grains would be removed for a given period of time. Then, grains would be added back while all dairy would be removed for a given period of time. Then, dairy would be added back while all legumes would be removed.

How do you know how long to remove the foods? The best person to ask is yourself. Use the method we shared in Practical Bite #49 regarding how to listen to your body. Ask your body which food group it wants you to remove. Then, remove that food group. After a few weeks, ask your body if it wants to eat that food again. If it doesn't, refrain from eating that food group until your body gives you a "yes."

If you aren't currently able to communicate with your body then remove a food group for at least two weeks – a month if possible. After a minimum of two weeks, add that food group back into your diet and remove a different food group. Pay attention to how your body feels when you cycle. If you feel better after removing a food group and then you feel worse after adding those foods back then you didn't wait long enough before re-introducing the food into your food cycle. Remove the food again.

Why?

Joel: I'll go a bit out on a limb here and admit that I haven't done this much. But then again, I haven't eaten the Standard American Diet. But by eating from our own garden, seasonally, I automatically cycle. I can just about live on lettuce, tomatoes, peppers, and cucumbers in the height of the summer. But come winter, I'm into heavy stews, lots of meat and root vegetables like sweet potatoes.

The fact is that most modern Americans eat similarly every meal. Oh, the name might change. It might be frozen pizza one night and macaroni and cheese the next, but the basics in both those meals is practically identical. The difference in ingredients between Hot Pockets® and Campbell's® vegetable soup is pretty minimal. When it comes to snacks, of course, the similarities are even more profound. The difference in the ingredient list between different chips or different candy bars is inconsequential.

The result of this similarity is that while our ancestors did indeed cycle through different foods throughout the year - they didn't eat strawberries in the winter - today we eat similarly every single day. Eating seasonally is one way to enjoy cycling by default. In fact, even meat was part of this cycling. Poultry was consumed more in the summer because it's not a heating protein; whereas beef does bring more heat.

That meshes really well with the natural ebb and flow of chickens. Chickens lay more eggs in the spring, which offers enough excess to grow out for boilers to eat. In the winter, egg production is so low it's hard to save any eggs for hatching meat birds since we need all the eggs for eating. Cattle numbers naturally want to be high in the summer when the grass is growing and then drop going into winter when grass stops. Harvest time, then, to mesh with ecology is in late summer or early fall.

Pigs typically birth in the spring, although they are happy to birth anytime it's warm. In most cultures, pork is the favorite meat to cure, meaning it's preserved with salts or smoking and stabilized to last a long time without refrigeration. Spain, of course, is the world leader in this and routinely keeps specialty hams 5 years without refrigeration. So, they enjoy pepperonis any time. Fresh milk was a summer gig. Cheese was winter, when the cows weren't milking. These seasonal ebbs and flows, prior to modern technology, forced people to cycle through different foods. Today, we have to think more about it, and here to coach us is Sina.

Sina: Like Joel said, most Americans eat the same foods every day. We eat as though seasons do not exist. In fact, I didn't even know which foods grew during each season until I started gardening. I never even thought about it. But I've learned that cycling your food is critical for your health and longevity.

Cycling your food reduces your chance of developing an autoimmune disease or food sensitives/allergies. We know there's been a dramatic rise in both autoimmune diseases and food sensitivities/allergies during our lifetime. One plausible theory behind this phenomenon is leaky gut, which we previously discussed.

To recap, the gut lining becomes leaky and large particles of food pass through the gut and eventually end up in the blood stream where they are not supposed to be. Consequently, the immune system attacks the food, as though it's a foreign invader. That process can lead to food sensitivities and allergies. It's like the immune system puts a tag on that food as a reminder to attack it if it is eaten in the future. And, if you continue to eat those foods, your body can get confused between the protein in the food and the protein in your tissues because they look structurally similar. That process is called molecular mimicry. It's like a case of mistaken identity where your body mounts an immune response to your tissues because it thinks it is a foreign invader. Over time, that mistaken identity can lead to the development of a disease, such as: diabetes, heart disease, or rheumatoid arthritis. This mechanism of leaky gut is becoming well known and accepted. But, there's a missing piece to the puzzle that's critical to know if you want to prevent food sensitivities and disease.

Health care practitioners often recommend you add variety into your diet to prevent disease. For example, instead of only eating that one vegetable you can tolerate, eat many different types of vegetables. Or, instead of only eating sandwiches for lunch, try a salad or soup. That's great advice, but it's just one side of the coin.

On the other side of the coin is food scarcity. In addition to adding variety into your diet, you must also temporarily remove foods from your diet. I call it food cycling.

Let's use gluten as an example. We know that the gene for non-celiac gluten sensitivity has been triggered by gluten and it's making itself well known in our modern culture. In fact, our society has turned gluten into a villain. Case in point: you can buy nearly any type of "gluten free" food these days, from pizza to cereal to donuts and noodles. "Gluten free" is one of the fastest growing segments in the marketplace. But I contend there's nothing special about gluten. Think about this for a moment: why would gluten be the ONLY food that can turn on a gene and trigger inflammation? That doesn't make sense.

I have the genotype for non-celiac gluten sensitivity, which means that if I eat gluten, my body becomes inflamed. Some gluten "experts" have stated that even one crumb of a gluten-containing food will cause my body to become systemically inflamed for up to two months! They also say I can never eat any gluten again, unless I want to develop a disease again. That statement sounds logical because gluten is the trigger that turns on the gene for non-celiac gluten sensitivity. Thus, in order to keep the gene turned off, you have to remove the trigger i.e. gluten. But, why is it only gluten? Why does roughly 30% of the population have non-celiac gluten sensitivity, but other foods are not triggering disease in large portions of the population?

The truth is that other foods can turn on genes and trigger inflammation too. In fact, that assumption is built into the leaky gut theory. According to the theory, when the lining of the gut is compromised, large particles of food can pass through and enter your blood stream. It's not specific to gluten. When the gaps in your gut lining are large enough, any food particle can pass through. Hence, you can develop a sensitivity to any food. I developed a sensitivity to bay leaf! And, some children have developed a sensitivity to pepper. Both bay leaf and pepper can modify your gene expression and cause inflammation, like gluten can. So, why isn't there a movement for "bay leaf-free foods" or "pepper-free foods"?

The answer largely lies in food scarcity. Specifically, the population at large doesn't eat bay leaf or pepper in mass quantities like we eat gluten. Likewise, cruciferous vegetables can cause inflammation, but how many cruciferous vegetables do you eat in one week? How much spinach or lettuce do you eat in one week? Compare those numbers with how much corn you eat in one week. For the typical American, corn wins every single week, hands down.

If you recall from Practical Bite #22, the typical American eats corn every single day in the form of genetically modified, synthetic corn byproducts. You may not recognize corn on the food label because it has been processed into hundreds of different synthetic chemicals, such as: vitamin C, dextrose, and MSG. But, when you walk into the grocery store, corn surrounds you on all sides.

Corn can be in cookies, cakes, pies, crackers, cereals, baking powder, some spices, bread, dressings, soups, pudding, sauces, some meats, soda, vitamins, and even the wax that coats produce. Imagine you're standing in the frozen food section deciding between Mexican and Italian for dinner. What you may not realize is that the decision has already been made for you. You are really choosing between processed corn byproducts and processed corn byproducts. Both frozen dinners are just variations of the same foodstuffs: synthetic, genetically engineered, subsidized corn byproducts.

Now think of how much wheat you eat every week. How many bowls of cereal, pieces of bread, or handfuls of crackers or cookies do you eat each week? And, as you know from Practical Bite #39, gluten is not just in corn and wheat. Gluten, or gluten-mimicking compounds, are in rice, quinoa, barley, rye, oats, millet, buckwheat, and a whole slew of other foods. Take a moment and really think about how much grain you eat every week. Is it the majority of your calories? Do grains make up at least half of your plate?

Most Americans are bombarding their gut and immune system with grains every day. I ate the Standard American Diet most of my life, which meant I consumed grains every day – in every meal. And, gluten was one of my main triggers – perhaps the primary dietary trigger – for the autoimmune disease.

To top it off, I ate conventional grains most of my life, which means I was also eating glyphosate. Gluten can trigger leaky gut by itself. But when you add glyphosate into the mix, the damaging effects are more severe. That's one reason why some studies have reported a dramatic increase in the incidence of Celiac Disease in step with the dramatic increase in the use of glyphosate on our food crops.

Here's a question I have pondered: do you think I would have developed an autoimmune disease if I hadn't eaten grains every day?

Joel: Interesting question. Like you, I wonder sometimes if our current problems with celiac and gluten - this whole grain-based issue - isn't as much about volume as anything else. The sheer volume of grains consumed by the average human is far higher than it's ever been historically. Imagine if a loaf of bread cost $10. Would that slow down your consumption? Of course, it would. Until extremely recent times, grain was so difficult to plant, produce, harvest, and store that it was extremely expensive compared to other things like meat and milk (not poultry).

Because meat and milk could be produced without tillage, without planting, without weeding, and often without harvesting, it was the go-to foundation nutritionally and people ate more of it. The Native Americans who developed corn, for example, would eat 10 pounds of bison a day per person when they could get it. They didn't have small grains at all; that came with the Europeans. And so, the animal-centric diet enabled people to receive sustenance without planting annuals.

When your tools are a hoe made out of a bison clavicle tied to a piece of wood with sinew cordage, how much corn are you going to plant? And when harvested, where are you going to store it? You have to keep mice out and keep it dry; two difficult things to do in crudely constructed buildings. Cheap grain is a modern invention. It came along with mechanization, cheap energy, sheet metal storage and price subsidization. One of the big reasons for government subsidies early on was to help give railroads enough freight to be economically viable. It's a tangled web, this food system, and often reality is stranger than you can imagine.

From cereal to crackers to pastries to bread, the amount of grain in the modern American's diet is astronomically higher than it was just two centuries ago. Goodness, back then it was actually cheaper to raise a pig on skim milk than on grain. Why? Because the dairy cow could convert perennials into highly nutritious milk. Harvesting the grass with an herbivore, converting it to milk, and then feeding it to pigs made more economic sense than feeding grain to pigs like we do today. This is why it's critical to pasture pigs today on grain-based rations, in order to get the pigs a much larger variety of food in their diet.

Had we never started gorging on so much grain, perhaps this manifestation of consumption would not have reared its ugly head.

Sina: Exactly! It is highly likely that I could have avoided developing a disease, along with food sensitivities, if I had cycled my food (and had a robust microbiome). Cycling your food gives your immune system a break, which allows it to calm down. Without a break, your immune system wears down. Have you ever been "on the go" to the point where you became exhausted? But, after taking a break you felt re-energized? The same concept holds true for your immune system. If you overstimulate it with the same foods, it can reach a point of exhaustion – that's when food sensitivities and disease can set in. Just like you have to schedule breaks for yourself so you don't completely wear yourself down, you also have to schedule breaks for your immune system.

The power of cycling your food cannot be overstated. Any food can be toxic at high enough doses, even if you don't have leaky gut. But, when eaten in small doses on a cyclical basis, the "poison" can become a benefit. For instance, apricot kernels contain cyanide. In small doses, the cyanide kills cancer cells. In fact, apricot kernels have been successfully used to reverse cancer. But, in large doses, it can kill a person. Likewise, raw kale can help protect you from inflammatory diseases, like cancer and heart disease. But, consumed in large doses, raw kale can damage the thyroid gland and even contribute to the development of hypothyroidism. Hence, a little "poison" is good for us. In small doses it's beneficial; it makes us more resilient. But, in large doses, it's toxic.

Joel, we know a diet predominantly filled with grains makes a cow sick. However, your pasture-raised cows eat a small amount of grain because they nibble the tops of certain plants. Do they nibble on grains year round? Or does nature cycle the grains for the cows?

Joel: Absolutely. They only eat grains (seed heads) when they are available, which would only be for about 60 days during late summer. In spring, the grass hasn't made seed heads yet, so none are available. It's about balance. In an incessantly indulgent culture, it's a crazy concept, I know, but it sure has wisdom built in. Anything to excess can cause problems. As soon as you come off processed foods, it's easier to cycle because you can actually tell what you're eating. When it's just one box or another from a mainline manufacturer, it's all pretty much the same thing and harder to differentiate.

But when you see lettuce, or slice the cheese, or dice the onions, you can really see the item. If you want to take a break from something, take a break. That doesn't mean switching from Cheerios® to Lucky Charms®. That's no break. In my whole life, I think I can remember only about 5 days in which our house contained a packaged breakfast cereal. I kind of rotate along between sausage and eggs, bacon and eggs, oatmeal, and grits as my breakfast staple. Once in a while pancakes smothered in maple syrup, with eggs and bacon on the side. Now that's a breakfast, but it's heavy. My body tells me it doesn't like wheat too much. So about once a quarter is enough, but I do like it. It just doesn't like me.

My one indulgence is bananas. Oh my, do I like bananas, which of course don't grow in Virginia. Although I see an outfit in Ontario growing bananas in green houses. Maybe I need to check into that. Wow, 300 bananas from one tree in a year. Sounds too good to be true. At Christmas, we indulge ourselves with several crates of citrus. When it's gone in early February, we don't really eat any citrus against until next Christmas. Sometimes cycling can be meshed with an indulgence. We don't grow grapefruits here, either. This is more than just seasonal and local; it's switching out your daily food foundation to create balance.

Sina: Precisely! I used food cycling to reverse my food sensitivities. For instance, when I had an autoimmune disease, my body was very sensitive to all dairy and eggs, which is not surprising because those are two of the top food triggers for people with inflammatory conditions. According to my test results, I had the "strongest" immune reaction possible to those foods. In fact, each time I ate dairy or eggs, my right forearm was riddled with debilitating pain.

Because the response was so strong, my functional medicine doctor said I would never be able to eat those foods again. He's a leading expert in the area of food sensitivities and, in his practice, he very rarely sees people reverse those food triggers when the reaction is that strong.

But I chose to believe that all of it would reverse; my body just needed a break. So, I removed all traces of dairy and eggs from my diet for 3.5 years. Then, I retested and my lab results came back NEGATIVE for any type of reaction to dairy and eggs! Consequently, I reintroduced those foods, one a time, and had no issues! I've been eating them for almost a year without a problem. But, of course, I cycle those food groups. My body tells me when it's time to remove them from my diet and when it's okay to reintroduce them. On average, I eat dairy for a few days and then I remove all traces of dairy from my diet for roughly a month. Likewise, I eat eggs for a few days and then remove eggs from my diet for 2-4 weeks, depending on my body's needs. Using that strategy, I'm still healthy and pain-free but now I can eat dairy and eggs.

Joel: Sina is an off-the-charts example, but I know from my travels and conversations she's not alone. I can't imagine the kind of debilitating sickness she's gone through. In the last 40 years, literally, I can only remember being sick - cold, flu - a couple of times. Now I could certainly die tomorrow, but I can't help but think that all those gallons of raw milk, all those meals straight from the garden, and never having soft drinks in the house are paying off as I enter old-man geezer hood.

The remarkable thing about Sina's story is the capacity of the body to heal. I've met people with autistic children who nearly restore normalcy by changing diet. I've met people with all sorts of debilitating diseases that got relief from moving away from the Standard American

Diet. Changing from Classic Coke® to Diet Pepsi® is not cycling, folks, just to remind you. Switching from high caffeine to low caffeine coffee is not cycling. I've never tried going without milk. Maybe I should. I'm getting the shakes just thinking about it; and it's not milk shakes. Although that is a great way to drink milk.

Sina: I love milk shakes! But yes, cycle them. I think eating "seasonally" can be confusing. What does eating "seasonally" mean? Is it referring to the season where I currently live, in Virginia? That implies I can only eat freshly harvested foods that are grown in the Virginia climate. If that were true, I'd never be able to eat an avocado again. And, Joel would have to live without his beloved bananas!

In addition, I've only lived in Virginia for 7 years. What if that's not long enough for my genes to adapt to the foods grown in Virginia? Should I eat based on the seasons of my ancestors in Europe? How far back does seasonality go from the perspective of our genes? For all we know, eating "seasonally" might stretch back to the beginning of the human race when we all came from the Garden of Eden or Africa, depending on your world view.

My point is that nobody knows what eat "seasonally" means to your genes. In that sense, it's an over-simplified catch phrase. And, most of us are going to eat foods from other climates or foods that are now available year-round thanks to the modern food supply. A better approach is to listen to your body; let your body tell you what it needs and when it needs it.

Generally speaking, when it comes to fruits and vegetables, I eat what's grown locally, in season, as much as possible. That way, nature creates food cycling for me. However, when eating processed foods, meat, or foods grown in other climates (like bananas and avocados), I create artificial cycling for myself. That way, I'm receiving benefits offered from local foods while not depriving myself. But, I'm also cycling my foods so I stay healthy and thrive.

SECTION 4:

Meet Your Neighbor

CHAPTER 6

Shift From Whole Food To Locally Grown Whole Food

You've now replaced some processed foods with whole foods, and that's a remarkable achievement! High five!

Let's move a little closer to your goals by acknowledging that most whole foods purchased in a grocery store still contain weaknesses, including: nutrient loss and addition of chemicals due to traveling long distances to arrive at your grocery store, lack of an optimally healthy microbiome, and the loss of adaptive advantages that locally grown food provides. The next category helps you fill those holes.

Moving along the road map, we find ourselves arriving at locally grown whole foods, which includes foods you buy from a local farmer, either directly or in a store, that are whole or minimally processed. Buying local food supports your local economy and small family farmers, but it also helps you move toward maximal health, trust, and freedom.

In terms of health, locally grown fruits and vegetables are generally picked when ripe, which insures the proper pH and nutrient ratios. In addition, locally-adapted plants contain significantly higher levels of functional molecules, or health-promoting compounds. As previously discussed in Chapter 5, plants produce health-promoting compounds in response to various stressors, such as changes in the environment or pathogen/herbivore attack.

Those functional molecules help protect the plant against disease. When you eat those functional molecules, they also help protect you against disease.

Crops grown using commercial or industrial agriculture often contain low levels of functional molecules because they are typically selected for productivity. When varieties that are not productive enough for commercial standards are discarded, it indirectly leads to loss of biodiversity and disease-fighting compounds. In contrast, locally-adapted plants can contain significantly higher levels of functional molecules. For example, studies have reported higher amounts of carotenoids, flavonoids, and anthocyanins in local produce when compared with commercially available produce. These compounds are associated with decreased susceptibility to inflammatory diseases, including cancer and heart disease.

In Chapter 5, we also learned that when you eat whole foods, you consume microRNAs. It is theorized that eating locally grown plants can help you adapt to your local environment in order to optimize your health because you receive genetic adaptations, in the form of microRNAs, from the plants that have thrived in the conditions where you live. While the exact mechanism is not known, we've all heard that eating local honey can reduce your immune response to local pollen. Eating local plants may provide similar health benefits. However, more research is needed to shed light on the adaptive benefits of eating locally grown foods.

In terms of trust, buying whole foods directly from your local farmers increases trust in your food supply because it's easier to hold them accountable compared with a large company located distantly. You can talk with your local farmer face-to-face, and visit the farm to see how your food is grown. Plus, if you don't like something your local farmer is doing to the food, you can more easily shift the market by asking friends and family to place a call or visit the farmer and kindly request changes. Trying to do that within the industrialized food system is like trying to scale the Empire State Building with ice skates on your feet.

Buying directly from your local farmers also increases your trust in your food because when you buy whole foods at a grocery store, you are still relying on the product label and you are still trusting that the regulations around that label are enforced. That's not always a good idea. For example, we previously mentioned that most of the organic grain fed to livestock in the U.S. is imported. And, recently, it was revealed that the U.S. bought more "organic" grain from Turkey then Turkey can produce. That's mathematically impossible! Nonetheless, the U.S. has become the dumping ground for fake "organic" grains because the organic regulations are not adequately enforced.

In addition, the current state of government certified organic affairs takes no notice of anything but a minimal dos and don'ts list that most people would find grossly inadequate to address the concerns of the average buyer. Add to that the current state of adultery in the program, from soilless systems to factory farming and you realize quickly that a simple "Government Organic" label is woefully lacking. In order to sell at a big box store, all the questionable nuances surrounding the idea originally espoused in the word organic must be either dismissed or watered down. This is why we now have numerous non-profits routinely suing the USDA over its failure to enforce the requirements. Even the makeup of the National Organic Standards Board is a mockery of what Senator Patrick Leahy originally envisioned and articulated in the original enabling legislation.

To narrate this point, let's use an example. At Polyface Farm, broilers are raised on pasture in portable shelters, just 75 to a shelter and they are moved every single morning to a fresh salad bar. They get fresh grass, bugs, and manure-free lounge area. Here in the Shenandoah Valley, just down the street from Polyface, is a large government certified organic outfit that raises their broilers in factory houses. For the most part, these are houses that failed to upgrade when the conventional industry said they needed to.

These chickens do not see sunshine, fresh air, or grass, and they live in their toilet all day. Their feed, at least some if not most of it, comes through Istanbul from Kazakhstan or any of the other "-stan" countries. But because it has an organic stamp on the paperwork, these factory chickens are government certified organic.

They are in and Polyface is out. What value is sunshine? Small groups? Fresh pasture? Bugs? Does that not count for anything? In government certified organics, no, it doesn't. It's quite a game that doesn't recognize some of the most salient aspects of animal welfare, husbandry, and respect. Neither does it recognize whether workers are fairly treated or have happy work environments. But, when you buy direct from your farmer, you break free from these loopholes and inadequacies that have become par for the course in the industrialized food system – even in the organic arena.

In addition, buying local allows you to break free from your dependence on the industrialized food system for your survival. For example, if you buy produce from a grocery store and there is a power outage or natural disaster that prevents trucks or planes from delivering food to that store, you go hungry. But, if you are relying on your local farmer, you can drive or walk down the street to get your food from the farm.

By making the shift to buy whole foods from your local farmers, you are one huge step closer to maximal health, trust, freedom, happiness, and personal responsibility.

Practical Bite #51: Choose Local In The Grocery Store

How? Buy locally grown organic products in the grocery store instead of their non-local counterparts. You can identify locally grown products by looking at the company address that is listed on the product label. Also, there is typically a sign in front of locally grown produce stating it's from local farmers.

Why?

Joel: Connecting with our food and communicating about it are two key elements in both authenticity and auditing. If you can't know about its provenance, you can't affect it. The modern industrial food system bathes in obscurity; in fact, being opaque is the main reason it survives. Remove that and it crumbles.

The shorter the chain of custody, from field to plate, the easier transparency becomes and the more likely both buyer and seller can influence each other. This is very much a two-way street. I know that because at Polyface, since we direct market our farm products, we're sensitive and responsive to customer feedback.

Perhaps the single biggest reason, though, to look for local is that it preserves your own foodshed proximate to your life. The quickest way to create food vulnerabilities is to lengthen the distance between producer and consumer. When your area loses its food production and processing capabilities so that everything must be imported from afar, it enters the place called food insecurity.

I read a fascinating book in the last year written by the family that housed Anne Frank's family during the Nazi occupation of the Netherlands during the second world war. While the Franks were holed up in secrecy upstairs, their protectors had to scrounge food for everyone. Thousands upon thousands of Dutch folks starved . . . in the cities. Although the book was not about food, what to eat every day became an all-consuming task. Without fuel for automobiles, they could only go as far as they could get on a bicycle. The folks who survived the occupation were the folks who had connections to the country or who grew things themselves. Starvation in a land as plenteous as the Netherlands claimed countless lives in the cities while people in the country got along fine. The closer your connection to your food, the more resilient your sustenance.

Sina: An easy way to start eating locally is to buy locally grown foods in the grocery store. It takes minimal effort and you still have the convenience of shopping in the grocery store. There is, however, a catch.

Where I live, most locally grown foods sold in the grocery store are not organic. Occasionally, I can find organically grown local foods, but it's the exception and not the rule. When that situation occurs, you must decide for yourself which principle is more important: organic or local.

For me, hands down, organic is more important. I understand the many benefits of buying local. However, I believe it's more important for my health to not eat pesticides, especially glyphosate. So, when faced with the choice of local versus organic, I choose organic.

I do, however, call the farm that is selling locally grown food in my grocery store and ask if they use organic methods. Sometimes the farmer follows organic practices, but can't afford the USDA Organic seal or they understand the loopholes in the label and don't want to support it. So, I always call the farmer and ask. If they do follow organic practices then I buy their product, even without the organic label.

Joel: That's charitable and reasonable, Sina. If you've gotten to this point in the book, you know I have a government certification rock stuck in my craw, but I agree with Sina. Nothing about local makes something necessarily grown well. But the beauty of local is that you can go visit the farm. A rule of thumb is that if you spend more than 2 minutes on the phone with the farmer and he or she does not invite you to come visit the farm, don't buy from that farm. That's a transparency litmus test.

A true-blue farm has no problem with people visiting. In fact, it wants you to visit. If a farm has no trespassing signs or seems in the least reluctant for you to visit, like requiring a time or funneling everyone to a certain date, beware. And be sure to not demand personal escorts and tours. You should be able to wander around at your own pace, breathe in, smell, look, contemplate. You can't always process what your senses are telling you when someone is jawing in your ear and things seem to be in a hurry. You need time to process, to take it in. That's where accountability develops. But if you aren't ready to visit a farm, buying local in the grocery store is a great start.

Practical Bite #52: Eat Ecologically Grown Produce From Your Local Farmer

How? Go to the website www.localharvest.org/organic-farms. Enter your zip code and farms in your area will pop up. Visit or call the farm and ask questions, such as: What is your fertilizer program? What is your pest control program? What is your weed control program? Do you till the soil? Do you apply biosolids to your land? Where does the water come from that is used to irrigate your crops? Do you wax your produce?

Why?

Joel: Many small producers can't or won't go through the time and complexity of getting the organic license partly because there's a long list of questionable practices allowed in organics.

For example, let's take an organic carrot grown under government organic certification. It can be hybrid or open pollinated. The soil can be prepared with tillage, biological oil for herbicide, deep mulch, double digging, cardboard. The soil can be fertilized with fish emulsion from the ocean, off-farm compost from industrial concentrated animal feeding operations (CAFOs), on-farm compost from manures and carbon sources on site, earthworm castings, manure tea, or cover crops. The labor can be provided by paid family, unpaid family, legal labor, nonlegal labor, well paid labor, poorly paid labor. Weeds can be handled by hand pulling, tillage, decomposable mulch, plastic mulch, or propane burners.

Does any of this matter to you? None of it does to government organic certification. What the label does NOT tell you is far more than it tells you.

Sina: I'll add that the USDA Organic certification does not require testing of the soil for heavy metals either. And, neither the FDA nor the USDA have set any limits on the amount of heavy metals allowed in organic foods. That's a problem because heavy metals can be present in the water used to irrigate the crops, and in the soil, partly from fertilizers. And, those heavy metals can be absorbed into the produce that you eat. In fact, toxic levels of heavy metals have been found in organic whole foods. That's bad because too many heavy metals in your body can contribute to the development of inflammatory conditions, such as: ADHD, autism, diabetes, arthritis, and cancer.

So, if you rely on the USDA Organic label when buying fruits and vegetables, you don't know if they contain high levels of heavy metals. And, you can't track it to find out.

Joel: So, what's the solution? Find your local farmer who grows produce using ecological practices.

Whether you use a website or just start asking around, finding a local farmer that direct markets is not difficult. These local farms come and go so don't be discouraged if a recommendation ends up being a dry hole. Stay with it. It's a whole subculture and you'll find it quickly.

Another way to find these farms is through your state's ecological farming society. Nearly every state has one. Here are a few to show you what I'm talking about:

- Ohio Ecological Food and Farming Association (OEFFA)
- New England Organic Farming Association (NOFA)
- Carolina Farm Stewardship Association (CFSA)
- Virginia Association for Biological Farming (VABF)
- California Organic Farming Association (COFA)
- Pennsylvania Association of Sustainable Agriculture (PASA)
- Texas Organic Farming and Gardening Association (TOFGA)

I won't list them all, but you get the idea. As easy as it is to Google® things these days, you can find out what's going on in your state and then zero in on your area. These organizations are committed to helping you source clean products and they'll love to send you to their members.

Sina: When I decided to buy food from my local farmers, the biggest hurdle was actually finding the farms. I was willing to pay higher prices because I understood the value, but I couldn't easily find my local farmers. In fact, after doing many Google® searches, I became overwhelmed. Many of the farms I was able to find did not have websites. Or, the websites were difficult to navigate. Or, they advertised organic practices but they really did spray with synthetic pesticides.

But then I learned about the website localharvest.org and it was a game changer! Not only does this website list the farmers in your area, it connects you to farmers' markets, food coops, u-picks, farm stands, and community-supported agriculture (CSA) programs. And, it's free!

I used that website to find my local farmers, and then I called each of them. I introduced myself and then asked questions based on my food principles, such as:

1. Do you spray pesticides or herbicides on your crops?
2. Do you till the soil?
3. Do you cover the soil?
4. What fertilizers do you use on the crops?
5. Where does the water come from that is used to irrigate your crops?
6. Do you apply biosolids to your land?
7. Do you wax your produce?

Joel: You're looking for a farmer who uses practices that are as natural as possible, including: no spray, no till, no biosolids or sludge, no bare soil, no wax, and clean fertilizer and water. My preference for water sources is: pond, roof run-off, well, then municipal. In terms of fertilizer, ideally it would be generated on site from carbon and manure in situ. However, I would not crucify someone for bringing in compost; some people (like Vermont Composting) make really super compost. But if the farmer is bringing it in from outside, you want it to be as clean as possible.

For direct access to your food and the highest level of integrity, nothing beats your local farmer. You'll build a relationship over time, become friends, and you'll be able to sleep comfortably at night in the complete freedom that your food provenance is the best that it can be. And if you'd like to see a change, you can talk about it face to face. You'll both learn something but you'll both feel validated in the process rather than feel like you're being ignored.

Practical Bite #53: Eat Ecologically Raised, Pastured Chickens From Your Local Farmer

How? Find your local pastured poultry producer. You can do a shout out on the American Pastured Poultry Producers Association (APPPA) website. (www.apppa.org) Once you find your local pastured poultry producer, visit the farm or give them a call. Ask if the chickens are ecologically raised, including: raised in mobile housing; no GMOs, pesticides, or herbicides present in the feed or on the land; no antibiotics administered; and the chickens are not disinfected with chemicals during processing.

Why?

Joel: If you want to eat the best chicken, make sure you get pastured poultry. Not organic, not natural, not animal welfare or any other orthodox certification. The American Pastured Poultry Producers Association (APPPA) is a trade organization for those who move their poultry around on green grass. The chickens are not living in their excrement; they get exercise, fresh air, sunshine, and most important, a few blades of grass and clover each day. Pastured poultry, whether you get it local or shipped to your doorstep, is the gold standard for healthy terrain birds.

Sina: It makes sense to move the chickens in terms of both the chicken's health and our health. Moving the chickens increases the microbial diversity and the available nutrients in the chicken's diet. By consistently providing fresh pasture, the chickens are consuming more bugs as well as grasses that are richer in vitamins, minerals and antioxidants compared to chickens standing still. In addition, the chickens are exposed to a new ecosystem each time you move them – including new microbes in the soil, bugs, and grasses.

When that type of variety is offered in their diet, as opposed to eating from a moonscape, it increases the bird's microbial number and diversity, which increases the health and resilience of the bird.

Joel: Exactly. Now, it can be tricky finding truly pasture-raised poultry. 99 percent of APPPA members use mobile housing. The only reason I didn't say 100 percent is to give myself wiggle room. The whole association is devoted to mobile housing. I suggest you visit the farm. Or, look at the farm website and see if the birds live in mobile shelters.

A stationary house cannot offer fresh pasture to chickens. The house must move. If you can get aerial pictures, you should see a mosaic. Regular satellite pictures will tell the tale. At our farm, anyone can see what we call the "jet stream" the chicken shelters leave as they traverse the pasture. Right behind the shelters, the grass is eaten and tromped down, but count back a week of moves and the grass is dark, vibrant green. That's the telltale signature of movement.

Sina: That's so cool. And, after you've found a farmer who raises truly pastured chickens, call or visit the farm to ask if the land is sprayed with any pesticides or herbicides. Also ask about the feed. It's not enough to be pasture-raised because up to 85% of the chicken's diet can come from supplemental sources. So, you need to know what the farmer is feeding the chickens. You're looking for feed that is non-GMO, has not been sprayed with pesticides or herbicides, and was not irradiated.

Also, ask the farmer if their chickens are given antibiotics and if they are disinfected during processing. You don't want to go through the trouble of finding pasture-raised chickens and end up serving your family a helping of synthetic chemicals and a disinfected microbiome.

The goal is pasture-raised chickens that are not exposed to GMOs, pesticides, herbicides, or antibiotics and are not irradiated or disinfected with chemicals.

Joel: Agreed. And, obviously, when I say "ecologically raised," I'm assuming the pasture is fertilized with manure and compost and that it has not been sprayed with weed killers. Manure tea is fine. The point is that if you can't find it in regular ecology, you might not want to use it.

And, one more thing. Pastured poultry producers are all over the U.S., and many of them are desperate for a handful of additional customers so they can quit their town commute and farm full time. You could be just that tipping point for them, the key patron (saint?) who enables them to reach enough critical sales to come home. Now wouldn't that be a cool thing to do?

Practical Bite #54: Eat Ecologically Raised, Pastured Eggs From Your Local Farmer

How? Find your local pastured poultry producer using the American Pastured Poultry Producers Association (APPPA) website. (www.apppa.org) Then, visit the farm or give them a call. Ask if the chickens and eggs are ecologically raised, including: raised in mobile housing; no GMOs, pesticides, or herbicides present in the feed or on the land; no antibiotics administered; and the eggs are not disinfected with chemicals during processing.

Why?

Joel: As your integrity food radar becomes more refined, you'll find out that all marketers try to tout their product as the best. The buzzwords are obvious: fresh, safe, nutritious, free range, happy, sanitary. You get the idea. If it sounds good, use it. That's the theme. I think by now you realize that a little skepticism on all these phrases is a good thing.

The proof is in the eating. And in the testing. Are differences real? Yes. Several years ago, our farm participated, along with about 11 others in the nation, in a Mother Earth News magazine-sanctioned test to put to rest, once and for all, the naysayers' notion that food is food is food and it doesn't really matter how it's raised. They chose eggs. We sent some into the lab and here are the results, per egg:

NUTRIENT	USDA	POLYFACE FARM
Vitamin E (mg)	0.97	7.37
Vitamin A (IU)	487	763
Beta-carotene (mcg)	10	76.2
Folate (mcg)	47	1,200
Omega-3's (g)	0.033	0.71
Cholesterol (mg)	423	292
Saturated Fat (g)	3.1	2.31

Now I want you to look at that chart carefully, again. Don't skim over this. Do you see the differences? They're not little deviations of a couple percent. They're hundreds of percents! This is not the same food. This is not about organic certification in a factory house; it's about fresh grass, fresh salad bar in the diet. This can only be achieved when birds are rotated very frequently onto fresh, vegetative pasture.

I wish we could afford to run tests like this on everything, but they are extremely expensive and we appreciate Mother Earth News magazine fronting the costs for it. Most farmers will not have this empirical data for their products. But the difference between factory organic and pastured GMO-free is night and day. Now do you think this food is worth more?

Sina: I love this chart because the numbers speak for themselves. You don't need to hide behind fancy marketing and clever wordsmithing. Consumers, like me, can see the difference for ourselves. When I look at these numbers, I'm reminded of why we are heavier than ever before in the history of our nation, yet we are malnourished. Our food doesn't contain the nutrients we need. From processed foods to factory raised poultry and meat, our food is sick – deficient in many nutrients that are essential for our health and longevity. It's no wonder micronutrient deficiency diseases are rearing their ugly head again. As someone who developed two diseases from micronutrient deficiencies, I can assure you that it costs more money and time to diagnose and treat the diseases, as well as the complications from the diseases, than buying nutrient dense food in the first place.

Just like we cautioned in the previous Practical Bite, once you find a pastured poultry farmer, visit the farm or call and ask questions. The goal is to eat pasture-raised eggs from chickens that were not administered antibiotics or exposed to GMOs, pesticides or herbicides through the feed or the land. And, that were not disinfected with chemicals during processing.

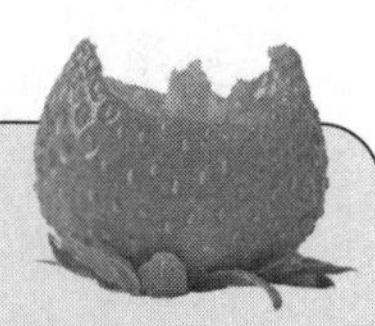

CHEW ON THIS

Lots of folks wonder how they can tell if a farmer is raising the kind of eggs that are safe to eat. Here's an easy litmus test: go sit with the chickens. If you wouldn't want to eat a sandwich sitting there with the chickens, something is wrong. Another test: take your 5-year-old. If she wrinkles her nose and says "this is gross" then that farmer just failed. This is not rocket science. Good farming is aesthetically and aromatically sensually romantic.

Practical Bite #55: Buy Ecologically Raised, Grass-Finished Beef From Your Local Farmer

How? Find your local grass-finished beef farmer using the website www.eatwild.com. Then, visit the farm or give them a call. Ask if the cows are ecologically raised, including: rotated on pasture; no GMOs, pesticides, or herbicides present on the land; no antibiotics or hormones administered; and the meat is not disinfected with chemicals during processing.

Why?

Joel: The operative term here is grass-finished. Not grass fed. The grain-fed feedlot industry takes the position that if a beef animal has one day on grass, then it's grass-fed. Technically, that's correct, but it sure isn't what a person using this designation thinks. The person making the grass component distinction is thinking no grain, no feedlot, grass only right up until the day of processing. Yes, that's what I'm thinking. Clever speak is everywhere, as we know.

During the mad cow mayhem after the turn of the century, consumer pressure mounted on the USDA to ban feeding all animal slaughter waste products to herbivores. The industry routinely cooked dead cows and fed them to living cows. It looked for a time like a comprehensive ban would be implemented, but as the initial paranoia from consumers wore off, the prohibitions were worded carefully to allow some glaring continuations. One was feeding dead chickens to cows. Back in the 1980s, land grant universities developed a protocol for feeding chicken manure to beef in feedlots as a way to cheapen the cost of beef production and to do something with the burgeoning problem of chicken manure from factory houses. It was a perfect scientific two-for. Of course, the industry and its lackey PhDs at the universities touted the normal "no scientific evidence" that this affected the taste, texture, or toxicity of the beef. Interestingly, during this time, the owner of the slaughter house we used to get our own animals processed quit buying Virginia beef because he said he got tired of walking into the meat cooler and the whole thing smelling like chicken manure. I guess "scientific evidence" depends on who's paying for the research.

At any rate, today, beef cattle feedlots are still feeding chicken manure to their animals. While it is called chicken litter in polite and academic circles, you must remember that this manure contains quite a few dead chickens. In a 20,000-bird factory house, mortalities don't all get picked up by the farmer; some invariably find their way into the litter and out the door and then to the feed trough over at the cattle yard. You don't hear about this much, but it's being done today even though a lot of people think they "won" this battle a decade ago. Appreciating the ability of the industry to present itself as something it's not can hardly be overestimated.

Grass-finished beef may or may not be government certified organic. But in order to grass finish, the farmer must exercise some real management finesse. Grass-finished beef is equivalent to making wine. It's an artisanal thing and requires a healthy confluence of several components: genetics, maturity, mineral, brix index (a measure of forage sugar), stress, and fat cover. These are all pieces of the pie that inform a good eating experience. Beyond the farmer, it includes proper cooking technique.

Grain can cover up a multitude of sins. Some people wonder if grass finishing is so superior to grain finishing, why does anyone feed grain? The answer is simple: any dummy can finish a beef with grain. It takes the craft out of it and makes it easy. Grass finishing has a lot of moving pieces to coordinate. With grain you just put it in front of them, they get soft and fat, and then you process; easy peasy.

Grass-finished is never as fat as grain-finished, but the flavor is far beefier. Because the grass-finished animal eats as many as 40 different kinds of plants each day - all that pasture diversity - all those different phyto-chemicals and compounds make for a highly nuanced nutritional experience. You're not just eating second hand corn. You're eating second hand plantain, chicory, clover, fescue, orchard grass, and a host of others. That's why here at Polyface we coined the term *Salad Bar Beef*, to help capture all those essences.

Just like the eggs, grass finishing stimulates and protects a host of variant nutrients. The ongoing work of Jo Robinson, who wrote the book *Pasture Perfect*, keeps us abreast of new findings about the superiority of treating herbivores like herbivores. According to her research, it only takes 14 days of grain feeding to chase most of the conjugated linoleic acid out of a beef animal. As we discussed in Practical Bite #11, conjugated linoleic acid consumed in its natural state (through grass-finished meat) is associated with reduced risk of heart disease, diabetes, cancer and weight gain when compared to grain-fed beef. Since most grain finishing regimens require at least 90 days and many 150 days, which is way longer than 14 days, the conjugated linoleic acid content is drastically reduced in grain-finished beef.

Sina: That's one reason there is conflicting dietary advice around meat, particularly beef. Not all researchers fully understand the far-reaching consequences of the cow's diet. "Cows are herbivores, so does it matter if they eat grass or grains – they are both plants? And, if I feed them grass most of their lives, will it really make a difference if they eat grains for 90 days?" The answer is a resounding yes!

There are also researchers who don't take diet into account when designing a study. Or, if they do, the researcher does not know how to adequately control for diet intake. And, as previously discussed, some scientists are bought and paid for by industry. Consequently, there is conflicting data, making it difficult to discern the truth.

To Joel's point, we know that *every* meal makes a difference – for a cow and for us. Every meal has a profound effect on your microbiome, hormones, biochemistry, and mood. That's why grass-finished meat has a vastly different nutrient profile than grain-finished meat. Consequently, they both have entirely different effects on your body. I would never feed my family grain-finished meat because it generally contains a nutrient profile that is inflammatory. I will, however, feed them grass-finished meat; in moderation, of course.

Once you have found a farmer who grass-finishes, just like we encouraged you to do in the two previous Practical Bites, visit the farm or call and ask questions. The goal is to eat grass-finished meat from cows that were raised on healthy pasture and not administered antibiotics or growth hormones, or exposed to GMOs, pesticides or herbicides. Also, ask if the meat was sterilized upon processing.

Joel: Yes, sterilization occurs at initial slaughter. An anti-microbial "kill step" is required between slaughter and placing the carcass in the chill room. This is to make sure any pieces or flecks of manure left on the carcass are sterilized. At T&E, an abattoir I co-own, we use super-hot water. Some places use chlorine and other toxic agents. I think in general the industry is moving toward hot water - not to protect the consumer, but to keep from having yet another hazardous condition for worker exposure and hence liability considerations. Regardless, it is important to ask the question so you know what you are getting in your next bite of hamburger.

Practical Bite #56: Eat Ecologically Raised, Pastured Pork From Your Local Farmer

How? Find your local pastured pork farmer using the website www.eatwild.com. Then, visit the farm or give them a call. Ask if the pigs are ecologically raised, including: rotation on pasture; no GMOs, pesticides, or herbicides present on the land; no antibiotics or hormones administered; and the meat is not disinfected with chemicals during processing.

Why?

Joel: Pigs raised in the industrialized food system are generally confined in factory houses, in tiny pens on slatted floors. Nothing to root in, no fresh air, no sunshine, crowded with a manure/urine slurry pit under their slats. This is why farmers cut off their tails - to make a sore nub there so that if a pig begins nipping on it, it hurts and the pig moves away quickly before drawing blood. If blood starts, all the other pigs jump on it and eat the pig - they are omnivores.

Of course, they get no forage whatsoever; just grain and water. Thousands in one house, each group of perhaps 100 in a little cell. If you've ever encountered a happy, contented pig, these confinement houses are the most despicable horrendous environments you can ever imagine. To take an inquisitive, responsive, socially interactive pig and put it in such a disrespectful environment is evil and unconscionable. So please, do not buy pork from f actory farms.

Pigs are notoriously stinky and filthy, but they are actually fairly fastidious animals. They pick toilet areas carefully and, like all animals, love new ground. But unlike other animals, they have an onboard plow, meaning they can do a lot of landscape disturbance. I'm not opposed to pigs inside as long as they have deep, clean bedding and get a steady diet of supplemental forage, either as green material or hay. If the pigs stink to high heavens, something is wrong. Certainly, some residual odor may be apparent, but it shouldn't knock you over. In the dead of winter, we bring our pigs into hoop houses on deep bedding so they and we can be more comfortable. And to protect outdoor paddocks from being torn up in the winter.

Nothing here is about scale. Some of the worst pig production scenarios I've seen have been in extremely small outfits. It's not about scale; it's about management. During the spring, summer, and fall, of course, the pigs should be outdoors either in woods or on pasture. Silvo-pasture is ideal (widely spaced trees with forage underneath). In any case, the area where the pigs are located should not be denuded of vegetation.

Because pigs can churn up an area, the farmer needs to be mindful about duration of stay and total area offered at a time. In general, wetter areas can get by with smaller paddock sizes and drier areas need larger areas. This is due to fragility of the landscape. How fast can disturbed vegetation grow back? The faster it can grow back, the more it can handle disturbance; the slower it can grow back, the less it can handle disturbance.

What we call a moonscape is NOT what you want to see. That indicates that the pigs have been there too long or the paddock is too small for the number of pigs. An excellent pastured pig farmer will be able to show you a mosaic of progression: paddocks the pigs have been through that are in various stages of recuperation, and paddocks ahead of their rotation that are extremely vegetated (salad bar) and awaiting their turn to be eaten (pruned). Everything else is less important.

Some farmers use self-feeders and others feed them every day. Some use nipple waterers and some use bowls. Some use trees for shade and others use portable shelters. Those are all personal preferences and not worth fighting about. But the landscape mosaic IS worth fighting about. On our farm, we move our pigs every 5-12 days so they are never in an area more than two weeks. Ideally, it's more like 8-10 days. More frequent moves are fine, of course.

In a good production scenario, pigs are content (they'll come up and nibble on your shoelaces), and pettable, meaning they don't stink and they're relatively clean. Beyond that, GMO-free feed, no chemicals, and water are all they need to be happy and healthy.

Much like the broiler chickens, pigs are omnivores so you probably won't find someone who uses no grain whatsoever. Some breeds of pigs can almost live on forage, but they are very slow growing, small, and have a low meat-to-bone ratio, all of which requires an extremely high price. The most popular of these breeds is the Kune Kune from New Zealand and the Guinea hog.

For a lot of reasons, at our farm we use the traditional British breeds that have been raised in America since colonial times. They grow a bit faster, put on fat easier, and tend to be easier to handle, which includes keeping them home. A wandering pig can do a lot of damage before you finally get him herded back to his paddock.

Here again, mobility is key. Mobile shelter and constant movement are the secret to sanitation and hygiene. The ration is a bit different than the broilers' but all the provenance desires are the same.

Sina: I sound like a broken record! Again, just like we cautioned in the three previous Practical Bites, once you find a farmer who raises pastured pigs, visit the farm or call and ask questions. The goal is to eat meat from pigs that were rotated on healthy pasture, not administered antibiotics or growth hormones, and not exposed to GMOs, pesticides or herbicides through the feed or the land. Also, ask if the meat is sterilized upon processing.

Practical Bite #57: Meet Your Local Farmers

How? Now that you found your local farmers and they passed your litmus test, if you haven't done it already, go meet them! Start with one farmer so you're not overwhelmed. Drive to the farm. Walk around and ask questions so you can make sure they really do practice what they claim.

Why?

Joel: Time. It's a scapegoat for a lot of things. "I don't have time to . . .." Yes, I'm like you. I use it all the time. I spend half an hour reading the newspaper but don't have time to do something for my lovely bride. I get it. We tend to make time for what's important and nobody has more than 24 hours a day.

My favorite story on this comes from Toronto. I did a seminar up there one year and the other speaker was a high-powered attorney who lived in a fifth-story condominium in the heart of Toronto. She and her husband decided to start a family and during her pregnancy, she started thinking deeply about her responsibilities to this little life growing inside of her. And not just inside, but what about after the birth, growing up, teenage years? She found the thought of her responsibility for this life sobering indeed.

She and her husband sat down and charted out a plan for offering the best care possible. It started with sustenance. Against plenty of advice from peers and career-minded friends, she decided the first and most important thing she could do was breast feed. Pull the plug on the formula industry, take full responsibility, and nourish the baby with the best stuff on earth. Check.

But what next? After much soul searching, she and her husband decided to set aside one year and devote it to finding integrity food in their region. This story dates to about 2005 so electronics were not quite as ubiquitous as today, but their goal was still totally revolutionary: "we will not have a bar code in our house at the end of the year." That is drastic, folks. How to accomplish that? They decided to look at their entertainment time and spend one year investing all that recreation/entertainment time in finding their local food provenance.

No theater. No concerts. No vacation in the typical sense. No trips. It was a one-year sabbatical from personal fun to find their life's food. They visited farms, lots of them. They invested in a hand-cranked grain mill for the kitchen. They made new friends. Over the year, they found their meat guy, their grain guy, their vegetable guy, their seasonal fruit guy (strawberries, blueberries, raspberries) and their dairy guy. Some might have been gals, but you get the idea. She stood proudly at that podium and told those University of Guelph students "we did it!"

I was never so proud of somebody in all my life. And more challenged. If she, a high-powered attorney in a high-rise condo in Toronto expecting her first baby, could find the time to find her farmers, what was my excuse? The whole room erupted in applause; I'll never forget it. Chances are today she has some barcodes in her pantry because even little farms like ours now have barcodes on things. But the exploration and the objective are no less admirable. I repeat, if she could do it, what's my excuse?

Sina: The first farmer my children officially met was Joel, and they did NOT want to do it. I wanted to bring my children to the farm because I wanted to connect them with their food supply. But my kids hate driving in the car and the farm is one hour and 40 minutes from our house. You can imagine how much push back I got from my boys when I asked them to join me on the long trek. But then I mentioned that Joel is the reason they have Polyface hot dogs. And suddenly, my boys started jumping up and down saying, "We want to go to the farm. Let's go meet the hot dog guy!"

I couldn't believe how excited they were. They didn't even complain once during the entire drive! When we got to the farm and walked up to Joel, both of my boys became very nervous – as though they were meeting a rock star. My 5-year old stood next to Joel and softly said, "Thank you for making Polyface hotdogs."

In that moment, my heart melted. I wasn't expecting them to appreciate their farmer at such a young age. But they did. Once they connected the hot dogs with Joel, he became their hero and I became the most grateful Mom alive. I can't think of a better role model for a child than a regenerative farmer.

Joel: Farming is a lonely business. Most of us spend a lot of time alone. With the vegetables. With the animals. With the chain saw or bumping along on the tractor. And most of us feel like second class citizens.

You tell me; when's the last time you heard a guidance counselor tell a bright rising high school senior "wow, Mary, your grades are wonderful. You are so smart you should become a farmer!" That's right, think back. Think a little harder. Never heard it, did you? That's because society has a fairly marginal condescending attitude toward farmers, and we all feel it.

Whenever I do a big media event the press wants me to walk in with hay seeds dangling off my bib overalls and wearing a goofy straw hat like Junior Samples on Heehaw. When I walk in with a suit and tie, they get all bewildered, like I'm out of costume and threatening their stereotypes. They get all "aw shucks" on me and let me know in no uncertain terms that they were hoping I'd walk in like the redneck hillbilly we all know that I am. I smile and say I have country clothes and town clothes; "today, I'm wearing my town clothes."

The point is that farmers need affirmation just like you do. But society does not reward farmers, generally, with accolades and "best, brightest, most likely to succeed" commendations. The peasant class is still alive and well. Farmers crave your support, your "atta boy" and "atta girl" encouragement. Farmers feel besieged by a lot of things in society, especially good farmers. And it means the world to be affirmed.

I know as our children were growing up whenever a patron took them aside and told them how important it was for our family to produce their food, our children felt like a million dollars. Suddenly they were participating in noble, sacred, important work and they walked with chin up, back straight, and a spring in their step. Freeing farmers from the shackles of societal condescension is one of the most valuable ministries you can ever perform to protect your food. Do you have time for that? You be the judge.

Practical Bite #58: Thank Your Farmers

How? Send an email, a letter, or pick up the phone and call your local farmers to tell them "thank you." It doesn't have to be complicated or long. A simple "thank you" will suffice.

Why?

Joel: As previously mentioned, farming is kind of lonely. But beyond that, farmers are the first and most important stewards of our resource base. Farmers, for the most part, decide whether we're going to have a civilization or not. They decide if we're going to have enough soil to grow food or not. They decide if we're going to have pollinators or not. They're the bridge between us and starvation.

I spoke at a large gathering of the Nature Conservancy a few years ago in a beautiful setting near the Atlantic Ocean. The large annual gathering in a wetland included a session showcasing all the spots the organization had protected.

Unfurling a large map, a couple of folks walked the crowd through sites protected for some various reasons: endangered plants; endangered animals; endangered insects or just rare ecologies. All of these sites were relatively small, encompassing a few acres. Each of these areas, colored in on the large map, looked like little spots, or blotches. Most of the map was colorless, indicating private land.

When I spoke, I pointed to the map and said "thank you for protecting these areas. That's quite an accomplishment. But if we destroy all this uncolored land - 99 percent of the map - nobody anywhere can hang onto whatever is special about these sites. So, I'm going to talk to you about all this uncolored land." The point is that just like no man is an island, no ecosystem is an island either. You can't have a pristine special place continue to function if the surrounding area is destroyed.

Farmers are the ultimate arbiter of what happens on all that uncolored land. When you find a good one, and patronize a good one, that farmer can use some encouragement. Most farmers who actually build soil and hydrate the landscape and create more breathable air are ostracized by the conventional agricultural community. I've been called a Typhoid Mary and a bioterrorist for letting animals roam outside unvaccinated. Really good farmers are few and far between but they suffer the same emotions and have the same needs as anyone else. They aren't superman and superwoman.

Sina: I agree with Thomas Jefferson when he said that farmers are "the most valuable citizens:"

> "Those who labour in the earth are the chosen people of God…cultivators of the earth are the most valuable citizens. They are the most vigorous, the most independent, the most virtuous, & they are tied to their country & wedded to its liberty & interests by the most lasting bonds."

Farmers are the key to our food freedom. They are the foundation upon which our freedom is built – the last stronghold in the preservation of our liberty. It's important that farmers know we appreciate them and the sacrifices they make so that we can be free. So, please take a moment out of your day to thank your farmer for standing firm in their principles so that your family can continue to eat healthy, healing food in the land of the free.

Practical Bite #59: Say No To Subsidies

How? Eat one meal that does not contain any of the six most subsidized crops (corn, soy, wheat, rice, sugar and cotton). For instance, instead of processed spaghetti noodles made from wheat, try spaghetti squash. Or, leave the bun off your burger and add a vegetable to your plate. Alternatively, buy from your local farmer. By default, when you buy from your local farmer, you are withdrawing your support of and participation in the commodity pricing cartel.

Why?

Joel: Most people don't realize that only a handful of crops get subsidies - actually called crop insurance these days. The word subsidies has fallen into disrepute, so now these programs are called crop insurance; it sounds more politically palatable.

Here are the market protected commodities: corn, soybeans, wheat, rice, sugar cane, cotton. Notice you don't see any vegetables or animals or fruit. It's a fairly short list. But because these few crops have enjoyed special treatment for a long, long time, they have grown to dominate the American agricultural landscape. If you wonder why these crops seem to enjoy sacred status, look no further than government agricultural policy.

Sina: Subsidies are the reason corn surrounds you on all sides in the grocery store, as described in Practical Bite #22. Subsidies are also why your food supply is filled with wheat, rice, soy, sugar, and cotton. Yes, you eat cotton! It's commonly used in fast food chains for deep frying, but can also be found in some processed foods.

In America, we have a centralized food program that allows the government to pick winners and loser. Using the Farm Bill, the government incentivizes farmers to grow government-selected crops. Farmers grow that handful of crops, which produces a surplus. The surplus is converted into cheap, synthetic byproducts – like high fructose corn syrup. Businesses are incentivized to add those byproducts to our foods because they are cheaper than the natural counterparts. And, consumers are incentivized to eat the processed foods containing those byproducts because they are inexpensive.

Since you literally become what you eat, each time you eat subsidized food, you are consenting to allow the government to decide which chemicals you are made of. In doing so, you are allowing the government to determine, in part, your long-term health and well-being. It's a scary predicament we find ourselves in, especially when you realize that the CDC has declared subsidized foods to contribute to disease. In 2016, the CDC published a study in *JAMA Internal Medicine*, one of the most reputable scientific journals. According to the study, "People who ate more of these subsidized foods were more likely to be obese, register high levels of bad cholesterol, and have high blood sugar and inflammation."

But, don't worry. If you choose to eat lots of subsidized, synthetic byproducts and you get sick, the government has a plan: government funded healthcare is available in the form of Medicare, Medicaid and the Affordable Care Act in the event that the government subsidized food makes you sick.

Welcome to the new "circle of life" in modern day America, where taxpayers foot the bill to make cheap processed food. Then, taxpayers foot the bill again to heal the people who get sick from the subsidized food. All of us have already bought into this system on some level. It's a system that uses our own tax dollars against us by making healthy food expensive and potentially unhealthy food cheap. And, it's built on hypocrisy.

For instance, our government-issued dietary guidelines recommend we eat less junk food, including processed food. The former Surgeon General, Dr. Richard Carmona, linked processed food to our current obesity epidemic. According to Dr. Carmona, "Obesity is the terror within" and "unless we do something about it, the magnitude of the dilemma will dwarf 9-11 or any other terrorist attempt." Do you see the hypocrisy?

The government tells us that processed foods lead to disease and we should eat less of them, but they subsidize the very same food that they claim is making us sick. They create and enforce agricultural policies that are in direct opposition to their own dietary recommendations. For instance, our government guidelines suggest you fill half of your plate with fruits and vegetables. However, historically, less than 1% of the Farm Bill budget has been set aside to support these crops. Instead, the money supports the commodity crops that are used to make cheap junk food.

In addition, while propping up a system that creates cheap junk food, our government drives up the price of fruits and vegetables. For instance, incentivizing farmers to grow a handful of commodity crops discourages them from growing fruits and vegetables because the guaranteed money is in subsidized crops. To put it another way: would you plant the crop that guarantees you money or would you plant the crop that could bankrupt you if it fails? Less fruits and vegetables are grown in the United States partly because the guaranteed source of income is dangled over the farms that produce commodity crops.

That's largely why fruits and vegetables are relatively more expensive than junk food. In fact, the indexed price of fruits and vegetables has increased 40% since 1980. In contrast, the price of soda dropped 30% during the same time period.

Joel: To be sure, not all farmers who grow these crops receive a government check. Farmers who participate in the government organic certification program, or grow GMO-free, seldom receive any government payments. Just because the chicken you buy, for example, ate corn, does not mean that corn participated in these government programs.

Sina: That's exactly right. Most of the government aid for farm subsidies goes to giant agribusinesses and wealthy farmers while the small family farms are squeezed out. So, our tax dollars are paying Big Ag to stay big.

Joel: Generally, if you're buying from a local farmer, by default you're withdrawing your own support of and participation in the commodity pricing cartel. If all of us would simply withdraw our patronage from the farmers and crops sucking on the government nipple, it would completely revamp the program. Never underestimate the power of your food patronage as a vote for a different system.

Practical Bite #60: Eat Mindfully

How? Instead of eating while distracted (i.e. watching TV, working, or reading), sit down at a table and focus on your food. Observe the various colors and shapes, and then notice the smell of each food. Say a few words of gratitude, out loud, for your food. Then, place one bite in your mouth and chew slowly, paying attention to the flavors and texture. Chew that piece of food 30 times and notice how it changes. Repeat this for each bite of food. If you are eating with someone, you can enhance your experience by describing the smell, taste and texture to each other.

Why?

Joel: Any American who travels to foreign countries learns quickly that food is different there. I don't mean just the types of recipes, but the spirit of it, the soul of it. For me, the hardest country to do seminars in is Spain. I don't know how they do it. After my first trip, I made a stipulation on my subsequent visits: we have to be sitting down to supper by 8 p.m. Since instituting that requirement, my hosts have been mindful of it but we're always - I mean always - the first ones into the restaurant. And just about the time we leave at 10 p.m. folks are filtering in.

In other countries, dining is not just a pit stop between more important activities. It is THE activity. Lingering at the table is expected. Prince Charles says a culture is defined by its architecture, its food, and its religion. When anyone asks what the food culture is in the U.S., the answer is always the same: fast. Or McDonald's®. That's a sad commentary on the respect and honor bestowed on the fuel for our bodies, brains, and babies.

A famous Roman Catholic priest said eating is a conscious act. The blandness, homogenization and amalgamation of food takes away its identity. A typical fast food hamburger contains pieces of 600 cows. You can't think about the lives of 600 cows as you chew that burger. But if you get ground beef from a local farmer and fix that burger in your home, it'll no doubt come from one cow. Now you can focus on one cow. Her color, the fields she was in (that you've visited), the farmer who handled her (because you've met him and know him by name).

Some research indicates that we actually release digestive enzymes commensurate with memories we have regarding the food we're eating. In other words, if we eat something that conjures up a memory, it digests better. The ideal memory is having stood in the pasture with the cow before she went into your burger, for example. Or weighing out the carrots at the farm store. Or even walking through the carrots in the garden before they matured enough to adorn your plate. These are all visceral but profound memories that influence how our bodies metabolize food.

Sina: This Practical Bite boils down to awareness: are you present when you eat? Or, are you gobbling down your sandwich during a lunch meeting or standing at the kitchen counter inhaling your cereal so you can get the kids off to school on time?

I used to eat in my car while running errands and I'd gobble down my dinner so I could finish the dishes and get the kids to bed on time. Since I was eating organic, homemade "healthy" food, I didn't think it mattered *how* I ate. But I was wrong. *How* you eat is just as important as *what* you eat.

Joel, when I say the word "digestion," what comes to mind?

Joel: I think of meditation. I think of contemplation, of provenance and provision. Of abundance, sufficiency, and ecological righteousness. I view digestion as exactly what happens in a compost pile. Decomposition, decay, and digestion are nuances of the same thing. It's a beautiful thing, because out of it springs regeneration, new life, vitality and new energy. It's not a deadening, but an enlivening. It's not an ending but a beginning. It's not a loss but a profound gain. Death wraps up in life. These meditations force accountability in the whole process.

As soon as we head down this path toward mindfulness, we can no longer discount the ramifications of our food choices. We can no longer dismiss provenance as bothersome. It forces us to evaluate not just for ourselves but our ecological nest and even our unborn descendants, what kind of wellness context we're going to leave. Indeed, recent studies in epigenetics reveal that how I eat can influence descendant's susceptibility to things down to the fifth generation. That's some real responsibility.

It begs the question: do I have time today to invest in my great, great, great, great granddaughter? The answer had better be yes. Anything else is sacrilege.

Sina: Most of us think of digestion as being isolated to our gastrointestinal tract, starting in your mouth and ending with your anus. But, that's not actually true. At least 60% of your digestion begins in your brain! That means, if you aren't present when you eat, you are not allowing yourself to properly digest your food and absorb the nutrients from that meal. In fact, if you are stressed out while eating, even the healthiest meal can inflame your body.

Think about this: when you are stressed, you are in a state of fight-or-flight. And, if your body thinks there's a tiger in the room, it's not going to spend energy digesting your food! It's going to spend energy on what it needs to do in order to survive the perceived threat. So, digestion gets pushed to the side: the peristaltic contractions that are needed to move your food along your gastrointestinal tract get dampened, so the food you just ate moves ever so slowly through your digestive tract. In addition, the enzymes, bile, and acid that are required to properly digest and absorb your food are suppressed. So, your food essentially rots inside of you, resulting in a buildup of toxins and inflammation.

Hence, how you eat is just as important as what you eat. In fact, when I know a stressful situation is coming up, such as giving a talk, I will fast prior to that event.

Joel: Amazing, Sina; that's exactly what I do. If you recall the famous mongoose Rikki-Tikki-Tavi in Rudyard's Kipling's story by that name, he trained himself to fast before encountering the king cobra so he would be quick and not lethargic. I got onto fasting before speeches when I was on the intercollegiate debate team in college. It was certainly not by design, but by accident. Before a tournament we always pulled all-nighters getting our evidence and cases put together and we found it was more important to prepare than to eat.

One time we were especially behind and I did not eat for 36 hours. We did really well that tournament and put two and two together, realizing that my sharpness was partly because I didn't have any blood going to digestion. I still practice this today and eat as little as possible when I'm doing seminars.

Sina: That's so cool! My husband was right; you are the male version of me!

So, how do you become mindful when eating? Single-task. You cannot be fully present if you are multi-tasking. You have to slow down and bring awareness to the present moment. In other words, pay attention to what is happening right now. By directing your focus to the present moment, you shift your nervous system away from fight-or-flight (where digestion is not a priority) toward rest and digestion.

In our home, we practice mindful eating with every meal. I have two young children, so some attempts are more successful than others. But we always sit down at the table together and pray before we begin to eat. We thank God for allowing our bodies to digest and absorb all of the nutrients in our food. That expression of our gratitude is proactive because if you thank your body in advance, it aids in the digestive process and sets your body up to receive the nutrients more efficiently. So, we pray as though it already happened. After our prayer, we each say three things we are grateful for. Practicing gratitude shifts your energy by helping you focus on the positive so you can get out of fight-or-flight.

Joel: We practice the blessing prior to eating in our home too, Sina, and I think it helps us appreciate that something bigger than us nourishes us. You know that hilarious scene from the iconic Jimmy Stewart Civil War movie Shenandoah when he asks the blessing over the meal? He's not very religious and he starts the blessing with "if we hadn't planted it, it wouldn't have grown and if we hadn't harvested it, it wouldn't be here but we thank You just the same." Of course, Jimmy Steward drawls out the lines like only Jimmy Stewart can do.

Giving obeisance to something bigger than us who placed soil, water, oxygen and the sun here to care and nurture us, puts us in a frame of reference to appreciate a hand bigger than our own; a plan bigger than ours; a mission bigger than our lifetime. That's a good way to view our nourishment, our significance, and our dependence on things outside our control.

Sina: So, stop eating on the go. Slow down and actually taste your food. You are worth the time it takes to sit and enjoy a meal.

Practical Bite #61: Meditate Daily

How? Spend 5 minutes each day practicing meditation. Don't let man define meditation for you. Meditation might include: mindfulness, guided meditation, nature walks, hiking, sitting in silence, petting your dog, prayer, deep breathing, chanting, or practicing loving-kindness. The intention behind meditation is to develop better concentration, clarity of mind, calmness, emotional positivity and stability, and a connection with your higher self.

Why?

Joel: I've heard that all great leaders spend an hour a day by themselves, walking. Something wonderful happens when we are alone with our thoughts. In the solitude and quiet of aloneness we get inspiration and illumination. One of the most enjoyable parts of my farm life are the hours I spend alone, walking, thinking. No ear buds. I don't even have a smart phone. No radio. Just nature. It's a powerfully refreshing thing.

Sina: I used to think meditation was a waste of time. Why would I sit around chanting to myself when there's so much to do? Besides, I didn't know anyone who meditated. I thought it was something only Buddhists did. But then, one day, I opened myself up to the idea of meditation and it changed my life.

Once I began researching the healing powers of meditation, I was floored. Did you know that meditating on a regular basis can *reverse* the aging process by at least 15 years? It works through increasing the length of your telomers. Telomeres are located on the end of each strand of your DNA. They are like protective caps. Each time a cell divides, the telomeres get shorter. Consequently, the length of your telomeres is used as a marker for aging – the shorter your telomeres, the more you have aged. Well, researchers from Harvard found that you can increase the length of your telomeres by practicing meditation. In other words, meditation has been scientifically shown to reverse aging! Do you really need another reason to start meditating?

Meditation has also been shown to relieve chronic pain. A study published in *The Journal of Pain* reported a significant decrease in pain following 8-weeks of meditation. Interestingly, the participants who did home-based exercise and no meditation, did not experience the same type of pain reduction.

In addition, numerous scientific studies have shown that meditation can help you feel energized, reduce stress, reduce blood pressure, improve heart and lung function, alleviate depression and anxiety, decrease irritability, increase fertility, increase focus and productivity, and help you sleep better. Meditation can also help heal the body from inflammatory diseases like rheumatoid arthritis and cancer, in addition to assisting with weight loss - partly by reducing the desire for binge eating and emotional eating. It sounds like a miracle drug! So why not try it?

Emergency responders, the military, and some corporations are utilizing the power of meditation. For example, it's been successfully used to treat post-traumatic stress disorder. In addition, meditation has helped soldiers stay calm and focused in battle while improving their overall mental and physical health. If meditation can help soldiers deal with the stress of battle, it can certainly help the rest of us deal with our daily stresses.

Meditation has become a pillar of my health and wellness program. I strive to meditate at least 5 minutes twice a day, every day – once in the morning and once in the afternoon. It helps me transcend the ego so I can more fully connect with God and receive His healing energy, sometimes called the Life Force. I largely credit that healing energy for my full recovery and my continued wellness.

When I meditate consistently, I feel unshakable peace. The kids can be screaming while the water on the stove is boiling over and the phone is ringing, yet I am able to remain calm and address each issue in a peaceful and compassionate manner. However, when I skip a day, everyone in my family knows because my entire disposition changes. I move from a space of peace and calm to one of anxiety feeling and overwhelmed. Everything seems harder. Everything takes longer. Everything is more draining. I'm easily irritated and, by the end of the day, I'm exhausted. For me, meditation is a gift that brings me closer to God and, consequently, closer to optimal health, wellness and happiness.

I used to think I didn't have time to meditate. It was one more thing added to my "to do list." But it's interesting because I feel like I gain time when I meditate. I'm more productive but I feel less stressed. In fact, my friends and family are constantly amazed at how much I'm able to achieve in one day while staying healthy, calm, and happy.

It was difficult to start the new habit of meditating. But, once I felt that unshakable peace, it was addicting. I never wanted to go back to my hectic life and stressed out self.

Meditation works on many levels, most of which we do not understand. We know it induces deep physical, mental, and spiritual healing. We believe it allows you to achieve a state of rest that is 5 times deeper than sleep! It works partly through deexciting the nervous system so you create order. And, we know it allows your body to release stress from the present moment, like with mindfulness or exercise, but it can also release stress from the past. That's what makes meditation so powerful and so important for health and wellness.

It's not bad to get stressed. We all get stressed and the body is equipped to deal with acute stress. But it can be bad to stay stressed. Chronic stress contributes to at least 95% of all diseases. And, stress can be anything from constantly checking email or text messages to sitting in traffic or even having negative thoughts and emotions. It's all stress and it can all contribute to disease if not managed.

For instance, when you stress, adrenaline and cortisol are released. Cortisol shrinks the memory center in the brain thereby increasing the risk of dementia. It's also acidic and leads to inflammation. As you know, inflammation sets you up for disease. Thus, by releasing your stress on a regular basis, you are practicing disease prevention. For example, meditation counters the problems caused by stress by releasing dopamine and serotonin, which are both alkaline so they change the pH of your body in a good way. Dopamine and serotonin are also known as "feel good" chemicals. Therefore, through meditation, the stress from the current moment, as well as the stress from the past, is able to be released from your body, which sets you free. Who wouldn't want that?

So, how do you meditate?

If you search online, you'll find many definitions of meditation. I choose not to limit myself to a man-made definition. For me, meditation is anything that helps me transcend my ego so I can connect with my higher self. It's how I connect with God on the deepest level. That may include sitting in silence with my eyes closed and praying to God, hiking with my dogs in the mountains, listening to a guided meditation, or participating in a Circle of Friends. Whatever it looks like for you is okay. Do what works for you and call it whatever you'd like. It's your journey.

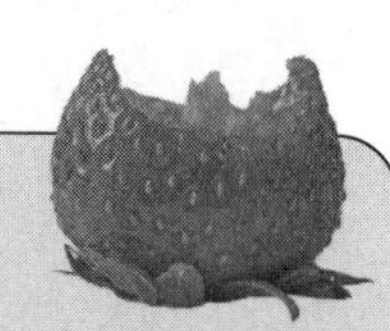

CHEW ON THIS

Meditation is often differentiated from mindfulness. We previously talked about practicing mindfulness when you eat. Mindfulness is commonly described as practicing awareness i.e. noticing the way your food smells, or tastes, or how the food effects your mood. Meditation is sometimes described as going beyond the ego to reach a higher level of consciousness.

SECTION 5:

Get Your Hands Dirty

CHAPTER 7

Shift From Locally Grown To Home-Grown Whole Food

The final category, home-grown whole foods, contains foods that are whole or minimally processed that you grow or raise yourself.

Choosing to grow or raise your own food brings you closer to maximal health, freedom, and trust. Growing your own food is as local as you can get, which means you receive the greatest health advantages IF you use ecological or regenerative practices. For example, picking and eating fruits and vegetables when fresh from your own garden provides your body with the optimal nutrient profile, plant microbiome, and adaptive advantages. Plus, getting your hands in the soil and breathing in the microbes through your lungs and nasal passages helps re-populate and diversify your own microbiome.

If you become self-sustaining, meaning you don't need inputs from companies or any outside sources, growing your own food ensures maximal trust in your food supply since you control and oversee everything. You don't have to trust that the labels or the companies are honest. There is peace of mind when you know exactly what is in the food you are eating and feeding your family.

When you do not depend on anyone for your basic needs, including food, you are truly free. You are no longer a slave because you are self-sufficient; nobody can control you if you can survive on your own without help from anyone. Since the beginning of time, food has been used to control and manipulate people. That ends when you can feed yourself.

Practical Bite #62: Grow One Herb In Your Kitchen

How? Pick an herb you like. If you don't have a favorite then start with mint. Buy organic herb seeds from your local nursery or purchase them online (www.southernexpsoure.com). Alternatively, make it easier by purchasing an herb plant that is already grown.

Keep the herb in your kitchen, making sure it receives sun light. Add the herb to your food. For cooking suggestions, refer to Practical Bite #46.

Why?

Joel: Mint is almost fool proof. Incredibly hardy and prolific, it's not picky about place, soil, pot or care. It's a great starter herb. Success breeds success, so the idea here is for you to have some success and start your progression. Around our farm mint actually grows wild down along the river.

Sina: My first success was with mint. When I was trying to garden outside and I kept failing, it was very frustrating. I would work really hard for weeks and then bugs would eat my crop, or the weeds would explode and overtake my garden faster than I could pick them, or it would become too humid for me to want to work outside (Yes, I'm spoiled regarding weather. What can I say, I'm from California!). I would end up getting worn-out and then I'd take a season off just to step away from it. Instead of a yo-yo dieter, I was a yo-yo gardener.

After failing miserably for the fourth time, I decided I was trying to do too much too fast. So, I dialed it way back and started again with just one plant. I bought an organic mint plant from my local grocery store (they are available in some stores seasonally). And, I decided to keep my precious plant in the kitchen so that I would remember I had it.

Seriously, I needed the constant reminder in order to make the plant a priority. My kids took turns watering it and I would sing to it and brush the leaves with my hand. If you've never done that before, please try it! The smell of the herb is transferred to your hand. It's wonderful!

My mint plant sat in the kitchen for weeks until I finally decided to do something with it. I picked a few leaves and added them to my smoothie. It was delicious! Fresh herbs add a unique flavor profile to your food that's hard to describe. It's like tasting flavors on a deeper level that are more complex and intricate than any flavor you've tasted before. And, they are packed with healing nutrients. Herbs are, after all, medicinal plants – God's medicine.

As soon as I tasted that smoothie, I was hooked! I wanted to grow more herbs. And, since I was successful at not killing my mint plant, my confidence grew and I felt ready for the next step.

So, my children and I went to our local grocery store and bought more organic herbs, already potted. Soon, half of our kitchen table was covered in herbs. We started adding herbs to everything. Sometimes our creations tasted good and sometimes they didn't. But that didn't matter. We had fun creating great memories while feeding our bodies healing plants.

Joel: I know this is about food, but I'm going to put in a plug for *Aloe vera*. We keep a couple on windowsills and they're the go-to medicinal for anything skin related. A burn, cut, abrasion - anything that creates an "owie" on the skin. You just break off a piece of it, squeeze the juice out on your wound, and it greatly speeds healing. These plants sit there seemingly eager to serve whenever you need them.

That's the spirit of herbs. They look innocent enough, but they pack big tastes and big nutrient concentrations, in small spaces, with generally easy care. What's not to love?

Sina: We also have an *Aloe vera* plant! That's another plant that thrives even when I neglect it. In fact, my husband jokes that the *Aloe vera* plant gets nervous when I walk by because, when I do pay attention to it, I overwater it and it doesn't do well.

Like you, I utilize *Aloe vera* for skin related issues, such as: cuts and burns and as a moisturizer. It's probably best known for its' ability to heal sunburns. I used to buy bottles of *Aloe vera* in the grocery store, but after growing my own, I stopped. Store-bought *Aloe vera* skin products do not contain the same healing properties as *Aloe vera* that is harvested fresh and unprocessed straight from your own plant. They may also contain preservatives or other ingredients intended to extend shelf life or improve the smell, texture or color.

Plus, if you grow your own, you can eat it as a medicinal food. You can add the gel to smoothies, salsas, salad dressing, etcetera. It's been reported to help lower blood sugar levels, decrease inflammation, boost memory, reduce dental plaque, heal canker sores, reduce wrinkles, and combat damage caused by free radicals, which are linked with inflammatory diseases.

The *Aloe vera* leaves consist of three parts: the skin, gel and latex. The gel is typically applied to the skin and eaten. Simply slice off the skin on the flat side of the leaf and remove the clear gel. Some herbalists recommend washing off the yellow liquid (latex) that is between the skin and the gel of the leaf because it can be bitter and it contains compounds with powerful laxative properties. In fact, products made with aloe were once regulated by the FDA as over-the-counter laxatives.

Again, my *Aloe vera* and my mint plants thrive inside my house and I hardly do anything to help them. So, gardening doesn't have to be hard and it doesn't have to be big or traditional. Meet yourself where you are. If one plant is all you can handle then go for it! Give it your all. Get to know that plant before you advance to the next. You never know where your journey will take you until you jump in and try.

Practical Bite #63: Grow One Edible Plant Indoors

How? Once you've successfully grown a single herb in your kitchen, challenge yourself to grow something larger indoors. You can buy one pot and grow one type of produce, such as: lettuce, arugula or kale. Or, if you're ready to grow multiple plants but don't have a lot of space, try growing a soil-based vertical garden.

Here are some simple steps to get you started:

To grow lettuce or arugula: Add organic potting soil to a pot; sprinkle 5-15 seeds on the surface and then cover the seeds with 1/8 inch of soil; mist with a spray bottle until the surface is damp; place in a sunny window and continue to keep the surface damp, but not soaking. Thin out the weaker, smaller seedlings as needed. When it's ready to be harvested, cut and eat the larger leaves while leaving the smaller leaves to grow for a later harvest. (Use lettuce varieties that are "cut-and-come-again" or "cutting lettuces" because you can harvest the leaves and the plant will keep growing back).

To grow kale: Plant a few seeds in a medium-size pot and cover with ½ inch organic potting soil. Keep moist. Thin to one plant per pot because kale can grow pretty large. When it's ready to be harvested, pick off and eat the bigger leaves while leaving the smaller ones to grow for a later harvest.

Why?

Joel: The reason you start with an herb or two is because these plants leverage freshness more than just about anything. In other words, the difference between store, stale, and fresh is bigger than it is for potatoes, let's say. So, you want to start with the food items that offer the greatest difference if you raise them yourself. Herbs are number one.

A close number two is leafy greens. Here are some reasons:

1. They're extremely fragile and perishable.
2. They're full of water. The percentage of water in leafy greens is higher than vegetables. From a transportation carbon footprint, we can't be delivering water everywhere.
3. They're fluffy and bulky. A box of lettuce or kale weighs a few pounds compared to a similarly sized box of beef, carrots, potatoes, or squash. This is related to number 2

above. If water is expensive to deliver, try keeping it fluffed up. Measuring shipping in both bulkiness and carbon footprint makes leafy greens the primary candidate to pull out of the industrial loop.

4. They're the most tolerant of cold. Long after your lawn has given up for winter, kale just keeps loving those cool late fall temperatures. Leafy greens extend the fresh food season like nothing else.
5. They're the most common vectors in food borne illness. About 95 percent of all food-borne bacterial contamination incidents stem from leafy greens. Why? Because by definition, leafy greens are cool, full of water, and fresh. Because they can't be frozen or cooked, they don't enjoy the forgiveness of what food safety engineers call "kill steps." Cool, moist conditions provide a perfect medium for a contaminant to grow. If you grow greens yourself, you can protect them from CAFO manure slurry contamination and harvest worker defecation.

Historically, nobody transported greens in long distance food commerce. People grew greens in their solariums and gardens. Distance transportation was reserved for spices, cheese, cured meats, and nuts. And wine and spirits. These nutrient dense food items could be reasonably transported. While greens are nutritionally important, they are not nutrient dense like these other things.

Sina: And, leafy greens can be grown inside your home. Growing an edible plant indoors is a great next step in your journey as a gardener. It's not as intimidating, time-consuming, or expensive as starting an outdoor garden. And, it's convenient because the plant lives in your house! So, you don't have to brave the weather to tend to your plant, or fight off bugs that want to eat your food.

Plus, if you have children or grandchildren, this can be a great family project. My children love sprinkling seeds in pots and watering the plants with a spray bottle. They actually fight over who gets to spray the plants!

Joel: The self-reliance movement developed a demand and market for all sorts of home-based planting infrastructure. For the solarium on the end of our house, I got Teresa a couple of planting boxes that have sub-irrigation plumbed in under the soil. They're pretty and practical. Sometimes a gizmo can be exciting enough to make you jump into something that otherwise would be intimidating.

I think most people don't appreciate how much food can be grown in a small space. Especially in the U.S. we're used to seeing monster tractors, fields, and processing facilities. The industry has done a great job of creating a national psyche that if it isn't big it isn't worth doing. Never underestimate the cumulative effect of lots of little things. They add up. Goodness, in Italy they don't have yards; they have gardens. Vines trellised up the side of houses. Expressway clover leaves aren't mowed with batwing mowers; they're gardens.

Sina: I've had a lot of success growing food inside my home. I use pots with soil, but hydroponic tower gardens are popular right now. They look cool and I have several friends who love theirs.

Hydroponics is a method of growing plants in water with a nutrient solution. The roots are supported using an inert medium, such as: clay pellets, peat moss, perlite, rockwool or vermiculite. Hydroponics can be appealing because the plants are touted to grow up to two times faster than they would in soil. In addition, there are no weeds to pick, no soil to get your hands dirty, and the environment is more controlled, which can result in less use of pesticides. It sounds great! But there's a potential downside.

Because there is no soil, plants grown in a hydroponic system may not develop the same diversity of beneficial microbes on their roots, stems, leaves and fruit. This is a recognized problem. In fact, attempts have been made to add microbial diversity back into hydroponics by using "organic" growing media such as coco coir and adding worm casting or using natural-made nutrients, such as: fish, bones, and alfalfa. But nothing you add will ever replace the biodiversity of *healthy* soil.

We don't even know all of the ingredients that make up healthy soil. So, how can you reproduce it? For instance, it's estimated that 90% of all organisms on the seven continents live underground, including: bacteria, fungi, protozoa, nematodes, mites, and microarthropods. There is so much diversity living under your feet that scientists think we've only discovered 1% of the microorganisms in soil! We still have a lot to learn, but we do know there are a lot of organisms in a small amount of soil. It's estimated that one gram of soil, which is roughly equivalent to ¼ teaspoon of sugar, contains one billion bacterial cells!

Thus, if you tried to add microbes to the hydroponic system to mimic healthy soil, you can only add the microbes that are known. What about the 99% of microorganisms that are still unknown? Even though the intention behind hydroponics is good, the method uses reductionist thinking. You cannot reproduce the microbial diversity nor the complexity of microbial interactions that exists in healthy soil.

Let's apply this concept to your health. A healthy soil sample can contain roughly three times the bacterial diversity of what is found in your gut. And, exposure to those microbes helps protect you from diseases like autoimmune disease, cancer, and diabetes. Consequently, when you eat plants grown without soil, you may deprive your body of the beneficial microbial diversity it needs to be healthy and thrive. Not to mention the adaptive advantages and nutrient profile that is developed in plants that interact with the soil and local environment.

Joel: The newest permutation on this theme, Sina, is aeroponics. This system delivers nutrients to the plants via the air so it's waterless. True, the air is extremely moist, but all the deficiencies true in hydroponics are perhaps even greater in aeroponics.

These non-soil systems enjoy excellent market messaging:

1. Freshness because it can be picked an hour before being eaten.
2. Local because it can be grown in our house or in the city.
3. Less water usage than soil requires; most of these systems have a water loop that re-uses the water so they're considered closed systems. This views the system as independent from the greater ecology of rainfall, transpiration, and overall landscape hydration. And the data points to impugn soil use industrial low-organic matter soils as benchmarks rather than compost-based high-water retentive soils.
4. Less disease because everything is in a controlled environment. You can exclude insects, fungus and other problems. That is true if everything is wonderful, but if something fails, the system is extremely fragile. The stories of complete devastation are legendary once you get past the veil of secrecy within the hydroponic industry. Disney's Epcott Center® has about four times as much space behind the public access space growing

replacement plants for the ones that show signs of weakness. It's not all what you think.

5. Extreme production per square foot due to environmental control: the temperature, moisture, and nutrients are always perfect, encouraging better growth. Does any biological entity perform best when it encounters zero stress? No. Every grape grower knows the secret to good wine is some stress on the vines; that enhances the flavors. We need some hardships and stresses to build healthy immune systems. And what is growth without nutrition? Cancer is growth.

Another offshoot of the hydroponics system is called aquaponics, which incorporates fish into the water loop. The fish generate manure which then fertilizes the plants, which purify the water so it can be returned to the fish. The running joke among aquaponics farmers is that you don't really learn the system until you've killed 10,000 fish. Again, when everything is perfect, the system is amazing. But it's extremely fragile: temperature, perfect mix of nutrients, perfect levels of oxygen. When your farming requires a dozen digital monitors and a computer control center, you might want to question its resiliency.

In order not to be a complete naysayer, I've come to a litmus test that allows a crack in the door of these non-soil systems. Introductions to numerous growers made me realize that just like every farming system, lots of permutations can exist under a broad umbrella. And, so it is with these non-soil systems. So, here's my test: if the medium the plants grow in supports active earthworm populations, I'm okay with it. Some systems use pebbles or even marbles that offer enough adhering surface to colonize microbes and organic matter. It becomes kind of a swamp. If I pull up a plant and it has earthworms clinging to the roots, that's good enough for me, even if the operator calls it a hydroponic system. That's my caveat.

Sina: Interestingly, we had some friends come to our home last weekend and their child tried my tomatoes, right off the vine. He eats freshly harvested tomatoes all the time because his Mom grows a hydroponic tower garden in her kitchen. But, this 10-year old kid could taste the difference! He was so inspired by the flavor of my tomatoes that he asked his Mom if he could grow his own inground garden! That says it all.

Practical Bite #64: Grow Your Sprouts

How? Purchase seeds that are organic, or that have not been genetically modified or sprayed with pesticides or herbicides. Soak the seeds overnight in a glass container. Then, put them in a glass jar in the windowsill, water them once a day, and in a week, you have a jar full of the most nutritious salad legs ever.

Why?

Joel: I remember the first time I saw mung bean sprouts in a quart jar. It looked like magic. It was, and still is. You can't believe that much material grows out of a simple little seed, but it does.

Sina: Sprouts add a new dimension of flavor, color, and texture to food, which is why they are used by many renowned chefs. I love adding sprouts to my salads, wraps, and sandwiches. Examples of sprouts include: broccoli, mung beans, radish, crimson clover, peas, and mustard.

Sprouts are also known as immature greens, which is a catch-all group for sprouts, bean sprouts, shoots, microgreens, baby greens, and soil sprouts. Studies suggest that immature greens can contain more nutrients and health-promoting micronutrients than their more mature counterparts. In fact, a study from the *Journal of Agricultural and Food Chemistry* reported that microgreens contained up to 40 times more nutrients compared to their mature counterparts. And, a 2018 study published in the same journal concluded that microgreens have a "potential use in diet-based disease prevention."

Plus, growing your own immature greens is less expensive then buying high-quality multivitamin and mineral supplements. And, they provide micronutrients in their natural state, which is easier for your body to digest and assimilate than manufactured supplements. So, why not try them?

The essence of this Practical Bite is to encourage you to grow your own immature greens. I favor using soil whenever possible. However, growing immature greens in a jar is easier, less messy, and still provides you with a nutrient dense food.

Joel: You can get sophisticated kits and exotic seeds. The sky is the limit on where you might want to take this, but if you want to eat well on pennies, few options afford more benefits than sprouting. You can buy sacks full of seeds for a few dollars and create mountains of incredibly nutritious sprouts. This is the most child-captivating food production project you can do, partly because it's clean and happens fast. It's not like waiting for a chicken to grow or a tomato to finally make ripe fruit. Sprouts take a few days start to finish; try some today.

Practical Bite #65: Start A Small Garden

How? Many books have been published offering a how-to guide on gardening. Below we provide some ideas to help you get started.

Why?

Sina: Growing plants inside is a great step forward in your health journey. As we've laid out, there are many health advantages to this practice and it's less overwhelming than growing a garden outside. But, if you are ready to scale up your food production or if you want to receive the health advantages that plants acquire as they adapt to the outside environment, take this next step and grow some plants outside.

I strongly encourage you to start small. When I first tried to garden outside, I bit off more than I could chew. I attempted to manage 20 rows that were each 20 feet long. I also had a young child and was pregnant! My intentions were good; I wanted to grow 75% of my family's food because I understood the health benefits of growing our own produce. But, by not setting a realistic expectation of myself, I ended up feeling like a failure; like organic gardening was just too hard. And, I walked away from it for quite some time.

So, be kind to yourself by starting out small. Bigger is not better if it stresses you out. You can always scale up once you know you can successfully manage the smaller garden. I currently have 4 beds that are each 10 feet long. It's only a fraction of my original garden, but now I don't feel resentful or obligated. I feel like a success because I can take care of my garden without feeling stressed or taxed.

Joel: I agree, the operative term here is "small." The most common mistake newbie farmers make is starting out too big. A simple 2 ft. X 5 ft. spot can grow lots of plants. Sina and I cannot begin to offer a comprehensive how-to section on gardening in this book. Goodness, libraries are full of gardening books. And everyone has their druthers.

I'll just introduce you to a few of the most common methods. If one of these strikes your fancy, you can research the intricacies more on your own.

1. **French Bio-intensive Gardening.** Developed by gardening guru John Jeavons, this method introduced double digging and raised beds. Based on research, this system

probably gets first place for being the most productive per square foot.

2. **Back to Eden**. Paul Gauchie popularized this system that uses no tillage whatsoever, but maintains as much as a foot of wood chips as a continuous cover. To plant, you push aside the wood chip mulch. It's a bit of a take-off from the iconic 1960s book The No Work Garden Book by Ruth Stout.
3. **Square Foot Gardening.** My understanding is that this book by Mel Bartholemew has sold more copies than any single gardening book in history. That's saying something. The idea is to segment your space in squares to reduce wasted space.
4. **SPIN Farming.** The acronym stands for Small Plot INtensive and is the brainchild of Wally Satzewich and Roxanne Christensen. From a foothold in Canada, it has now spread throughout the world as a way for tiny places to return big bucks.
5. **Permaculture.** I'm just using a generic notation on this one because it's so broad. Bill Mollison and Dave Holmgren invented the term and popularized it. A couple of years ago the one millionth permaculture certificate was issued for the basic design course. Many people call this "sloppy" gardening because it uses cardboard and mulch and spirals and water turrets. I think they're beautiful.
6. **Lasagna Gardening.** This technique uses layering to create a growing medium. One of the most common is simply to place a bale of hay or straw on the ground (don't worry about if the ground is a lawn or back alley) and then water it well for a couple of weeks. Put some compost on top and plant into it.
7. **Hugelkultur.** Developed in Germany, this technique utilizes wood scraps, heaped into a windrow then covered with a thin topping of soil. It greatly increases the surface area by creating mounds out of flat ground. The rotting wood underneath holds water, grows fungi, and maintains excellent aerobic conditions.

In this short list, I've certainly left out some of the current gurus of gardening: Eliot Coleman, J.M. Fortier, Ben Hartman, Singing Frogs Farm and the list could go on and on. When you get into it, you'll find this field far more fascinating than science fiction. Starting with a tiny plot outside your back door (or front door) is a crack into a world you'll never regret.

Sina: My garden sounds like a mixture of techniques. I essentially used the resources I had available. For instance, I currently use garden beds. I made the borders from trees that fell down during a few storms we had that year. I literally dragged them over to my garden and placed them in a rectangular shape as best I could. I held them in place by hammering wooden spikes into the ground.

Then, since I was building my garden on top of our lawn, I laid down cardboard (after removing tape or any spots that contained dye) because I didn't want to till the land – it seemed physically difficult to do by myself, and I didn't want to disturb the microorganisms. Next, I added layers of leaves and sticks, which had also fallen during storms. Then, I added soil from my big garden. I would like to make my own compost some day soon, but I'm not there yet. So, I bought organic compost. Finally, I covered the soil with organic mulch.

Joel: I'm a huge believer in garden beds, whether they have borders or are raised. The two primary reasons are psychological for the gardening and friendliness to kids. When you have beds of any kind, you can see the end when you start. A long row of anything seems unending. But beds give a clear idea of where you start and where you end. You can actually weed a bed in a few minutes. Each bed offers a task that you can start and stop within reason.

Now to the children. Few things are more fascinating to a child than a garden. Playing in the soil, watching plants grow, picking a cherry tomato straight off the vine and eating it - this is the stuff of legacy building. But children need to know where it's okay to run and where it's not okay. Clear lines of demarcation are the child's safety net and the gardener's frustration insurance. Nobody wants kids running willy nilly through the green beans. High beds two or three feet deep of course provide the most clarity as to where the garden is and is not. But even simple paths, whether they are grass or wood chips or even pebbles, between growing beds can work just fine. Children can see clearly the difference between walking areas and growing areas; the clearer those definitions, the more child friendly your garden.

Because small quantities make big differences, once again, herbs are often the best place to start if you want to grow some of your own food outside. The tendency is to start with staples like potatoes or tomatoes, but you can get a lot in a tiny space if you start with herbs. And herbs especially pop with zest if picked fresh. You can get hanging herb gardens made out of

PVC pipe with holes punched in it. You pack the pipe with soil and compost and plant your herbs in the pockets on the side. It hangs on your porch and offers fresh herbs anytime.

Nothing is easier to extend on the shoulders of the season than herbs. While a large greenhouse or solarium for broccoli and cabbage may be a stretch, even a tiny cold frame can offer lots of herbs during the winter. Historically, gardeners used cold frames to start plants in the spring.

Most cold frames are no larger than a couple of window panes. They're normally dug a foot or so into the soil so they take advantage of earth berming and ground warmth. Without an automatic window opener, it might take some babysitting to keep the temperature inside from getting too hot, but even a small one can offer many herbs deep into winter. Many herbs too are cold tolerant; very few are as cold-fragile as tomatoes or green beans. Don't mess with the fragile ones; plant the hardy ones, at least when you're starting out.

We've had a small herb garden right outside our back door for years. Whenever Teresa needs some garnishment, she steps out the door and picks what she needs. The whole thing only takes about 30 square feet - that's 3 ft. x 10 ft. or 5 ft. x 6 ft. It's a lot less space than a soccer goal. How about it? Is an herb garden as important as a soccer goal? Be honest, now.

Sina: Location ended up being a game changer for me. My original garden was roughly 50 yards from my house. So, I had to walk to my garden in the hot and humid Virginia summer. That probably sounds lazy! But, having the garden so far from my house was a huge deterrent for me. And, it was in the back of my house. So, I had to bring the kids with me each time I worked in the garden. My kids love gardening, but only in their own space and time. When I forced them to stay in the garden with me, they quickly got bored and became destructive. So, I moved my garden.

My current garden is next to my kitchen door, like Joel's herb garden. So, now I don't have to walk very far to tend to it. And, it's close to the yard where my children play, so I can garden while they have fun adventures of their own – without being dragged into mine. It's a win-win!

Practical Bite #66: Cover Your Soil

How? In your garden, cover any place where you can see soil. You can use any kind of organic material, preferably brown in color.

Why?

Joel: The most soil-damaging thing is nakedness. The sun bakes it and organic matter quickly dissipates.

Sina: Exactly. While driving down a road or flying in an airplane, you've probably seen rows and rows of farmland that are bare. Most of us don't think twice about it because bare rows are a common practice in industrial farming. But soil was not designed to be naked.

Think about a forest, for example. The ground isn't bare. It's covered with all different types of plant life and other organisms. Those plants protect the soil from sun burn, wind erosion, and water erosion. They also help increase water infiltration rates and decrease evaporation. In addition, by covering the soil, they help protect and build the microbiome of the soil. Consequently, covering the soil is a main tenant of regenerative farming because it helps regenerate the soil.

When you don't cover your soil, you hurt the microbes. They can actually die from the sun exposure and the change in temperature and moisture. Plants need those microbes to be healthy and thrive, just like you need microbes to be healthy and thrive. So, if you are going to put energy into growing your own organic food, cover the soil so you also benefit from the microbial diversity.

Joel: Mulching protects the soil moisture from evaporation and encourages an entire community of microflora and microfauna. Sourcing these mulches may take a bit of sleuthing. Obviously the easiest one is leaves, and most folks can get all they want from their neighbors. A nice big leaf pile in your back corner is the best garden equity you can imagine.

The best mulch I've ever used is pond weeds. We drained one of our ponds a few years back and it had hydrologic pond weeds all around it. I gathered it by the armload and wheelbarrowed it over to the garden, putting it on extremely thick (8-12 inches). Amazingly, within one month all of it had completely decomposed into the soil, and the soil looked like chocolate cake and smelled good enough to eat with ice cream. If you live anywhere close to a beach, kelp that washes up is an excellent mulch.

Every year my heart breaks to see city streets lined with leaves. Out here in the country, folks routinely burn their yard leaves. That's also a crime against the planet. Leaves are probably as forgiving a mulch as anything. Well-rotted wood chips or sawdust rotted enough to turn black are fine as well. Fresh sawdust is not good because it temporarily robs the soil of nitrogen while it breaks down. Whenever you see a chipper crew working in your neighborhood, ask them to dump at your place. We've cultivated relationships with a couple of utility rights-of-way chipper crews and an arborist who dump some 100 truckloads of chips at our house each year.

You can also use cardboard, newspapers, wool, cotton - if it's organic material, it's fair game. Be careful about sourcing from a place that fills it with chemicals.

Straw and old hay can also work, but be careful about seeds. For hay, I prefer something that's all moldy. That means it probably got hot and killed any seeds. Ditto for straw. Lawn clippings work fine as well. They'll break down rapidly since they are green and tender; don't put them on more than a couple of inches thick or they'll get anaerobic underneath, releasing formaldehydes.

You can also plant cover crops like buckwheat or clover in between the vegetables. That should be an option you use after developing some skill. Growing different kinds of plants together is trickier than growing a single one.

Sina: Covering your soil is also a time saver. Last spring was the first time I covered my soil and it made a huge difference. Not only did it help my soil retain moisture so I was able to water less frequently, but it kept the weeds to a minimum. The main reason I kept failing at organic gardening in previous years was because the weeds would get out of control. But, now that I've covered my soil, I only spend roughly 20 minutes each morning tending to my garden and 95% of that time is spent fighting pests while only 5% is spent pulling weeds.

Joel: Remember that each of these covers has a different Carbon: Nitrogen ratio and decomposes a little differently. That's fine. Just start with what you have and play with it. Years ago, I made a couple of extremely fertile garden beds by going out into the lawn and putting on a foot of leaves, then a layer of manure (only an inch thick), then another foot of leaves. One year later, without doing anything, I had a weed less earthworm-crawling black soil garden bed.

I did that after building a couple of beds by double digging. Each one worked, but the no-digging one was easier.

Sina: So, do yourself and your soil a favor by not leaving your soil naked. Put some clothes on your soil! It's worth the added expense.

Practical Bite #67: Create Your Own Compost

How? When building compost, there are many different methods available and there are different types of compost. Here's a very basic recipe for hot-compost:

- ❖ The general idea is to layer organic materials and add a dash of soil to create a mixture that will turn into humus.
- ❖ Buy a composting container or simply create a freestanding pile that is at least 3 feet x 3 feet x 3 feet (1 cubic yard).
- ❖ Collect brown items and green items.
- ❖ Brown items include: dry leaves, straw, hay, untreated sawdust, unbleached and undyed paper, corrugate cardboard (with no waxy/slick coatings), twigs, and dry pine needles.
- ❖ Green items include: vegetable and fruit scraps, coffee grounds/tea bags (unbleached), eggshells, seaweed, trimmings from perennial and annual plants, and annual weeds that have not gone to seed.
- ❖ Add your green items and your brown items, alternating green and brown. Add 3 times as much brown as green. Fold in a couple shovelfuls of garden soil.
- ❖ Regularly sprinkle water over the pile just until the consistency is of a damp sponge. If you add too much water, the pile will rot.
- ❖ Once a week, turn the pile using a garden fork or shovel. If the compost pile looks too wet and smells then add more brown items. If it looks very brown and dry then add green items and a little water to make it slightly moist.
- ❖ Your compost is ready to use when it has become dry, brown, and crumbly and no longer gives off heat. It may take 3-6 months. When it's done, add 1-2 inches of compost to your garden or flower beds at the beginning of each planting season to provide beneficial nutrients and microbes, as well as organic matter (compost can be a replacement for fertilizer).

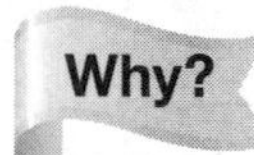

Sina: I've tried three times to create compost, and each time was not fruitful. The first two times, I had no idea what I was doing. I didn't want to spend time researching how to build compost, so I just started throwing food scraps, leaves and grass clipping on a pile. Needless to say, it did not turn into a beautiful pile of nutrient dense fertilizer filled with beneficial microorganisms.

However, knowing how important compost is for the health of the garden as well as the health of my family, I tried again last year. I was determined to make it work this time. I even got the whole family involved in building what I called "Our Family Compost Farm."

My husband found a spot for our compost farm right next to the garden. He even built a barrier around it, using poles and chicken wire, to protect it from wild animals. Every day, our entire family collected food scraps in a bowl that sat on our kitchen counter. When the bowl was full, I'd blend up the scraps in my Vitamix®; I thought I was being kind to the microbes by making their job easier. Then, my son and I would walk the slurry down to the compost pile and pour it on our compost farm. It felt good, like we were serving the microbes and the worms a healthy breakfast.

We even made sure to add both greens and browns – dried leaves made up most of the browns. My boys were in charge of collecting the leaves. When we used all of the leaves on our property, we asked our neighbor if we could remove the leaves from their lawn - they do not spray any chemicals either. Our neighbor was thrilled about the proposition! So, my boys and I grabbed a huge tarp, dragged it to our neighbor's house, piled leaves on top of it, and then enlisted my husband to drag it back to our house because it was so heavy.

For weeks, we cared for Our Family Compost Farm as if it was a newborn baby! We watered it, turned it, and talked nicely to it. And then, we left it alone to do its thing.

After anxiously waiting for about two months, I walked down to the compost pile to check on it. I expected to see a beautiful pile of dark, warm compost being created right in front of my eyes. But, when I arrive at Our Family Compost Farm, it was gone! The entire pile had disappeared! It didn't just shrink down from the decomposition process; it was literally ALL gone!

I stood there dumbfounded. Where could it have gone?

Then, out of the corner of my eye, I see my golden retriever, Daisy, waddling down the hill with a huge smile on her face. She walked right up to the compost farm, squished her face through an opening in the chicken wire, and started licking the ground where my compost farm used to be. Daisy had eaten all of my compost!

I was so upset with Daisy. All of that work, for nothing! But then I felt relieved. You see, Daisy had been gaining weight for several weeks. I restricted her calories and she still continued to balloon up. She seriously looked like she swallowed a balloon. When she walked through the house, she waddled from side to side as she tried to maneuver her massive stomach. I had already put her on probiotics, suspecting dysbiosis, and I was beginning to think she had developed a hormonal imbalance. But no, she simply ate every last crumb of our compost farm!

So, I will try again this year. Except this time, I will make sure we build a stronger barrier to keep Daisy out.

Joel: That's hilarious! Nothing creates ownership like participation. Few things are as freeing, or liberating, as doing something for yourself. Whether it's learning to play the piano well enough to not struggle at it with the teacher, or leaning how to read on your own, doing for yourself, or in modern parlance Do It Yourself (DIY), is a powerful antidote for dependency. For sure, we are all dependent on others, but to the extent that we can do things for ourselves, we gain independence emotionally and economically. I've been making compost since about the time I started reading, so to me this is literally as normal and perfunctory as brushing my teeth. I apologize beforehand if I sound over-simplistic or condescending in this tip. Sina's experiences, as smart as she is, show me that what I consider brainless is actually fairly cerebral.

Let me start with why you would want to complicate your life's schedule, clutter up your back yard, and handle non-delightful material. Perhaps the biggest lie of our modern techno-glitzy culture is that we're smart enough to artificial intelligence our way into some Star Trek® cosmic nirvana levitating above the earth extricated from an ecological umbilical tied to soil. That ubiquitous notion indicates a profound hubris and devolution into ignorance, not a newfound sophistication into artificial abundance. The most fundamental building block of ecology is the cycle of life and death: life, death, decomposition, regeneration. In order to live, something has to die. Everything is eating and being eaten. If you don't believe it, go lie naked in your flower bed for a week and tell me what gets eaten. Nowhere does that happen more dramatically, more graphically, than in a managed compost pile. It literally metamorphosizes from detritus to productive gold. If that isn't alchemy, I don't know what is.

Every time we humans engage with humus, the most important component of soil, we literally physically and spiritually touch our person-ness. If we never do, we go through life without the reverence and the gratitude that come from touching our roots. The singularly healing aspects of engaging in life's cycle, viscerally and tactilely, is well documented in every institutional setting imaginable, from brain injury to old-time insane asylums to prisons. The calming and gentling effect of engaging with soil is profound.

Any school garden project administrator will testify to the whole person impact of soil connectedness.

Finally, realize that as Bill McKibben is wont to say, "there is no away." When you put your kitchen scraps out for the garbage truck, where does it go? When you rake your leaves up and throw them away, where is away? The fact that 75 percent of everything that has ever gone into landfills, since we've had them, has been decomposable organic material should make us proclaim a day of prayer and fasting in sack cloth and ashes. It is a moral and ecological travesty that what was supposed to build soil, that what the sun grew through photosynthetic and chlorophyll activity, has been disrespected and violated this profoundly. The first step in planetary stewardship is to use our mechanical and intellectual ability to leverage biomass into fertile soil. That's the least we can do.

Time on this Practical Bite will not permit an exhaustive treatise on compost building, but plenty of information exists out there to make you successful—as long as you keep the dog out, Sina. The five essential components of compost are nitrogen, carbon, oxygen, water, and microbes. In addition, it needs an ambient temperature of about 50 degrees F and a mass of about one-yard square. The biggest problem with home compost piles is that we don't generate enough stuff fast enough to create enough mass to get it going. That's why I'm such a fan of 2 or 3 chickens. They will eat it before the dog, before the raccoon, before the rats.

And they will turn it immediately into eggs. What's not to love about that?

What most homeowners think of as a compost pile is really a static pile of decomposables. And that's actually okay as long as we remember a few things. In general, you want to put in about three times (by weight) as much brown stuff as we do green stuff. The brown tends to be high in carbon (C); the green high in nitrogen (N). This is called C:N ratio, and it should be somewhere around 25-30:1. Lawn clippings are kind of a hybrid. They're green, but they also have a lot of carbon in them, so mixing about twice as much brown (like leaves, straw, hay) would be appropriate.

Both carbon components and nitrogen components exist along a continuum as well. Sawdust is about 500:1; wood chips about 300:1 unless they came from deciduous trees with the green leaves on, in which case they might go as low as 75:1. Deciduous leaves when they fall in autumn run about 35:1, so it doesn't take much nitrogenous material to bring them into balance. Meat scraps are the most highly nitrogenous stuff you'll ever get out of your kitchen; most vegetable and fruit scraps will be around 20:1.

Don't get hung up on this stuff; it sounds a lot more complicated than you might think. And like any new endeavor, you'll learn a lot quickly. The difference between reading about riding a bike and actually getting on one is immense. You know way more in 5 minutes trying to ride a bike than you could know in a lifetime of reading books. All skill requires repetition and you learn most on the front end. Building compost is a little like a good soaking in the tub. Everyone has their recipe for water temperature, depth, length, time of day and suds. Consider your compost pile a caress of your earth womb. If that doesn't make you want to get out there and participate, I don't know what will.

Sina: Wow, now I'm more motivated than ever to make my own compost. I truly want to succeed at this Practical Bite because compost can add millions, and possibly billions or more, of beneficial microbes to your body. Simply touching the compost with your hands adds microbial diversity to your skin microbiome. Breathing in the aerosolized particles of the compost strengthens the microbiome that lives on your nasal passages and in your lungs. And, eating the tiny bits of compost and soil that remain on freshly harvested vegetables can add billions of beneficial microbes to your GI tract. Compost can be a game changer in your quest for optimal health and wellness.

So, I'll try again. But I'm not going to worry about all of the ratios you listed off – at least not at this point. That's like trying to do a wheelie when I'm still learning how to pedal the bike. I'll start with the basics and, like you said, learn as I go – one small step at a time.

Practical Bite #68: Add A Solarium On Your Home

How? This can be as simple as a couple of cattle panels (4 ft. x 16 ft. square-holed metal fencing pieces) bent in an arc against your house and covered with plastic. That might not appeal to a lot of people, but it's sure easy and cheap.

Why?

Joel: One of the biggest bangs for the self-reliance buck is a solarium on the sunny side of your house. Years ago, we sprang for a kit from Cedar-Built in Canada. It's beautiful and functional.

By attaching a solarium to the sunny side of your house, it can usually incorporate a window or two which allows you to open them up on sunny winter days and get some additional passive solar heat to reduce heating costs. With plants in there, you also get a rush of nice oxygenated fresh air in the winter when things usually get a bit stuffy indoors. Around this area, old-timers say that it was common practice to open all the doors for a minute or two, even on the coldest days, just to freshen up the stale air.

But the most important reason to have a solarium is to extend the growing season for plants. If you add heat to the solarium, then it becomes a true-blue green house and you can grow anything in there. But if you don't add a heat source, it's primarily for extending the season on the shoulders. Cool hardy things like kale, swiss chard, lettuce, carrots, beets, and peas can all handle hard frosts. If you plant in late summer, you can enjoy these kinds of vegetables well into winter.

At the other end of the season, of course, you can plant things much earlier than outside. You can enjoy fresh greens as much as two months before you could get them out of your garden. A little warming mat under some seeds can get you up and running very early. Tending green growing plants this early in the season ministers to your psyche, too.

In general, I think every single house in latitudes where it frosts should have a solarium. They are not expensive and add tremendous benefits to your life: physical, emotional, and mental. Like some of these other homestead type tips, this book is not a solarium how-to manual. You can get plenty of books on solariums. Our point here is to recommend it as one of the most efficacious ways to participate in your own food freedom and happiness.

Practical Bite 69: Catch The Rain

How? Whether you have nothing more than a rain barrel or you install a massive cistern, catching rain that falls on your roof is another empowering project.

Why?

Joel: Water that lands is typically wasted into storm drains through the municipal water system. It's an ecological liability because in nature, all raindrops want to stay where they land for as long as possible. The longer a raindrop stays put, the more beneficial it is to its surroundings. The faster a raindrop leaves the area and heads on its journey toward the sea, the less it can nourish its landing area. This is a basic tenet of permaculture.

Most people don't realize how much water comes off a roof. One inch of water on a square foot of surface is 10 cups, or 0.625 gallons. So, if you have a 1,500 square foot roof on your house, which is a modest size, a one-inch rain will give you nearly 1,000 gallons. If you live in a 30-inch rainfall area, which includes everything east of the Mississippi, that would be 45,000 gallons in a year. Many areas receive more than that, of course. That's a lot of water. When you consider your neighbor's house and the next neighbor's house and all the houses on the street . . . . You get the idea. It's a lot of water. I mean a lot of water.

Every drop you can hold and use on high ground, delaying its rush away from the area, reduces flooding potential and offers hydration options for dry times. Rain water is soft. It's not full of impurities like municipal water nor minerals like well water. It's what plants like most. Again, this book is not a how-to for cisterns and rain barrels; plenty of information exists out there to get you up and running when you're ready to pursue the catchment and storage.

Not that long ago, cisterns were cheaper to build than wells. Once drilling technology developed, wells became more competitive to install. That's a shame because excess water became a waste problem and instead, we poke holes in the aquifers and deplete the commons. Catching roof rain is a piece of that whole living responsibly puzzle.

Sina: This Practical Bite reminds me of playing in the rain as a child, and trying to catch raindrops on my tongue. Catching rain in containers is the supersized version of that fun, childhood experience. It's a great project to do with your children or grandchildren. Start small by putting any container outside to catch rain. Then use that water to nourish plants you are growing inside. Personally, I would filter the water first, especially if you plan to drink it. Rain water samples in some areas of the country have tested positive for glyphosate.

Practical Bite #70: Save Money By Preserving One Fruit Or Vegetable

How? Whether it's canning, dehydrating, or freezing, choose one fruit or vegetable to preserve. Start simple by washing some berries, placing them on a cookie sheet in a single layer, and freezing them. Once frozen, transfer the berries to a glass container and store in the freezer.

Why?

Joel: When Teresa sends me shopping, it's to the basement where some 800 quarts of glass canning jars await toting to the kitchen. This is my favorite way to shop. Canned vegetables, pickles and fruit don't require electricity. If the power goes out, they're fine. For years. We've canned meat too. Almost anything can be canned. Maybe not bureaucrats, but most everything else.

Preserving food is a skill like any other and the hardest part of the whole process is to jump in and start doing one thing. We tend to freeze things like blueberries, strawberries and occasionally some applesauce. I love it when it's not quite thawed; when it still has some cold crunchies in it. Wow, that's good. We freeze sweet corn too.

Sina: My children love frozen fruit! For them, it's a dessert, like ice cream. For me, it's peace of mind because I know the fruit is clean and healthy since it was picked from my garden. My oldest son also loves to eat frozen peas. He says they taste like, "cold flavor explosions" in his mouth. I don't grow all of my own fruit, so I buy fruit when it's on sale and freeze it. It's a huge money saver. We eat the frozen fruit raw, blended in smoothies, as fruit syrup over pancakes, or in desserts like cobblers.

Joel: We've also dehydrated apple slices but not much else. We should do more. You can purchase home-scaled dehydrators and make everything from fruit leather to raisins.

Sina: Dehydrating is a fun activity to do with your kids. My kids love washing the fruits and vegetables, slicing them, laying them on the trays and then periodically checking them for doneness. Dehydrating was one of the first methods I used to preserve the fruits we grow, as well as the fruits I buy on sale. It is easy and I don't have to stand in the kitchen waiting for it to be done cooking. Win-win!

Joel: The main point of preserving is to build your domestic storehouse. The personal satisfaction and peace of mind that come from developing your in-home food stash is hard to quantify in dollars, but it's real. One of my favorite visits is to Powhatan village near Jamestown, Virginia. These crude homes, made of bent over saplings and bison hides, did not have chimneys. A fire in the middle of the home sent smoke into the domed ceiling and eventually out the open hole. Food hung on all that upper smoky lattice work: meat, corn, squash, beans, fish. Imagine lying down with your beloved at night, staring up into that smoky canopy of food, knowing both the security and dependence of that inventory.

I think when we lie down with our beloved in a modern American house and know that proximate to the bedroom is a larder full of food that we've grown, sourced, processed, packaged and preserved, we have a similar serenity and satisfaction. We've acquired. We've invested. We've participated. Come merchant marine strikes or teamster unrest or power outages and catastrophes, we're prepared, calm, and happy. What's that worth?

I feel like in general our culture has become more a wandering, homeless maverick rather than a snug squirrel surrounded by nuts. We might be surrounded by nuts, but they aren't the eating kind.

Practical Bite #71: Adopt Chickens & Feed Them Kitchen Scraps

How? Rent the Chicken is a nationwide business that offers layers for backyard flocksters not wanting the full responsibility of owning chickens. Also, it's a nifty arrangement around some ordinances that preclude owning chickens. When the inspector comes, you just say "we're renting them; we don't own them." Chickens will eat virtually anything a human would eat, even if it's spoiled. Generally, kitchen scraps are not high enough in protein for chickens, unless you offer routine meat scraps and fat.

Why?

Joel: Oh my, this Practical Bite is near and dear to my heart. I call them Kitchen Chickens; it's a bit hard to say, but once you get the hang of it, it's a pretty catchy phrase. In this Practical Bite we've made a quantum leap from plants to animals. I'm an animal guy, but I also appreciate the big differences between plants and animals. Plants don't move. You'll never have a green bean wander over and scratch out your neighbor's rose bushes.

Second, plants don't need attention every day. Timely attention, to be sure, but they offer fairly wide caretaking time frames. Animals, on the other hand, need feed and water every day. Plenty of urban chicken enthusiasts have designed and built multi-day chicken coops so you can be gone for a few days without choring. I haven't seen any designs capable of chore-free function for more than a week.

Consider these chickens similar to a pet. You'll be surprised at their individual personalities and their social interest. If you jump off this cliff, you'll be in love with chickens before you know it. Like everything else Sina and I advocate, start small. A normal healthy chicken will generally lay about 4 eggs a week, so 3 would give you a dozen eggs a week.

Sina: I don't own chickens because my home owners association won't allow it. But, if I have chickens one day, I will feed them my kitchen scraps. Although my dogs would probably have something to say about that!

Joel: Chickens get a bum rap for being dirty and encouraging disease. Give me a break. It takes 11 chickens to generate the poop of one average dog, and dog manure is toxic. You can almost put chicken poop in cookies; it's great stuff. You can throw out the gerbil, boa constrictor, cat and dog and put in 3 or 4 chickens. You'll never regret it. They eat anything and will clean up your kitchen scraps - everything. And then they'll turn around and lay eggs to boot.

If you have teenagers in your house, a laying hen provides the best role model in the world. Chickens rise early; they're the first ones up on the farm. Cows are second and pigs like to sleep in. So, chickens are up and happy at the break of day. Then they spend all day happily working turning trash into treasure, chirping contentedly as they work, never complaining or whining. Then in the evening, as soon as the sun starts to go down, they don't go out on the town; they head straight for the roost, curl up, and go to bed. Now if that isn't a perfect role model for a teenager, I don't know what is.

If you're growing a garden, composted chicken manure is an excellent soil amendment. Don't put it in fresh because it's hot, meaning that the 7:1 C:N ratio is too high for plants. Good compost is about 25-30:1. Some wood shavings (yes, the curly ones) are an ideal bedding for the chickens. Let them build up past a foot deep and leave them in there for a long time (up to a year). Just keep adding some more shavings on top. The chickens will stir that bedding, injecting oxygen, which stimulates decomposition. When the material gets old and dark colored, it's okay to apply to your garden.

Practical Bite #72: Relocate To A Homestead

How? A homestead is a functional place, 1-5 acres, where you can grow almost all your own food, including maybe some beef or lamb. Certainly, chicken and eggs, fruit trees, grapes, and garden vegetables. Maybe a hive or two of honey bees. A nice big hoop house for season extension and maybe even a greenhouse fully heated would be doable.

Why?

Joel: I did not say "get a horse." That's the worst thing you can do. I don't hate horses, mind you, but they are hard on the ecology and they cost a lot of money.

If you aren't going to actually leverage the extra land to wean yourself from supermarkets and urban lifestyles (running from activity to activity for yourself and your kids) then don't go this route. But if the yearning in your spirit calls you and draws you to self-reliance and do-it-yourselfism, a small homestead can offer tremendous entertainment and security. As I've said in my other books about raising a family in rural settings, if you can't figure out how to get as excited about exploring the edges of a pond as you get about going to a movie, you have a creativity problem.

With a bit of room, too, you can explore some income-generating schemes like woodworking or other crafts, including culinary craft, that would be problematic in a more urban setting. And the kids can run wild. And have chores. And build forts in the woods, dams in the creek, and tree houses. They can catch fireflies on warm summer nights and enjoy being able to see stars. I don't think this life is for everyone, by any means. But I'm always amazed at how one thing leads to another and then to another. You start down a self-improvement path and the next thing you know you're milking a goat. I've seen it happen. Fortunately, most people don't end up here; if they did, our farm wouldn't have any customers.

SECTION 6:

Spread Your Wings

CHAPTER 8

Become Your Own Headliner

Sina: Thank you for joining us on this healing journey. We've shown you how to navigate the grocery store labyrinth and how to move beyond those labels - to a place where you can find foods that truly heal. You had a front-row seat into how Joel and I think about our food supply and how we make decisions based on common sense and acquired knowledge, as well as our principles and intuition.

We also demonstrated why more labels are not the answer. Labels do not connect you with your food. New labels bring new loopholes, exceptions, and confusion. To be truly healthy and free, you must look beyond those labels so you can re-connect with nature and re-connect with your own body.

We hope you have met with your local farmers and are enjoying the benefits of consuming foods that were grown ecologically. However, we understand that most of us will continue to buy foods from a grocery store – including Joel and me. And, all of us will continue to hear conflicting dietary advice, and experience social situations that challenge our principles.

That's why, we hope you have gained enough knowledge and trust in yourself to be able to discern any situation we did not directly cover in this book. The individual Practical Bites are important to understand and implement, but the main purpose of this book is to give you a glimpse into our thought process behind each Practical Bite. That's the real treasure because it provides you with a foundational approach that you can apply to practically any situation in order to harness your power.

When you encounter situations that we did not cover during our journey together, think about how Joel and I approached the food supply, the labels, and the situations; and then apply those concepts. It might help to refer back to the road map to see if it passes the litmus test:

1. Does it bring me closer to my health goal?
2. Does it give me more freedom?
3. Does it give me more trust in my food supply?

Joel: We deeply appreciate you investing your time and energy in traveling this continuum with us. I appreciate Sina pushing me to articulate things I often don't think about; we're all so close to our routines that we often just do things by rote. I found some inconsistencies in my own thinking. Bummer. I also enjoyed digging deeper into the why on some things I've kind of taken for granted. And that's the way this journey is; it's fraught with twists and turns, and a little inconsistency won't kill you. I'm thankful for that. (Don't tell anyone about my affinity for ice cream).

Sina is right about the thought process. Knowing how to think, how to decide, is more important than the ultimate decision. In the end, you need to live with the decisions and choices you make. Take the easy ones first; don't get ulcers worrying about the most difficult ones. And don't fail to start with the obvious ones just because you haven't figured out the hardest ones. Sometimes we can use that as an excuse to not get started. Just because you don't know how you're going to get those last two farthest apples at the top of the tree, don't assume you can't go ahead and pick the ones you can reach from the ground.

I always encourage folks to start with the biggest items first. Cut out the junk, and the junk snacks. Add healthy snacks. Now cut the processed and add whole. Attack the big budget items first. Gurus often say that plans never written down never get implemented. So, go ahead and make a list of what's in your refrigerator and pantry. What's on your grocery list? Now put a line through the stuff you know is bad. If there is a good substitute, write that next to it. Put a red dot next to the ones you're not sure about. If you have a list, you're well on the way to actually implementing changes because creating practical change from the whole pile of stuff in our pantry is too hard to do mentally. You have to build it on paper before you build it in reality.

Sina: And, if you slide back down the continuum from time to time, don't be hard on yourself; give yourself grace. It's human to cycle between periods of eating healthier and periods of eating less healthy. Consider retaking the quiz every 6-12 months to see which direction you are headed on the continuum. And, remember, slow and steady wins the race. If you slide back, don't change everything all at once. Pick your new health goal; visualize it, feel it, and speak positive affirmations over your mind, body, and spirit. Then, move forward by changing your diet one step at a time.

Joel: Simple things like taking the sugar bowl off the table can necessitate a whole series of actions in the right direction. Get juice and seltzer water and make your own carbonated beverage out of juice. Once you try that, you'll lose your appetite for soft drinks. You'll be surprised at the domino effect of just a few things. Goodness, a chicken plopped in the crock pot - wow, your family will love you.

I think the most amazing thing about all this, beyond your own health journey, is what thousands of changes like this would do to our whole farm and food system. As you withdraw support from the bad guys, you'll starve them out. As you throw support to the good guys, you'll bolster their success.

If everyone who reads this book would actually implement even half of what's in here, I guarantee you the food system would feel the change. Our farmland would feel the change. I'm assuming we're going to sell a million copies, of course. But even if we don't, every dime invested in the good guys bends the trajectory; every dime withdrawn from the bad guys weakens them. Make no mistake, in the food system we have good guys and bad guys. You now know who they are. And you know you're smarter than a label.

My greatest hope is that we've helped free you from the prison of inadequacy. You are completely capable of nurturing yourself and the ones you love. Enjoy the freedom.

Sina: We welcome you to continue your healing journey with us by connecting with us online (www.PolyfaceFarms.com and www.HandsOffMyFood.com). Through our websites, we strive to keep you updated on your food supply while providing commentary and solutions. I also post cooking videos to hopefully inspire and motivate you in the kitchen.

But now, without further ado, it's time for you to spread your wings and fly. You have the tools you need to thrive in any situation. Tap into your intuition and trust yourself. Believe in yourself. Become the headliner in your own life. And, always remember, you are not alone and you are worth it!

APPENDIX

Joel's Story

I was born Feb. 19, 1957 in Wooster, Ohio and at 6 weeks old flew Pan American Airlines back to our home and farm in Venezuela, South America. My dad always wanted a farm in a developing country. Mom always wanted adventure. After being discharged from the Navy after WWII, Dad got his business degree from Indiana University while Mom finished up her master's in health and physical education.

Dad then went to Middlebury in Vermont for a semester of Spanish, then hitchhiked to Mexico, where he stayed for a few months. He returned stateside and sat for the foreign civil service exam (Spanish), passed, and got hired on with Texas Oil Company (later Texaco) as a bilingual accountant in the developing oil fields off the coast of Venezuela.

He and Mom married a year later and returned to a high paying corporate job that gave him enough savings to purchase a 1,000-acre farm in the highlands of tropical Venezuela. The goal was to produce broiler chickens and have a dairy, two things the Venezuelans wanted but neither of which enjoyed efficient production at the time. We built a house and started raising chickens, selling them on the unregulated open market in the city square. Within a couple of years, unrest developed and the junta against Peres Jimenez was in full fury. By that time, our family had made enemies in the farming community because our chickens were clean and healthy and Dad stole the open market from the native farmers. They thought we were into witchcraft and black magic.

The social and political unrest gave room for anarchy and we became targets of the junta; essentially, we fled the back door as the machine guns came in the front door. Lost everything. After exhausting all efforts to get protection, the only solution was to walk away and return to the states, where we landed on Easter Sunday 1961. Dad still wanted to go back after things settled so he wanted to be within a day's drive of Washington D.C. and the Venezuelan embassy. We looked at farms in an arc from Lancaster, Pennsylvania, down the Shenandoah Valley, and into northern North Carolina.

Here in Augusta County we found the cheapest most worn-out, gullied rock pile of a place, but Dad knew it could be redeemed. Mom, 5 months pregnant with my sister, wanted the move-in ready house. My older brother (7) and I (4) liked the concrete swimming pool in the yard. So here we started over, Dad working as an accountant and Mom as a high school teacher; every extra penny went to the mortgage. Every spare minute went to experiments and conservation projects. We planted thousands of trees on eroded hillsides. We stacked brush in gullies. Dad sought both public and private counsel from agricultural experts; every one admonished him to build silos, plant corn, graze the forest, and buy chemical fertilizer.

My paternal grandfather was a charter subscriber to Rodale's *Organic Gardening and Farming Magazine* when it first came out in the late 1940s. His compost and magnificent garden are still monuments in my memory and played a key role in my love for production agriculture. He was also a master craftsman and tinkerer, inventing the very first walking garden sprinkler, the kind that roll up a garden hose as they move. Dad got his environmental kick from Grandpa and realized that all this advice he sought would send him into what he saw as an addiction treadmill financially and ecologically.

One Sunday afternoon he drove us somewhere to see a fellow he'd heard about that used portable shelters. I have no recollection of what animal was in these field shelters; all I remember is Dad's ebullience on the way home. The mobile infrastructure idea intrigued him as a way to farm without high capital infrastructure. At the time, he also read Andre Voisin, the French godfather of timed grazing management. Dad set to work inventing a portable electric fencing system so we could move the animals around. Mobile animal shelters followed: rabbits, lambs, veal calves and finally, my chickens.

When I was 10 years old, I ordered my first 50 chicks from Sears and Roebuck, out of the big catalogue, and started a laying hen business that I expanded throughout my high school years. As an economist, Dad realized right away that a small farm could not compete in the commodity business; the margins are too small. But if we created a brand and wore all the hats of the middlemen—processor, distributor, marketer—we could stand a fighting chance of making a go of it. By the early 1970s, Mom and Dad's off-farm salaries finished the mortgage and we were debt free, but Dad was slowing down. He never recuperated emotionally from his losses in Venezuela.

Vietnam was in full swing and spawned the back-to-the-land hippie movement of the early 1970s. I needed an outlet for my eggs and Dad saw potential in direct marketing. Our town, Staunton, had a leftover depression-era direct sales market called the Curb Market. A precursor of today's modern Farmers' Market movement, the curb market enjoyed broad regulatory exemptions. I could sell cooked chicken, yoghurt from our two Guernsey milk cows, cheese, butter, beef, pork and everything but fluid milk without any government licensing or inspections. We were one decade too early. We developed a loyal clientele, but people had not yet heard the word "organic" and the cultural awareness regarding junk food and industrial farming had not yet taken hold.

Throughout my high school years, I got up each Saturday morning—it was a year-round indoor market—at 4 a.m. to be there at the 6 a.m. opening. It closed about 11 a.m. When people wonder how I can be so militant about unregulated direct food sales to customers, it is this experience that frames my politics and perceptions. For decades this market operated for the community without any sickness and without any regulation. Farmers knew their customers. Customers knew their farmers. For many farmers during those early years it was the single most valuable avenue to finding cash for their farms. My wife Teresa's grandmother made some 40 pies every Friday night in a Majestic wood stove to sell at the Curb Market. If you come to Polyface today, you can see that wood stove in our sales building.

When I went off to college, we shut down that market stand and shortly thereafter the two elderly matrons decided to quit also. I wonder if my youthful enthusiasm kept those two matriarch mentors going a little longer than they would have otherwise. I had worked weekends during high school at the local newspaper and loved it; they liked me and promised me a job as soon as I graduated from college. One morning during my junior year of high school Dad and I had a conversation in the farm lane about the future of this farm.

He had a realtor accounting client who happened to mention to him how much the farm was worth. Land appreciation was accelerating at the time and Dad, always ready for a new adventure, and Mom not far behind, toyed with the idea of selling here and moving to a much bigger (cheaper land) in Arkansas or Missouri. I caught wind of it; hence the conversation. Dad asked me point blank if I wanted to make a career here and just as point blank I said yes. I still can't talk about that interchange without sobbing. That day he handed me the keys to the kingdom. He promised to never mention selling again and he never did.

But we had a problem: how do we make a salary? Nobody had made a salary from the farm. He hadn't. Mom hadn't. It was not a going concern. Creeks for kids to build dams in and woods for kids to build forts in and chores to do and a garden to weed—this is all well and good, but it did not a business make. I very much enjoyed milking the couple of cows we had and realized I could milk 10 cows by hand, sell the milk at regular retail prices (not high because it was grass-finished and organic) and make a good living. There was only one problem: it was illegal. I've never gotten over that. Government policy, encouraged by fearful, ignorant consumer voters, deprived me of an entrepreneurial farm income and deprived my neighbors from getting good food. Instead of locking up farmers who want to sell raw milk to their neighbors who voluntarily exercise freedom of choice to engage in consensual commerce, we should lock up the tyrants, both bureaucrats and voters, who criminalize such basic exercises in personal choice.

So, I went back to the newspaper. But by this time, the farm was beginning to show definite signs of improvement. The gullies filled with trees. Soil began growing over the rocks in the fields. Clover grew, sparsely, where weeds and broomsedge grew before. The land was responding to animal movement, compost, and multi-species. Teresa and I married Aug. 9, 1980 and moved into the attic of the farm house. We called it our penthouse. We lived on $300 a month, ate only what we grew in the garden, had no TV (still don't) and devoted ourselves to a dream: full-time farming.

Within a couple of years, we had saved enough to live for one year without much income. I wasn't too proud to do any kind of work, even washing dishes at a restaurant. I walked out of that newspaper office Sept. 24, 1982 to the profound amazement and prophecies of stupidity and ruination from all friends and co-workers. But we made it the first year. We made it the second year. We re-introduced direct marketing and added the broilers. We tightened up the cattle rotation to every day moves and added more composting with winter manure. The nest egg ran out but we hung on for year three. By the end of year four, we exhaled. It looked like we would make it. Dad passed away in our sixth year, but he was pleased: "You're going to be just fine," he said from his sickbed. And we were.

Our children pitched in and by the end of our first decade, we had a building stack of media attention. Everyone wanted to know how a young couple, with no money, on a small eroded farm, could make a living in modern America. Today, our son Daniel operates the farm's day to day activities; our daughter lives a few minutes away and runs an agri-tourism bureau. A cadre of non-family team members keep things humming to service 4,000 families, 50 restaurants, on-farm sales building, nationwide shipping and other sales venues. We lease some dozen properties and run a professional apprenticeship program to launch a new generation of entrepreneurial land caressing farmers. My daughter-in-law Sheri handles urban drop points we service monthly and each grandchild has an autonomous farm enterprise (duck eggs, lambs, exotic chickens).

Me? I just do whatever I want. At least that's what Daniel says. My official title is now "Chief Visionary." I like that. And chief chain saw operator. And chief negotiator. Dad taught my bride Teresa how to keep the books and she still handles all the financials. We have four generations living on the farm. As of this writing, Mom will soon be 96 years old and still driving (heaven help us all) and our oldest grandson will soon start (heaven help us all). I don't deserve this, but I'll take it.

What gets me up in the morning? Being able to step out the back-porch door and enter God's creation as a participant, a steward to heal and caress abundance from a loving nest. That is a privilege and an honor all of us can enjoy, either directly like I do or indirectly by patronizing a farm like ours that generates a legacy of soil, water, and abundant clean air. What a blessing. And welcome aboard.

Sina's Story

For the first 35 years of my life, my relationship with food was similar to most Americans. I ate the Standard American Diet, consumed fast-food on a regular basis, over-indulged on the holidays, and was addicted to sugar. Even after receiving a PhD in Nutrition, I still ate that way. And, even after working in the supplement industry, I still ate that way. Unlike Joel, who was groomed his entire life for his current role, my awakening occurred because of debilitating health challenges.

In 2015, I was diagnosed with an autoimmune disease - an advanced stage of Rheumatoid Arthritis *in my 30's*. It was accompanied by muscle wasting, like cancer patients can experience, arsenic poisoning, leaky gut and deficiencies in 15 nutrients. I took a vitamin and mineral supplement every day, yet my nutrient deficiencies were so severe that I was borderline for pellagra and beriberi – both of those diseases can lead to death, and both were eradicated in the U.S. by the mid-1900s.

The sickness began in my early 20's with gastrointestinal issues that progressed to chronic sinus infections, multiple food sensitivities, kidney stones, a tumor that developed on the white of my eye, chronic fatigue, hair loss and 5 miscarriages.

At rock bottom, I spent most of my time lying on the floor in pain. I was too weak to walk up the stairs without getting winded and too tired to stand long enough to finish doing the dishes after lunch. Some days my body hurt so badly that my 6-year old son had to hold a cup to my mouth just so I could take a drink of water.

My husband and I knew that if we didn't do something drastic, I wouldn't be around to see my kids grow up and graduate from high school or get married. But I had already seen countless medical doctors over the span of 20 years, and none of them knew what was wrong. They ran so many tests that I lost count. At one point, I even agreed to exploratory surgery out of desperation. But nobody had any answers, except for prescription drugs.

I refused to take the drugs. And, when the last medical doctor told me that my symptoms must be in my head, I knew that if I had any chance of healing, I had to find a different path. So, I broke out of the box of conventional medicine. That was over 4 years ago.

Today I'm disease free and have no pain! I'm healthy, happy, and free. I homeschool my two amazing children, run a company, consult, write when inspired, and hike with my dogs on the weekends. So, how did I do it? How did I go from lying on the floor in chronic pain to having more energy than ever before in my life?

First and foremost, I surrendered to God. He showed me a path that would lead me out of the conventional box of medicine and nutrition. Second, I finally took responsibility for my own health and happiness.

I became my own investigative journalist, starting with our food supply. I found so much corruption and deception that I ended up spending nearly 5 years investigating what's really in our food. I published my findings in my first book, *Hands Off My Food*, and provided easy solutions designed with the busy soccer Mom in mind.

At the same time, I studied how to reverse diseases. I listened to cutting edge health summits featuring "experts" in the medical field who were pushing the boundaries of our understanding of disease. It was common for me to spend 40 hours a week learning about the role of inflammation in disease and how to reverse it. Eventually, I saw a pattern; all of the practitioners who were successful in helping their patients reverse disease were using the same basic steps.

So, I created my own healing program by combining all of those steps. The program addressed physical aspects of disease, such as: nutrient deficiencies, food allergies and sensitivities, toxicities and infections, microbiome imbalance, stress, etcetera. I tested it on myself, and it worked! With help from God, I was able to reverse the disease without the use of medications!

Once I made the necessary changes to my diet and lifestyle, my healing was rapid. I was able to get off the floor in 3 days! Within 3 months, nearly all of the pain was gone. And, within one year, there were no signs of disease in my body. The autoimmune disease had disappeared!

However, I soon realized that the program did not go far enough. I still had gastrointestinal issues, including a sluggish colon, which resulted in constipation and gas. And, I kept hearing practitioners on various health summits describe the disease reversal as a "remission." In other words, their patients were never fully healed; they were only keeping the disease at bay knowing that it could come back. I didn't want to live in that fear, so I dug deeper.

What I learned changed my entire perspective on life: in order to fully heal from a disease, you have to address the root cause. But, the root cause of disease does not exist on the physical level. That's why practitioners who only address the physical realm will tell their patients they are in "remission," instead of declaring they are fully healed or that the disease is gone.

The root cause of all disease exists on the emotional or energetic level. Forgiveness, in particular, is essential for reversing disease and maintaining optimal health. So, I began the process of forgiving everyone, including myself – which was the hardest person to forgive.

While forgiveness is not the only component involved in reversing disease, it can be a game changer. Once I took full responsibility, including changing my diet, lifestyle, and perspective as well as practicing forgiveness, my healing was complete. The gastrointestinal symptoms disappeared. The autoimmune disease became a distant memory of a person who I no longer was. And, my energy level increased so dramatically that, at times, my kids can't keep up with me!

I wasn't surprised that the disease was gone; I always believed that complete healing is possible. But I was surprised at how free I felt. I reached a level of mental, emotional, spiritual, and physical freedom that I never imagined possible. And, with that freedom came immense joy – the type of joy you hear in a baby's laugh or see on a child's face on Christmas morning.

But, here's the really cool part!

You don't have to reverse a disease in order to experience that elevated level of freedom and joy. In fact, it's easier to receive those gifts if you start taking responsibility BEFORE you get a diagnosis.

So, please don't let sick become your norm. You can choose to be full of energy, filled with joy, and completely healthy starting right now. The power is inside of you, waiting to be harnessed. So, go ahead, give yourself the freedom to create the life you've always dreamed of. You're worth it!

A Farmer And A PhD Unite!

Joel: I met Sina first through her blockbuster book "Hands Off My Food." As a small government environmentalist, I don't find many people who share those normally contradictory values. As I read her book about government's ineptitude and indeed the collusion between regulators and the corporatocracy, I jumped up and down with excitement when I realized she did not ask for some sort of oversight committee.

Here she was shining the light of truth on a completely dysfunctional labeling, oversight, and market system without screaming for an agency, a law, or anything. She took complete responsibility for her own ignorance, for what she had delayed learning, and for what she was going to do about it. Normally a rant about these sorts of issues ends with the pipe dream of some government solution. But she didn't go there.

She went squarely to the consumer, including herself. Instead of a refrain asking for government intervention, she sang a chorus of "we have the power." I was almost in tears identifying with this highly articulate researcher who refused to give her freedoms to someone else. She understood true liberty and true responsibility and true self-empowerment.

The reason I read the book was because a mutual friend in the Virginia Independent Consumers and Farmers Association (VICFA) had scheduled both of us to headline a fundraiser rally in Richmond. I had not heard of Sina and wanted to find out who was going to share the stage with me. These events always combine information and entertainment; meaning spontaneous humor as well as good-natured ribbing add to the show. Who was this lady, anyway? So, it was in that context that I decided I'd better read her book and catch up on my evening's sidekick.

Well, what an evening. We had a fantastic turnout and soon Sina went onstage. I batted clean up. She was so powerful and profound I almost forgot I had to talk too. I wrote notes furiously during her whole presentation, sitting on the edge of my seat spellbound. Not only was she a captivating speaker, but she also had a way of putting complex ideas in simple terms that a peasant like me could understand. Because I travel and do a lot of speeches, I also get to hear a lot of speeches. This one was off the charts.

When we were both done, we found each other in the crowd and she said "let's do a book together." I might be foggy on the details and words, but that's the way I remember it. After that night we began talking about it and this project grew out of that encounter. Sina is a dynamo that makes her story one of the most compelling I've ever encountered. And she's smart. So, why wouldn't I want to do a book with her?

I tell folks all the time I'm not that bright, but if I have one enduring talent, it's figuring out who to hook my wagon to so I can get pulled farther than I would ever go myself. Thank you, Sina, for being the engine that could.

Sina: I remember that night vividly. I was so nervous to share the stage with you – the great Joel Salatin!

You have a depth of knowledge in both food and agriculture that is unmatched by anyone I know. You were featured in Michael Pollan's book *The Omnivore's Dilemma*, as well as several food documentaries, including Food Inc. You've published 12 books. You're the editor of *The Stockman Grass Farmer*. You've flown around the world teaching farmers how to apply regenerative practices to help heal our land, our food, and our bodies. To top it off, you've spoken in front of England's Prince Charles! Now that's an intimidating resume!

The first time I heard your name was from my husband. We had recently moved to Virginia and were looking for local poultry and meat. My husband remembered reading about a farm in Virginia called "Poly-something" in *The Omnivore's Dilemma*. He found your farm and we went to visit with our homeschool group. After that, we started buying Polyface meat and became loyal customers. In fact, my kids love you because Polyface hot dogs are the only hot dogs I allow them to eat. So, in my household, you're a rock star!

Needless to say, I was intimidated to share the stage with you that night at the VICFA event. I wanted to impress you because I was hoping you would agree to an interview for my website. However, a day before the event, I got the flu! But, VICFA needed me to take the stage. So, I spent the day taking vitamin C, fasting, and drinking herbal teas. The night of the event, I probably smelled like a candy cane from covering myself in peppermint essential oil to help keep me alert.

After my speech, I remember sitting down next to you and your wife, Teresa. I couldn't stop thinking that I blew it. But you leaned toward me and said, "You just thoroughly impressed me." I responded like a giddy school girl, "Really? I was so nervous because I really wanted to impress you." You laughed and Teresa said, "Are you kidding? His pen ran out of ink because he was taking so many notes."

In that moment, the Spirit came over me, and I decided to have a child-like faith. Instead of asking for an interview, I boldly asked, "Do you want to write a book with me? I don't know exactly what it would be about, but I have an idea." You paused for a moment and said, "Sure, why not!"

The rest is history in the making.

Trademark Acknowledgment

All product names, logos, brands, and other trademarks identified or referred to within this book are the property of their respective trademark holders. All company, product, logo, and service names used in the book are for identification purposes only. Use of these names and brands does not imply endorsement.

- Mountain Dew® is a registered trademark of PepsiCo, Inc.
- Pillsbury® is a registered trademark of The Pillsbury Company, LLC.
- Roundup® and Roundup Ready® are registered trademarks of Monsanto Company.
- NutraSweet® is a registered trademark of NutraSweet Property Holdings, Inc.
- Doritos® is a registered trademark of Frito-Lay North America, Inc.
- Frito-Lay® is a registered trademark of Frito-Lay North America, Inc.
- Gatorade® is a registered trademark of PepsiCo, Inc.
- McDonald's® is a registered trademark of McDonald's Corporation
- Chick-fil-A® is a registered trademark of CFA Properties, Inc.
- Panera® is a registered trademark of Pumpernickel Associates, LLC.
- Campbell's® is a registered trademark of Campbell Soup Company
- Kellogg's® is a registered trademark of Kellogg North America Company
- Chipotle® is a registered trademark of CMG Pepper, LLC.
- SaladWorks® is a registered trademark of Saladworks, LLC.
- Silk® is a registered trademark of WhiteWave Services, Inc.
- Horizon® is a registered trademark of WhiteWave Services, Inc.
- Domino's Pizza® is a registered trademark of Domino's Pizza, Inc.
- BurgerFi® is a registered trademark of Restaurant Development Group, LLC.
- ShakeShack® is a registered trademark of HealthWatch Group, Ltd.
- Wendy's® is a registered trademark of Wendy's International, LLC.
- Sonic® is a registered trademark of America's Drive-In Brand Properties, LLC.
- Burger King® is a registered trademark of Burger King Corporation
- In-N-Out® is a registered trademark of In-N-Out Burgers Corporation California
- Carl's Jr® is a registered trademark of Carl's Jr. Restaurants, LLC.
- Coke® is a registered trademark of The Coca-Cola Company

- Twinkies® is a registered trademark of Hostess Brands, LLC.
- Nabisco® is a registered trademark of Kraft Foods Global Brands, LLC.
- Equal® is a registered trademark of Merisant Company
- NutraSweet® is a registered trademark of Nutra Sweet Property Holdings, Inc.
- Sunett® is a registered trademark of Hoechst Aktiengesellschaft Corporation Fed Rep Germany
- Splenda® is a registered trademark of Tate & Lyle Public Limited Company
- Sweet 'N Low® is a registered trademark of CPC Intellectual Property, Inc.
- Sucralose is patented by Tate & Lyle Public Limited Company
- Acesulfame potassium is patented by Celanese Corporation.
- Jell-O® is a registered trademark of Kraft Foods Group Brands, LLC.
- Rice Krispies® is a registered trademark of Kellogg North America Company
- Morton's® is a registered trademark of Morton Salt, Inc.
- Real Salt® is a registered trademark of Redmond, Inc.
- Cheesecake Factory® is a registered trademark of TCF CO, LLC.
- P.F. Chang's® is a registered trademark of P.F. Chang's China Bistro
- Game of Thrones® is a registered trademark of Home Box Office, Inc.
- Uber® is a registered trademark of Uber Technologies, Inc.
- Airbnb® is a registered trademark of Airbnb, Inc.
- Amazon Prime® is a registered trademark of Amazon Technologies, Inc.
- GrubHub® is a registered trademark of GrubHub Holdings, Inc.
- Butcher Box® is a registered trademark of MASX, LLC.
- Thrive Market® is a registered trademark of Thrive Market, Inc.
- Fed Ex® is a registered trademark of FedEx Corporation
- UPS® is a registered trademark of United Parcel Service of America, Inc.
- Cascadian Farms® is a registered trademark of General Mills, LLC.
- Kroger® is a registered trademark of The Kroger Co.
- Pop Tarts® is a registered trademark of Kellogg NA Company
- Duncan Hines® is a registered trademark of Pinnacle Foods Group, LLC.
- Hot Pockets® is a registered trademark of Nestle USA, Inc.

- Dirty Dozen® is a registered trademark of Environmental Working Group
- Clean Fifteen® is a registered trademark of Environmental Working Group
- Target® is a registered trademark of Target Brands, Inc.
- Walmart® is a registered trademark of Walmart Apollo, LLC.
- Buffalo Wild Wings® is a registered trademark of Buffalo Wild Wings, Inc.
- Peanuts® is copyrighted by Peanuts Worldwide, LLC.
- Cheerios® is a registered trademark of General Mills, LLC.
- Lucky Charms® is a registered trademark of General Mills, LLC.
- Classic Coke® is a registered trademark of The Coca-Cola Company
- Diet Pepsi® is a registered trademark of Pepsico, Inc.
- Disney's Epcott Center® is a registered trademark of Disney Enterprises, Inc.
- Egg Beaters® is a registered trademark of ConAgra Foods RDM, Inc.
- Impossible Burger® is a registered trademark of Impossible Foods, Inc.
- Beyond Meat® is a registered trademark of Beyond Meat, Inc.
- DuPont® is a registered trademark of E.I. du Pont de Nemours and Company
- Teflon® is a registered trademark of The Chemours Company FC, LLC.
- Scotchgard® is a registered trademark of 3M Company
- Cornflakes® is a registered trademark of Kellogg Company
- Google® is a registered trademark of Google, LLC.
- Star Trek® is a registered trademark of CBS Studios, Inc.
- VELCRO® is a registered trademark of Velcro Companies BVBA.
- Froot Loops® is a registered trademark of Kellogg North America Company.

References & Permissions

Chapter 1: Personalize Your Roadmap

1. Electronic Code of Federal Regulations. Available at: https://www.ecfr.gov/cgi-bin/text-idx?c=ecfr&sid=3f34f4c22f9aa8e6d9864cc2683cea02&tpl=/ecfrbrowse/Title07/7cfr205_main_02.tpl
2. Turnwald, Bradley P et al. "Learning one's genetic risk changes physiology independent of actual genetic risk." *Nature human behaviour* vol. 3,1 (2019): 48-56. doi:10.1038/s41562-018-0483-4
3. Zinöcker, Marit K, and Inge A Lindseth. "The Western Diet-Microbiome-Host Interaction and Its Role in Metabolic Disease." *Nutrients* vol. 10,3 365. 17 Mar. 2018, doi:10.3390/nu10030365
4. Doaei S, Kalantari N, Mohammadi NK, Tabesh GA, Gholamalizadeh M. "Macronutrients and the FTO gene expression in hypothalamus; a systematic review of experimental studies." *Indian Heart J.* 2017 Mar - Apr;69(2):277-281. doi:10.1016/j.ihj.2017.01.014. Epub 2017 Jan 24. Review.
5. Dispenza, Joe. "Making Your Mind Matter." Hay House Online Learning.
6. Hay, Louise. "Loving Yourself: Online Video Course." Hay House Online Learning
7. Dispenza, Joe. "Becoming Supernatural." Hay House Inc., 2019.
8. Lydon-Staley DM, Kuehner C, Zamoscik V, Huffziger S, Kirsch P, Bassett DS. "Repetitive negative thinking in daily life and functional connectivity among default mode, fronto-parietal, and salience networks." *Transl Psychiatry.* 2019 Sep 18;9(1):234. doi: 10.1038/s41398-019-0560-0.

Chapter 4: Shift from Low to High Quality Processed Foods

1. Grocery Manufacturer Association. "GROCERY MANUFACTURERS ASSOCIATION POSITION ON GMOS. *The Facts About GMOs; A Project of The Grocery Manufacturers Association*".
Available at: http://factsaboutgmos.org/disclosure-statement?_ga=1.19384190.792219552.1483234931. Accessed December 31, 2016.

Harness Your Power

1. GMO Free News. Monsanto: A Sustainable Agriculture Company. *www.gmoinfo.blogspot.com.* 2013.
Available at: http://gmoinfo.blogspot.com/2013/09/monsanto-sustainable-agriculture-company.html. Accessed September 18, 2016.
2. Grocery Manufacturer Association. GROCERY MANUFACTURERS ASSOCIATION POSITION ON GMOS. *The Facts About GMOs; A Project of The Grocery Manufacturers Association.*
Available at: http://factsaboutgmos.org/disclosure-statement?_ga=1.19384190.792219552.1483234931. Accessed December 31, 2016.
3. Poti JM, Mendez MA, Wen Ng S, Popkin BM. Is the degree of food processing and convenience linked with the nutritional quality of foods purchased by US households? *American Journal of Clinical Nutrition.* 2015;101(6).
4. Corriher SC. Most Americans Are Eating Genetically Engineered Foods Several Times A Day. *The Health Wyze Report & Fidelity Ministry.* 2009. Available at: http://healthwyze.org/reports/281-most-americans-are-eating-genetically-engineered-foods-several-times-a-day.
5. U.S. FDA. Statement of Policy-Foods Derived from New Plant Varieties. *Federal Register.* 1992;57(no. 104).
Available at: http://www.fda.gov/Food/GuidanceRegulation/GuidanceDocumentsRegulatoryInformation/Biotechnology/ucm096095.htm.
6. World Health Organization. Frequently asked questions on genetically modified foods. *www.who.int.*
Available at: http://www.who.int/foodsafety/areas_work/food-technology/faq-genetically-modified-food/en/. Accessed December 17, 2016.
7. Commoner B. Unraveling the DNA myth: The spurious foundation of genetic engineering. *Harper's.* 2002.
8. Yang B, Wang J, Tang B, et al. Characterization of Bioactive Recombinant Human Lysozyme Expressed in Milk of Cloned Transgenic Cattle. *PLOS One.* 2011;6(3).
9. Gucciardi A. Scientists To Add Spider Genes To Human Genome To Create "Bulletproof Skin." *www.naturalsociety.com.* 2012.
Available at: http://naturalsociety.com/scientists-to-add-spider-genes-to-human-genome-to-create-bulletproof-skin/.
10. Li Z, Zeng F, Meng F, et al. Generation of transgenic pigs by cytoplasmic injection of piggyBac transposase-based pmGENIE-3 plasmids. *Biol Reprod.* 2014;90(5):93.
11. Rahman M, Mak R, Ayad H, Smith A, Maclean N. Expression of a novel piscine growth hormone gene results in growth enhancement in transgenic tilapia (Oreochromis niloticus). *Transgenic Res.* 1998;7(5):357–69.
12. Davis N, Rawlinson K. Scientists attempting to harvest human organs in pigs create human-pig embryo. *www.theguardian.com.* 2016.
Available at: https://www.theguardian.com/science/2016/jun/05/organ-research-scientists-combine-human-stem-cells-and-pig-dna.
13. U.S. Department of Health and Human Services. Animal & Veterinary Consumer Q&A. *www.fda.gov.* 2015.
Available at: http://www.fda.gov/AnimalVeterinary/DevelopmentApprovalProcess/GeneticEngineering/GeneticallyEngineeredAnimals/ucm113672.htm. Accessed September 18, 2016.
14. Cummins R, Lilliston B. *Genetically Engineered Food: A Self-Defense Guide for Consumers.* New York, NY: Marlowe & Company; 2000.
15. Sarjeet S, Cowles E, Pietrantonio P. The Mode of Action of Bacillus Thuringiensis Endotoxins. *Annual Review of Entomology.* 1992;37:615–634.
16. Noteborn HP, Bienenmann-Ploum JM, van den Berg ME, et al. Safety assessment of the Bacillus thuringiensis insecticidal crystal protein CRYIA(b) expressed in transgenic tomatoes. In: Engels KH, Takeoka GR, Teranishi R, eds. *ACS Symposium Series 605 Genetically Modified Foods - Safety Issues; American Chemical Society.* Washington DC; 1995:135–147.
17. Pusztai A, Bardocz B, Ewen SWB. Genetically Modified Foods: Potential Human Health Effects. In: D'Mello JP., ed. *CAB International; Food Safety: Contimainats and Toxins.;* 2003:347–372. Available at: http://www.bioemit.math.ntnu.no/meetings/pusztaibookK.pdf.
18. El-Shamei Z, Gab-Alla A, Shatta A, Moussa E, Rayan A. Histopathological change in some organs of male rats fet on genetically modified corn. *J Am Sci.* 2012;8(10):684–96.
19. Rinamore A, Roselli M, Britti S, et al. Intestinal and peripheral immune response to MON810 maize ingestion in weaning and old mice. *J Agric Food Chem.* 2008;56(23):11533–9.

20. Vázquez-Padrón, RI Gonzáles-Cabrera, J García-Tovar C, Neri-Bazan L, Lopéz-Revilla, R Hernández M, Moreno-Fierro L, de la Riva G. Cry1Ac protoxin from Bacillus thuringiensis sp. kurstaki HD73 binds to surface proteins in the mouse small intestine. *Biochem Biophys Res Commun.* 2000;271(1):54–8.
21. GMO Science. Are all forms of Bt toxin safe? *GMO Science.* 2015. Available at: https://www.gmoscience.org/is-bt-toxin-safe/.
22. Sasaki YF, Kawaguchi S, Kamaya A, et al. The comet assay with 8 mouse organs: Results with 39 currently used food additives. *Mutation Research - Genetic Toxicology and Environmental Mutagenesis.* 2002;519(1-2):103–119.
23. Lancaster F, Lawrence J. Determination of total non-sulphonated aromatic amines in tartrazine, sunset yellow FCF and allura red by reduction and derivatization followed by high-performance liquid chromatography. *Food Additives and Contaminants.* 1991;8(3):249–63. Available at: https://www.ncbi.nlm.nih.gov/pubmed/1778264.
24. Goldschmidt V. 12 Dangerous And Hidden Food Ingredients In Seemingly Healthy Foods. *www.saveourbones.com.* 2016. Available at: https://saveourbones.com/12-dangerous-ingredients/. Accessed November 12, 2016.
25. Lim T, Poole R, Pageler N. Propylene glycol toxicity in children. *J Pediatr Pharmacol Ther.* 2014;19(4):277–282. Available at: https://www.ncbi.nlm.nih.gov/pubmed/25762872.
26. Oikawa S, Nishino K, Inoue S, Mizutani T, Kawanishi S. Oxidative DNA damage and apoptosis induced by metabolites of butylated hydroxytoluene. *Biochem PHarmacol.* 1998;56(3):361–370. Available at: https://www.ncbi.nlm.nih.gov/pubmed/9744574.
27. Bauer A, Dwyer-Nield L, Hankin J, Murphy R, Malkinson A. The lung tumor promoter, butylated hydroxytoluene (BHT), causes chronic inflammation in promotion-sensitive BALB/cByJ mice but not in promotion-resistant CXB4 mice. *Toxicology.* 2001;169(1):1–15. Available at: https://www.ncbi.nlm.nih.gov/pubmed/11696405.
28. Bauer K, Dwyer-Nield L, Keil K, Koski K, Malkinson A. Butylated hydroxytoluene (BHT) induction of pulmonary inflammation: a role in tumor promotion. *Exp Lung Res.* 2001;27(3):197–216. Available at: https://www.ncbi.nlm.nih.gov/pubmed/11293324.
29. Mikkelsen H, Larsen J, Tarding F. Hypersensitivity reactions to food colours with special reference to the natural colour annatto extract (butter colour). *Archives of Toxicology Supplementation.* 1978;1:141–3. Available at: https://www.ncbi.nlm.nih.gov/pubmed/150265.
30. Be Food Smart. Polysorbate 60. *www.befoodsmart.com.* 2011. Available at: http://www.befoodsmart.com/ingredients/polysorbate-60.php. Accessed November 12, 2016.
31. Conley M. Flame Retardant in Your Mountan Dew? Yep. *www.abcnews.go.com.* 2011. Available at: http://abcnews.go.com/blogs/health/2011/12/15/flame-retardant-in-your-mountain-dew-yep/.
32. Frito-Lay. DORITOS® Nacho Cheese Flavored Tortilla Chips. *www.fritolay.com.* 2016. Available at: http://www.fritolay.com/snacks/product-page/doritos/doritos-nacho-cheese-flavored-tortilla-chips. Accessed November 13, 2016.
33. U.S. Food and Drug Administration. *Preliminary Regulatory Impact Analysis for the Proposed Rules for Current Good Manufacturing Practices and Hazard Analysis and Risk-Based Preventive Controls for Human Food, Docket No. FDA-2011-N-0920.* 2013. Available at: http://www.fda.gov/downloads/Food/GuidanceRegulation/FSMA/UCM334117.pdf
34. Committee of Five. *Declaration of Independence.* Philadelphia; 1776. Available at: http://www.archives.gov/exhibits/charters/declaration_transcript.html.

Say No To Antibiotics When Eating Out

1. Hudson W. CDC: "Nightmare bacteria" spreading. CNN.com. 2013. Available at: http://www.cnn.com/2013/03/06/health/super-bug-bacteria-spreading/.
2. Bittman M. *A Bone to Pick: The good and bad news about food, with wisdom and advice on diets, food safety, GMOs, farming and more.* New York: Pam Krauss Books; 2015.
3. United States Department of Health and Human Services, Centers For Disease Control and Prevention; Antibiotic Resistance Threats in the United States 2019. Available at: https://www.cdc.gov/drugresistance/pdf/threats-report/2019-ar-threats-report-508.pdf
4. Martin, Michael J et al. "Antibiotics Overuse in Animal Agriculture: A Call to Action for Health Care Providers." *American journal of public health* vol. 105,12 (2015): 2409-10. doi:10.2105/AJPH.2015.302870
5. Ipci K, Altıntoprak N, Muluk NB, Senturk M, Cingi C. "The possible mechanisms of the human microbiome in allergic diseases." *Eur Arch Otorhinolaryngol.* 2017 Feb;274(2):617-626. doi: 10.1007/s00405-016-4058-6. Epub 2016 Apr 26. Review.
6. Centers for Disease Control and Prevention. "Biggest Threats and Data: 2019 AR Threats Report. Available at: https://www.cdc.gov/DrugResistance/Biggest-Threats.html
7. Zinöcker, Marit K, and Inge A Lindseth. "The Western Diet-Microbiome-Host Interaction and Its Role in Metabolic Disease." *Nutrients* vol. 10,3 365. 17 Mar. 2018, doi:10.3390/nu10030365

Look For The 100% USDA Organic Label

1. Electronic Code of Federal Regulations. "Title 7 – Agriculture, Subtitle B – Regulations of the Department of Agriculture." Available at: https://www.ecfr.gov/cgi-bin/text-idx?c=ecfr&sid=3f34f4c22f9aa8e6d9864cc2683cea02&tpl=/ecfrbrowse/Title07/7cfr205_main_02.tpl
2. Organic Consumers Association. "It's Time to Talk (Again) about Sewage Sludge on Farmlands." July 11, 2017. Available at: https://www.organicconsumers.org/news/it%E2%80%99s-time-talk-again-about-sewage-sludge-farmland
3. Environmental Working Group. "Dumping Sewage Sludge On Organic Farms?" April 30, 1998. Available at: https://www.ewg.org/research/dumping-sewage-sludge-organic-farms
4. EPA. "Biosolids Laws and Regulations." Available at: https://www.epa.gov/biosolids/biosolids-laws-and-regulations
5. Rodale Institute. "The Real Beef with Biosolids." Available at: https://rodaleinstitute.org/blog/the-real-beef-with-biosolids/
6. USDA. "Organic Labeling Standards." Available at: https://www.ams.usda.gov/grades-standards/organic-labeling-standards
7. USDA. "Organic 101: What the USDA Organic Label Means." Available at: https://www.usda.gov/media/blog/2012/03/22/organic-101-what-usda-organic-label-means
8. USDA. "Organic Regulations." Available at: https://www.ams.usda.gov/rules-regulations/organic
9. USDA. "The National List." Available at: https://www.ams.usda.gov/rules-regulations/organic/national-list
10. USDA. "National Organic Standards Board (NOSB). Available at: https://www.ams.usda.gov/rules-regulations/organic/nosb

11. Zinöcker, Marit K, and Inge A Lindseth. "The Western Diet-Microbiome-Host Interaction and Its Role in Metabolic Disease." *Nutrients* vol. 10,3 365. 17 Mar. 2018, doi:10.3390/nu10030365
12. USDA "Organic 101: Strengthening Organic Integrity through Increased Residue Testing." Available at: https://www.usda.gov/media/blog/2013/02/20/organic-101-strengthening-organic-integrity-through-increased-residue-testing

Mirror, Mirror

1. Dispenza, Joe. "Making Your Mind Matter." Hay House Online Learning.
2. Hay, Louise. "Loving Yourself: Online Video Course." Hay House Online Learning

Switch to Organic Eggs

1. USDA Agricultural Marketing Service, National Organic Program; Guidelines for Organic Certification of Poultry. Available at: https://www.ams.usda.gov/sites/default/files/media/Poultry%20-%20Guidelines.pdf
2. USDA Agricultural Marketing Service, National Organic Program; Organic Livestock and Poultry Practices Final Rule, January 2017. Available at: https://www.ams.usda.gov/sites/default/files/media/OLPPExternalQA.pdf
3. USDA; Guidelines for Organic Livestock Producers. Available at: https://www.ams.usda.gov/sites/default/files/media/GuideForOrganicLivestockProducers.pdf
4. USDA Natural Resources Conservation Service; Animal Feeding Operations. Available at: https://www.nrcs.usda.gov/wps/portal/nrcs/main/national/plantsanimals/livestock/afo/
5. Gerwyn Morris, Michael Berk, André F. Carvalho, Javier R. Caso, Yolanda Sanz and Michael Maes, "The Role of Microbiota and Intestinal Permeability in the Pathophysiology of Autoimmune and Neuroimmune Processes with an Emphasis on Inflammatory Bowel Disease Type 1 Diabetes and Chronic Fatigue Syndrome", Current Pharmaceutical Design (2016) 22: 6058.
6. Clapp, Megan et al. "Gut microbiota's effect on mental health: The gut-brain axis." Clinics and practice vol. 7,4 987. 15 Sep. 2017, doi:10.4081/cp.2017.987
7. Srikantha, Piranavie, and M Hasan Mohajeri. "The Possible Role of the Microbiota-Gut-Brain-Axis in Autism Spectrum Disorder." *International journal of molecular sciences* vol. 20,9 2115. 29 Apr. 2019, doi:10.3390/ijms20092115
8. Mu, Qinghui et al. "Leaky Gut As a Danger Signal for Autoimmune Diseases." *Frontiers in immunology* vol. 8 598. 23 May. 2017, doi:10.3389/fimmu.2017.00598
9. Ipci K, Altıntoprak N, Muluk NB, Senturk M, Cingi C. "The possible mechanisms of the human microbiome in allergic diseases." *Eur Arch Otorhinolaryngol.* 2017 Feb;274(2):617-626. doi: 10.1007/s00405-016-4058-6. Epub 2016 Apr 26. Review.
10. Rizzetto L, Fava F, Tuohy KM, Selmi C. "Connecting the immune system, systemic chronic inflammation and the gut microbiome: The role of sex." *J Autoimmun.* 2018 Aug; 92:12-34. doi: 10.1016/j.jaut.2018.05.008. Epub 2018 Jun 1. Review.
11. Cani PD. "Human gut microbiome: hopes, threats and promises." Gut. 2018 Sep;67(9):1716-1725. doi: 10.1136/gutjnl-2018-316723. Epub 2018 Jun 22. Review.
12. Thursby E, Juge N. "Introduction to the human gut microbiota." *Biochem J.* 2017 May 16;474(11):1823-1836. doi: 10.1042/BCJ20160510. Review.
13. Zinöcker, Marit K, and Inge A Lindseth. "The Western Diet-Microbiome-Host Interaction and Its Role in Metabolic Disease." *Nutrients* vol. 10,3 365. 17 Mar. 2018, doi:10.3390/nu10030365
14. Macfarlane S., Macfarlane G.T., Cummings J.H. "Review article: Prebiotics in the gastrointestinal tract." *Aliment. Pharmacol. Ther.* 2006;24:701–714. doi: 10.1111/j.1365-2036.2006.03042.x.
15. Martinez K.B., Leone V., Chang E.B. "Western diets, gut dysbiosis, and metabolic diseases: Are they linked?" *Gut Microbes.* 2017;6:1–13. doi: 10.1080/19490976.2016.1270811.
16. Singh, Rasnik K et al. "Influence of diet on the gut microbiome and implications for human health." *Journal of translational medicine* vol. 15,1 73. 8 Apr. 2017, doi:10.1186/s12967-017-1175-y
17. Shelly A. Buffington et al., "Microbial reconstitution reverses maternal diet induced social and synaptic deficits in offspring." *Cell;* doi: 10.1016/j.cell.2016.06.001, published online 16 June 2016.
18. Lloyd-Price, Jason et al. "The healthy human microbiome." *Genome medicine* vol. 8,1 51. 27 Apr. 2016, doi:10.1186/s13073-016-0307-y

Say No To Chlorinated Eggs

1. See References for "Switch to Organic Eggs."

Choose Organic Chicken

1. See References for "Switch to Organic Eggs."
2. Guarner F., Malagelada J.R. "Gut flora in health and disease." *Lancet.* 2003;361:512–519. doi: 10.1016/S0140-6736(03)12489-0.
3. Eckburg P.B., Bik E.M., Bernstein C.N., Purdom E., Dethlefsen L., Sargent M., Gill S.R., Nelson K.E., Relman D.A. "Diversity of the human intestinal microbial flora." *Science.* 2005;308:1635–1638. doi: 10.1126/science.1110591.
4. Mondot S., de Wouters T., Dore J., Lepage P. "The human gut microbiome and its dysfunctions." *Dig. Dis.* 2013;31:278–285. doi: 10.1159/000354678.
5. Vulevic J., Juric A., Tzortzis G., Gibson G.R. "A mixture of trans-galactooligosaccharides reduces markers of metabolic syndrome and modulates the fecal microbiota and immune function of overweight adults." *J. Nutr.* 2013;143:324–331. doi: 10.3945/jn.112.166132
6. Fava F., Gitau R., Griffin B.A., Gibson G.R., Tuohy K.M., Lovegrove J.A. "The type and quantity of dietary fat and carbohydrate alter faecal microbiome and short-chain fatty acid excretion in a metabolic syndrome "at-risk" population." Int. *J. Obes.* 2013;37:216–223. doi: 10.1038/ijo.2012.33.
7. Tuohy K.M., Conterno L., Gasperotti M., Viola R. "Up-regulating the human intestinal microbiome using whole plant foods, polyphenols, and/or fiber." *J. Agric.* Food Chem. 2012;60:8776–8782. doi: 10.1021/jf2053959.

8. Gibson G.R., Roberfroid M.B. "Dietary modulation of the human colonic microbiota:introducing the concept of prebiotics." *J. Nutr.* 1995;125:1401–1412.
9. Martinez K.B., Leone V., Chang E.B. "Western diets, gut dysbiosis, and metabolic diseases: Are they linked?" *Gut Microbes.* 2017;6:1–13. doi: 10.1080/19490976.2016.1270811.

Choose Your Disinfectant On Your Chicken

1. See References for "Switch To Organic Eggs."
2. Ipci K, Altıntoprak N, Muluk NB, Senturk M, Cingi C. "The possible mechanisms of the human microbiome in allergic diseases." *Eur Arch Otorhinolaryngol.* 2017 Feb;274(2):617-626. doi: 10.1007/s00405-016-4058-6. Epub 2016 Apr 26. Review.
3. Rizzetto L, Fava F, Tuohy KM, Selmi C. "Connecting the immune system, systemic chronic inflammation and the gut microbiome: The role of sex." *J Autoimmun.* 2018 Aug; 92:12-34. doi: 10.1016/j.jaut.2018.05.008. Epub 2018 Jun 1. Review.
4. Cani PD. "Human gut microbiome: hopes, threats and promises." *Gut.* 2018 Sep;67(9):1716-1725. doi: 10.1136/gutjnl-2018-316723. Epub 2018 Jun 22. Review.
5. Thursby E, Juge N. "Introduction to the human gut microbiota." *Biochem J.* 2017 May 16;474(11):1823-1836. doi: 10.1042/BCJ20160510. Review.
6. Electronic Code of Federal Regulations. Available at: https://www.ecfr.gov/cgi-bin/text-idx?c=ecfr&sid=3f34f4c22f9aa8e6d9864cc2683cea02&tpl=/ecfrbrowse/Title07/7cfr205_main_02.tpl
7. Belizário, José E, and Mauro Napolitano. "Human microbiomes and their roles in dysbiosis, common diseases, and novel therapeutic approaches." Frontiers in microbiology vol. 6 1050. 6 Oct. 2015, doi:10.3389/fmicb.2015.01050

Don't Waste Your Money on "Free Range" Or "Pasture Raised"

1. See References for "Choose Organic Eggs."

Eat 100% Grass-Fed, Organic Beef

1. USDA. "Organic 101: What Organic Farming (and Processing) Doesn't Allow." February 21, 2017. Available at: https://www.usda.gov/media/blog/2011/12/16/organic-101-what-organic-farming-and-processing-doesnt-allow
2. McAfee AJ, et al. "Red meat from animals offered a grass diet increases plasma and platelet n-3 PUFA in healthy consumers." *Br J Nutr.* 2011 Jan;105(1):80-9.
3. Daley CA, Abbott A, Doyle PS, Nader GA, Larson S. "A review of fatty acid profiles and antioxidant content in grass-fed and grain-fed beef." *Nutr J.* 2010 Mar 10;9:10.
4. Van Elswyk ME, McNeill SH. "Impact of grass/forage feeding versus grain finishing on beef nutrients and sensory quality: the U.S. experience." *Meat Sci.* 2014 Jan;96(1):535-40. doi: 10.1016/j.meatsci.2013.08.010.
5. Dhiman TR, Anand GR, Satter LD, Pariza MW. "Conjugated linoleic acid content of milk from cows fed different diets." *J Dairy Sci.* 1999 Oct;82(10):2146-56.
6. Castro-Webb N, Ruiz-Narváez EA, Campos H. "Cross-sectional study of conjugated linoleic acid in adipose tissue and risk of diabetes." *Am J Clin Nutr.* 2012 Jul;96(1):175-81.
7. Smit LA, Baylin A, Campos H. "Conjugated linoleic acid in adipose tissue and risk of myocardial infarction." *Am J Clin Nutr.* 2010 Jul;92(1):34-40.
8. Blankson H, Stakkestad JA, Fagertun H, Thom E, Wadstein J, Gudmundsen O. "Conjugated linoleic acid reduces body fat mass in overweight and obese humans." *J Nutr.* 2000 Dec;130(12):2943-8.
9. USDA Argicultural Marketing Service. Grass-Fed Beef and Naturally Raised Labels: Understanding Our Withdrawal of Two Voluntary Marketing Claim Standards. Available at: https://www.ams.usda.gov/content/grass-fed-beef-and-naturally-raised-labels
10. Electronic Code of Federal Regulations. Available at: https://www.ecfr.gov/cgi-bin/text-idx?c=ecfr&sid=3f34f4c22f9aa8e6d9864cc2683cea02&tpl=/ecfrbrowse/Title07/7cfr205_main_02.tpl

Eat What You Can Pronounce

1. Weise E. Experts who decide on food additives conflicted. *USA Today.* 2013. Available at: http://www.usatoday.com/story/news/nation/2013/08/07/food-additives-conflict-of-interest/2625211/.
2. Environmental Working Group. EWG's Dirty Dozen Guide to Food Additives: Generally Recognized As Safe-But Is It? *www.ewg.org.* 2014. Available at: http://www.ewg.org/research/ewg-s-dirty-dozen-guide-food-additives/generally-recognized-as-safe-but-is-it.
3. The Pew Charitable Trusts. *Fixing the Oversight of Chemicals Added to Our Food: Findings and Recommendations of Pew's Assessments of the U.S. Food Additives Program.* 2013. Available at: http://www.pewtrusts.org/en/research-and-analysis/reports/2013/11/07/fixing-the-oversight-of-chemicals-added-to-our-food.
4. Poti JM, Mendez MA, Wen Ng S, Popkin BM. Is the degree of food processing and convenience linked with the nutritional quality of foods purchased by US households? *American Journal of Clinical Nutrition.* 2015;101(6). Available at: http://doi.org/10.3945/ajcn.114.100925.
5. Goldschmidt V. 12 Dangerous And Hidden Food Ingredients In Seemingly Healthy Foods. *www.saveourbones.com.* 2016. Available at: https://saveourbones.com/12-dangerous-ingredients/. Accessed November 12, 2016.
6. Oikawa S, Nishino K, Inoue S, Mizutani T, Kawanishi S. Oxidative DNA damage and apoptosis induced by metabolites of butylated hydroxytoluene. *Biochem PHarmacol.* 1998;56(3):361–370. Available at: https://www.ncbi.nlm.nih.gov/pubmed/9744574.
7. Bauer K, Dwyer-Nield L, Keil K, Koski K, Malkinson A. Butylated hydroxytoluene (BHT) induction of pulmonary inflammation: a role in tumor promotion. *Exp Lung Res.* 2001;27(3):197–216. Available at: https://www.ncbi.nlm.nih.gov/pubmed/11293324.
8. Bauer A, Dwyer-Nield L, Hankin J, Murphy R, Malkinson A. The lung tumor promoter, butylated hydroxytoluene (BHT), causes chronic inflammation in promotion-sensitive BALB/cByJ mice but not in promotion-resistant CXB4 mice. *Toxicology.* 2001;169(1):1–15. Available at: https://www.ncbi.nlm.nih.gov/pubmed/11696405.

9. Sasaki YF, Kawaguchi S, Kamaya A, et al. The comet assay with 8 mouse organs: Results with 39 currently used food additives. *Mutation Research - Genetic Toxicology and Environmental Mutagenesis.* 2002;519(1-2):103–119.
10. Hamishehkar H, Khani S, Kashanian S, Ezzati Nazhad D, Eskandani M. Geno- and cytotoxicity of propyl gallate food additive. *Drug & Chemical Toxicology.* 2014;37(3):241–6. Available at: https://www.ncbi.nlm.nih.gov/pubmed/24160552.
11. Han Y, Moon H, You B, Park W. Propyl gallate inhibits the growth of calf pulmonary arterial endothelial cells via glutathione depletion. *Toxicol in Vitro.* 2010;24(4):1183–9. Available at: https://www.ncbi.nlm.nih.gov/pubmed/20159035.
12. Foti C, Bonamonte D, Cassano N, Conserva A, Vena G. Allergic contact dermatitis to propyl gallate and pentylene glycol in an emollient cream. *Australas J Dermotol.* 2010;51(2):147–8. Available at: https://www.ncbi.nlm.nih.gov/pubmed/20546226.
13. Pandhi D, Vij A, Singal A. Contact depigmentation induced by propyl gallate. *Clin Exp Dematol.* 2011;36(4):366–8. Available at: https://www.ncbi.nlm.nih.gov/pubmed/21564173.
14. Eler G, Peralta R, Bracht A. The action of n-propyl gallate on gluconeogenesis and oxygen uptake in the rat liver. *Chem Biol Interact.* 2009;181(3):390–9. Available at: https://www.ncbi.nlm.nih.gov/pubmed/19616523.
15. Routledge E, Parker J, Odum J, Ashby J, Sumpter J. Some alkyl hydroxy benzoate preservatives (parabens) are estrogenic. T*oxicol Appl PHarmacol.* 1998;153(1):12–9. Available at: https://www.ncbi.nlm.nih.gov/pubmed/9875295.
16. Darbre P, Aljarrah A, Miller W, et al. Concentrations of parabens in human breast tumours. *J Appl Toxicol.* 2004;24(1):5–13. Available at: https://www.ncbi.nlm.nih.gov/pubmed/14745841.
17. Barr L, Metaxan G, Harbach C, Savoy L, Darbre P. Measurement of paraben concentrations in human breast tissue at serial locations across the breast from axilla to sternum. *J Appl Toxicol.* 2012;32(3):219–32. Available at: https://www.ncbi.nlm.nih.gov/pubmed/22237600.
18. Government Accountability Office. *FOOD SAFETY: FDA Should Strengthen Its Oversight of Food Ingredients Determined to Be Generally Recognized as Safe (GRAS).* 2010:74.
19. Curtis N. Harmful if swallowed-The dangers of food irradiation. *www.naturalnews.com.* 2013. Available at: http://www.naturalnews.com/041878_food_irradiation_harmful_nutrition.html.
20. Neltner TG, Kulkarni NR, Alger HM, et al. Navigating the U.S. Food Additive Regulatory Program. *Wiley Online Library.* 2011. Available at: http://onlinelibrary.wiley.com/doi/10.1111/j.1541-4337.2011.00166.x/full. Accessed August 13, 2016.
21. United States Food and Drug Administration. Food Irradiation: What You Need to Know. *www.fda.gov.* 2016. Available at: http://www.fda.gov/Food/ResourcesForYou/Consumers/ucm261680.htm. Accessed August 19, 2016.
22. U.S. House of Representatives. *Food Additives Amendment of 1958.* U.S. House of Representatives; 1958:1784–1789.
23. Neltner T, Maffini M. Generally Recognized as Secret: Chemicals Added to Food in the United States. *Natural Resources Defense Council.* 2014. Available at: https://www.nrdc.org/sites/default/files/safety-loophole-for-chemicals-in-food-report.pdf.
24. Michael Farris. Personal Communication.
25. U.S. Department of Health and Human Services Food and Drug Administration Center for Food Safety and Applied Nutrition. *Guidance for Industry: Considerations Regarding Substances Added to Foods, Including Beverages and Dietary Supplements.* 2014:5. Available at: http://www.fda.gov/downloads/Food/GuidanceRegulation/GuidanceDocumentsRegulatoryInformation/IngredientsAdditivesGRASPackaging/UCM381316.pdf.
26. Anon. Generally Recognized as Safe (GRAS). *U.S. Food and Drug Administration Website.* 2015. Available at: http://www.fda.gov/Food/IngredientsPackagingLabeling/GRAS/default.htm. Accessed July 7, 2015.
27. National Archives. Guide to the Records of the U.S. House of Representatives at the National Archives, 1789-1989 (Record Group 233). *www.archives.gov.* 1989. Available at: http://www.archives.gov/legislative/guide/house/chapter-22-select-food-and-cosmetics.html. Accessed August 21, 2016.
28. FDA. Significant Dates in U.S. Food and Drug Law History. FDA.
29. American Heart Association. Trans Fats. *www.heart.org.* 2015. Available at: http://www.heart.org/HEARTORG/HealthyLiving/HealthyEating/Nutrition/Trans-Fats_UCM_301120_Article.jsp#.V7XzFDf7bII. Accessed August 18, 2016.
30. United States Food and Drug Administration Department of. *Final Determination Regarding Partially Hydrogenated Oils.* 2015. Available at: https://s3.amazonaws.com/public-inspection.federalregister.gov/2015-14883.pdf.
31. Fitzgerald R. *The Hundred-Year Lie: How Food and Medicine Are Destroying Your Health.* New York, NY: Penguin Group; 2006.
32. Winters D. The FDA's Determination On Artificial Trans Fat: A Long Time Coming. *healthaffairs.org.* 2015. Available at: http://healthaffairs.org/blog/2015/06/23/the-fdas-determination-on-artificial-trans-fat-a-long-time-coming/.
33. United States Food and Drug Administration. FDA Cuts Trans Fat in Processed Foods. *www.fda.gov.* 2015. Available at: http://www.fda.gov/ForConsumers/ConsumerUpdates/ucm372915.htm. Accessed August 18, 2016.
34. Morris S. Personal Communication with Steve D. Morris, Director-Food Safety and Agriculture. 2016.
35. Sciammacco S. Analysis Finds Hormone Disruptor Used in Cosmetics In Nearly 50 Different Foods. *www.ewg.org.* 2015. Available at: http://www.ewg.org/release/analysis-finds-hormone-disruptor-used-cosmetics-nearly-50-different-foods. Accessed August 19, 2016.
36. Feingold.org. Some Studies on BHT, BHA & TBHQ. *www.feingold.org.* 2012. Available at: http://www.feingold.org/Research/bht.php.
37. Feingold B. Dietary Management of Juvenile Delinquency. *International Journal of Offender Therapy and Comparative Criminology.* 1979;23(1). Available at: http://www.feingold.org/Research/PDFstudies/Feingold-delinq79.pdf.
38. Stokes J, Scudder C. The effect of butylated hydroxyanisole and butylated hydroxytoluene on behavioral development of mice. *Dev Psychobiol.* 1974;7(4):343–50.
39. U.S. Department of Health and Human Services. *Report on Carcinogens, Butylated Hydroxyanisole.* 2014. Available at: https://ntp.niehs.nih.gov/ntp/roc/content/profiles/butylatedhydroxyanisole.pdf.
40. General Mills. BHT statement. *www.generalmills.com.* 2015. Available at: http://www.generalmills.com/en/News/Issues/BHT-statement. Accessed November 12, 2016.
41. Seaman A. Industry influence found in food additive report. *Reuters Health.* 2013. Available at: http://www.reuters.com/article/us-influence-food-additive-idUSBRE9760MZ20130807.
42. Benson J. Reading food labels more important than ever after FDA admits it isn't doing its job. *Natural News.* 2015. Available at: http://www.naturalnews.com/048352_FDA_labels_food_industry.html.

43. Chassaing, Benoit et al. Dietary emulsifiers impact the mouse gut microbiota promoting colitis and metabolic syndrome. *Nature.* 2015;519.
44. Lerner A, Matthias T. Changes in intestinal tight junction permeability associated with industrial food additives explain the rise in incidence of autoimmune disease. *Autoimmunity Reviews.* 2015;14(6):479–489.
45. Feller S. Food additive may be cause of many allergies, researchers say. *www.upi.com.* 2016. Available at: http://www.upi.com/Health_News/2016/07/14/Food-additive-may-be-cause-of-many-allergies-researchers-say/4591468513168/.
46. Campbell A. Autoimmunity and the Gut. *Autoimmune Diseases.* 2014;152428. Available at: http://doi.org/10.1155/2014/152428.
47. Che J. Campbell Soup Will Cut Artificial Ingredients From Its Foods. *www.huffingtonpost.com.* 2015. Available at: http://www.huffingtonpost.com/entry/campbell-soup-artificial-ingredients_us_55b15a5ee4b0224d8831945e.
48. Kaplan J. Campbell to Cut Artificial Flavors, Colors by End of 2018. *www.bloomberg.com.* 2015. Available at: http://www.bloomberg.com/news/articles/2015-07-22/campbell-soup-to-cut-artificial-flavors-colors-by-end-of-2018.
49. Sewalt VP. *GRAS Notification-Exemption Claim.* Palo Alto; 2015. Available at: http://www.fda.gov/downloads/Food/IngredientsPackagingLabeling/GRAS/NoticeInventory/UCM441510.
50. Keefe D. Agency Response Letter GRAS Notice No. GRN 000567. *U.S. Food and Drug Administration Website.* 2015. Available at: http://www.fda.gov/Food/IngredientsPackagingLabeling/GRAS/NoticeInventory/ucm449888.htm. Accessed July 8, 2015.
51. Benson J. "Safety assessments" on nearly all common food additives found to be manipulated by processed food industry: Study. *Natural News.* 2013. Available at: http://www.naturalnews.com/041703_safety_assessments_food_additives_processed_industry.html.
52. Giammona C. Papa John's Is Spending $100 Million a Year to Clean Up Menu. *www.bloomberg.com.* 2015. Available at: http://www.bloomberg.com/news/articles/2015-06-23/papa-john-s-is-spending-100-million-a-year-to-clean-up-its-menu.
53. Anon. History of the GRAS List and SCOGS Reviews. *U.S. Food and Drug Administration Website.* 2013. Available at: http://www.fda.gov/Food/IngredientsPackagingLabeling/GRAS/SCOGS/ucm084142.htm. Accessed July 7, 2015.
54. Gaynor, Paulette PD. How U.S. FDA's GRAS Notification Program Works. *www.fda.gov.* Available at: http://www.fda.gov/Food/IngredientsPackagingLabeling/GRAS/ucm083022.htm. Accessed June 19, 2016.
55. Nicole W. Secret Ingredients: Who Knows What's in Your Food? *environmental Health Perspectives.* 2013. Available at: http://ehp.niehs.nih.gov/121-a126/. Accessed August 13, 2016.
56. United States Food and Drug Administration Department. Substances Generally Recognized as Safe; Docket No. FDA-1997-N-0020 (formerly 97N-0103). Federal Register. 2016;81(159). Available at: https://www.regulations.gov/document?D=FDA-1997-N-0020-0126.

Avoid Artificial & "Natural" Flavor

1. The Pew Charitable Trusts. *Fixing the Oversight of Chemicals Added to Our Food: Findings and Recommendations of Pew's Assessments of the U.S. Food Additives Program.* 2013. Available at: http://www.pewtrusts.org/en/research-and-analysis/reports/2013/11/07/fixing-the-oversight-of-chemicals-added-to-our-food.
2. Weise E. Experts who decide on food additives conflicted. *USA Today.* 2013. Available at: http://www.usatoday.com/story/news/nation/2013/08/07/food-additives-conflict-of-interest/2625211/.
3. Government Accountability Office. *FOOD SAFETY: FDA Should Strengthen Its Oversight of Food Ingredients Determined to Be Generally Recognized as Safe (GRAS).* 2010:74.
4. U.S. House of Representatives. *Food Additives Amendment of 1958.* U.S. House of Representatives; 1958:1784–1789.
5. Government Accountability Office. *FOOD SAFETY: FDA Should Strengthen Its Oversight of Food Ingredients Determined to Be Generally Recognized as Safe (GRAS).* 2010:74.
6. Nicole W. Secret Ingredients: Who Knows What's in Your Food? *environmental Health Perspectives.* 2013. Available at: http://ehp.niehs.nih.gov/121-a126/. Accessed August 13, 2016.
7. United States Food and Drug Administration Department. Substances Generally Recognized as Safe; Docket No. FDA-1997-N-0020 (formerly 97N-0103). *Federal Register.* 2016;81(159). Available at: https://www.regulations.gov/document?D=FDA-1997-N-0020-0126.
8. Oaklander M. The Soy Milk Ingredient That's Getting the Axe. *time.com.* 2014. Available at: http://time.com/3162074/carrageenan-whitewave/.
9. Food Babe. Breaking: Major Company Removing Controversial Ingredient Carrageenan Because of You! *foodbabe.com.* 2014. Available at: http://foodbabe.com/2014/08/19/breaking-major-company-removing-controversial-ingredient-carrageenan-because-of-you/comment-page-4/.
10. International Agency for Research on Cancer. *Alcohol drinking.* 1998. Available at: https://web.archive.org/web/20070927120656/http://monographs.iarc.fr/ENG/Monographs/vol44/volume44.pdf.
11. Andrews D. Synthetic ingredients in Natural Flavors and Natural Flavors in Artificial flavors. *www.ewg.org.* Available at: http://www.ewg.org/foodscores/content/natural-vs-artificial-flavors.
12. Hallagan JB, Hall RL. FEMA GRAS- A GRAS Assessment Program for Flavor Ingredients. *Regulatory Toxicology and Pharmacology.* 1995;21(3):422–430.
13. National Toxicology Program. *Toxicology and Carcinogenesis Studies of Isoeugenol.* Research Triangle Park; 2010. Available at: https://ntp.niehs.nih.gov/ntp/htdocs/lt_rpts/tr551.pdf.
14. R.L. SMITH, et al. *GRAS Flavoring Substances* 24. 2009. Available at: http://www.ift.org/knowledge-center/focus-areas/product-development-and-ingredient-innovations/~/media/Food Technology/pdf/2009/06/0609feat_GRAS24text.pdf.
15. Zinöcker, Marit K, and Inge A Lindseth. "The Western Diet-Microbiome-Host Interaction and Its Role in Metabolic Disease." *Nutrients* vol. 10,3 365. 17 Mar. 2018, doi:10.3390/nu10030365

Choose Preservative Free

1. Hamishehkar H, Khani S, Kashanian S, Ezzati Nazhad D, Eskandani M. Geno- and cytotoxicity of propyl gallate food additive. *Drug & Chemical Toxicology.* 2014;37(3):241–6. Available at: https://www.ncbi.nlm.nih.gov/pubmed/24160552.
2. Han Y, Moon H, You B, Park W. Propyl gallate inhibits the growth of calf pulmonary arterial endothelial cells via glutathione depletion. *Toxicol in Vitro.* 2010;24(4):1183–9. Available at: https://www.ncbi.nlm.nih.gov/pubmed/20159035.

3. Foti C, Bonamonte D, Cassano N, Conserva A, Vena G. Allergic contact dermatitis to propyl gallate and pentylene glycol in an emollient cream. *Australas J Dermotol.* 2010;51(2):147–8. Available at: https://www.ncbi.nlm.nih.gov/pubmed/20546226.
4. Pandhi D, Vij A, Singal A. Contact depigmentation induced by propyl gallate. *Clin Exp Dematol.* 2011;36(4):366–8. Available at: https://www.ncbi.nlm.nih.gov/pubmed/21564173.
5. Eler G, Peralta R, Bracht A. The action of n-propyl gallate on gluconeogenesis and oxygen uptake in the rat liver. *Chem Biol Interact.* 2009;181(3):390–9. Available at: https://www.ncbi.nlm.nih.gov/pubmed/19616523.
6. Knoblauch, Jessica A., "Some Food Additives Mimic Human Hormones." *Scientific American;* March 27, 2009. Available at: https://www.scientificamerican.com/article/food-additives-mimic-hormones/
7. Amadasi, Alessio et al. "Identification of xenoestrogens in food additives by an integrated in silico and in vitro approach." *Chemical research in toxicology* vol. 22,1 (2009): 52-63. doi:10.1021/tx800048m
8. Ferrero, Maria Elena. "Rationale for the Successful Management of EDTA Chelation Therapy in Human Burden by Toxic Metals." *BioMed research international* vol. 2016 (2016): 8274504. doi:10.1155/2016/8274504
9. Khan, Abdul Rehman, and Fazli Rabbi Awan. "Metals in the pathogenesis of type 2 diabetes." *Journal of diabetes and metabolic disorders* vol. 13,1 16. 8 Jan. 2014, doi:10.1186/2251-6581-13-16
10. Zinöcker, Marit K, and Inge A Lindseth. "The Western Diet-Microbiome-Host Interaction and Its Role in Metabolic Disease." *Nutrients* vol. 10,3 365. 17 Mar. 2018, doi:10.3390/nu10030365
11. Reardon, Sara. "Food preservatives linked to obesity and gut disease." *Nature;* February 25, 105. Available at: https://www.nature.com/news/food-preservatives-linked-to-obesity-and-gut-disease-1.16984

Don't Fear The Fat Label

1. United States Department of Agriculture. Dietary Guidelines For Americans 2015-2020. *www.choosemyplate.gov.* 2016. Available at: https://www.choosemyplate.gov/dietary-guidelines. Accessed September 18, 2016.
2. Teicholz N. The scientific report guiding the US dietary guidelines: is it scientific? *BMJ.* 2015;351. Available at: http://www.bmj.com/content/bmj/351/bmj.h4962.full.pdf.
3. Committee DGA. *Report of the Dietary Guidelines Advisory Committee on the Dietary Guidelines for Americans,* 1995. 1995. Available at: https://health.gov/dietaryguidelines/dga95/pdf/DGREPORT.PDF.
4. Fan S. The fat-fueled bran: unnatural or advantageous? *www.blogs.scientificamerican.com.* 2013. Available at: https://blogs.scientificamerican.com/mind-guest-blog/the-fat-fueled-brain-unnatural-or-advantageous/. Accessed November 10, 2016.
5. United States Department of Health and Human Services and United States Department of Agriculture. *Dietary Guidelines for Americans 2015-2020 8th Edition.* Washington DC; 2015. Available at: https://health.gov/dietaryguidelines/2015/guidelines/.
6. United States Department of Agriculture. Become a MyPlate Champion. *www.choosemyplate.gov/kids.* 2015. Available at: https://www.choosemyplate.gov/kids-become-myplate-champion. Accessed November 10, 2016.
7. United States Department of Agriculture. Teachers. *www.choosemyplate.gov/teachers.* 2016. Available at: https://www.choosemyplate.gov/teachers. Accessed November 10, 2016.
8. Teicholz N. *The Big Fat Surprise: Why Butter, Meat & Cheese Belong in a Healthy Diet.* New York, NY: Simon & Schuster Paperbacks; 2014.
9. American Heart Association. How the Heart-Check Food Certification Program Works. *www.heart.org.* 2016. Available at: http://www.heart.org/HEARTORG/HealthyLiving/HealthyEating/Heart-CheckMarkCertification/How-the-Heart-Check-Food-Certification-Program-Works_UCM_300133_Article.jsp#.V-UaTDf7blI. Accessed September 23, 2016.
10. National Heart Lung and Blood Institute. Conquering Cardiovascular Disease. *www.nhlbi.nih.gov.* Available at: https://www.nhlbi.nih.gov/news/spotlight/success/conquering-cardiovascular-disease. Accessed November 10, 2016.
11. Keys A. Atherosclerosis: A Problem In Newer Public Health. *Journal of Mt. Sinai Hospital.* 1953;2:134.
12. Page I, Stare F, Corcoran A, Pollack H, Wilkinson C. Atherosclerosis and the fat content of the diet. *Circulation.* 1957;16(2):163–178.
13. Page I, Allen E, Chamberlain F, et al. Dietary Fat and Its Relation to Heart Attacks and Strokes. *Circulation.* 1961;23(1):133–136.
14. Time. Ancel Keys. 1961. Available at: http://content.time.com/time/covers/0,16641,19610113,00.html. Accessed November 10, 2016.
15. Keys A. The Seven Countries Study Publications. 2016. Available at: http://www.sevencountriesstudy.com/study-findings/publications/. Accessed November 10, 2016.
16. Sarri K, Kafatos A. Letter to the Editor: The Seven Countries Study in Crete: olive oil, Mediterranean diet or fasting? *Public Health Nutrition.* 2005;8(6):666.
17. Sarri K, Linardakis M, Bervanaki F, Tzanakis N, Kafatos A. Greek Orthodox fasting rituals: a hidden characteristic of the Mediterranean diet of Crete. *British Journal of Nutrition.* 2004;92(2):277–84.
18. Keys A, Aravanis C, Sdrin H. The diets of middle-aged men in two rural areas of Greece. *Voeding.* 1966;27:575–586. Available at: https://www.cabdirect.org/cabdirect/abstract/19671404963.
19. Menotti A, Kromhout D, Blackburn H, et al. Food intake patterns and 25-year mortality from coronary heart disease: cross-cultural correlations in the Seven Countries Study. The Seven Countries Study Research Group. *European Journal of Epidemiology.* 1999;15(6):507–15.
20. Torrens K. The truth about low-fat foods. *www.bbcgoodfood.com.* 2016. Available at: http://www.bbcgoodfood.com/howto/guide/truth-about-low-fat-foods. Accessed November 10, 2016.
21. Hyman M. The Fat Summit. In: ; 2016.
22. American Heart Association. The American Heart Association's Diet and Lifestyle Recommendations. 2016. Available at: http://www.heart.org/HEARTORG/HealthyLiving/Diet-and-Lifestyle-Recommendations_UCM_305855_Article.jsp#.V-UZkDf7blI. Accessed September 23, 2016.
23. Crisco. Crisco Our Heritage. *www.crisco.com.* 2016. Available at: http://www.crisco.com/our-heritage. Accessed November 10, 2016.

24. Blasbalg T, Hibbeln J, Ramsden C, Majchrzak S, Rawlings R. Changes in consumption of omega-3 and omega-6 fatty acids in the United States during the 20th century. *American Journal of Clinical Nutrition.* 2011;93(5):950–62. Available at: https://www.ncbi.nlm.nih.gov/pubmed/21367944.
25. United States Food and Drug Administration; Department of Health and Human Services. Final Determination Regarding Partially Hydrogenated Oils; Docket No. FDA-2013-N-1317. *Federal Register.* 2015;80(116):34650–34670. Available at: https://www.gpo.gov/fdsys/pkg/FR-2015-06-17/pdf/2015-14883.pdf.
26. Fryar C, Carroll M, Ogden C. *Prevalence of Overweight, Obesity, and Extreme Obesity Among Adults: United States, 1960-1962 Through 2011-2012. 2014.* Available at: https://www.cdc.gov/nchs/data/hestat/obesity_adult_11_12/obesity_adult_11_12.pdf.
27. Centers for Disease Control and Prevention. Heart Disease Fact Sheet. 2016. Available at: http://www.cdc.gov/dhdsp/data_statistics/fact_sheets/fs_heart_disease.htm. Accessed November 11, 2016.
28. Schweikart L. *What Would The Founders Say?* New York: Penguin Group; 2011.
29. The Staff of the Select Committee on Nutrition and Human Needs United States Senate. *Dietary Goals for the United States.* Washington DC; 1977. Available at: http://zerodisease.com/archive/Dietary_Goals_For_The_United_States.pdf.
30. Burros M. In the Soda Pop Society-Can the American Diet Change for the Better? *Washington Post.* 1978:E1.
31. United States Congress. National Nutrition Monitoring and Related Research Act of 1990 (Public Law 101-445 - Oct. 22, 1990). 1990. Available at: https://www.gpo.gov/fdsys/pkg/STATUTE-104/pdf/STATUTE-104-Pg1034.pdf. Accessed September 22, 2016.
32. American Heart Association. The American Heart Association's Diet and Lifestyle Recommendations. *www.heart.org.* 2016. Accessed November 10, 2016.
33. Horowitz R. *Putting Meat on the American Table.* Baltimore: Johns Hopkins University Press; 2000:11–17.
34. Daniel C, Cross A, Koebnick C, Sinha R. Trends in meat consumption in the United States. *Public Health Nutrition.* 2011;14(4):575–583. Available at: https://www.ncbi.nlm.nih.gov/pmc/articles/PMC3045642/pdf/nihms-253312.pdf.
35. Wiest E. The Butter Industry In The United States: An Economic Study of Butter and Oleomargarine. In: The Faculty of Political Science of Columbia University, ed. *Studies in History, Economics and Public Law.* New York; 1916:202.
36. Ogden C, Carroll M, Fryar C, Flegal K. *Prevalence of Obesity Among Adults and Youth: United States, 2011-2014; No. 219.* Hyattsville; 2015. Available at: https://www.cdc.gov/nchs/data/databriefs/db219.pdf.
37. Centers for Disease Control and Prevention. Heart Disease Facts. *www.cdc.gov.* 2015. Available at: http://www.cdc.gov/heartdisease/facts.htm. Accessed September 23, 2016.
38. Grynbaum M. New York's Ban on Big Sodas Is Rejected by Final Court. *The New Tork Times.* 2014.
39. Sahadi J, Smith A. Philadelphia passes a soda tax. *www.money.cnn.com.* 2016. Available at: http://money.cnn.com/2016/06/16/pf/taxes/philadelphia-passes-a-soda-tax/.
40. Bjerga A, Bloomfield D. Tax on Sugary Foods Proposed by U.S. Panel to Fight Obesity. *Bloomberg.* 2015. Available at: http://www.bloomberg.com/news/articles/2015-02-19/tax-on-sugary-foods-proposed-by-u-s-panel-to-help-fight-obesity. Accessed September 23, 2016.
41. Lee B. 5 More Locations Pass Soda Taxes: What's Next for Big Soda? *www.forbes.com.* 2016.
42. Weiner J. Larry Summers: It's time to tax carbon and treats. *Washington Post.* 2012. Available at: https://www.washingtonpost.com/blogs/she-the-people/wp/2012/11/23/larry-summers-its-time-to-tax-carbon-and-treats/.

Throw Out Artificial Sweeteners

1. Smith JM. *Seeds of Deception: Exposing Industry and Government Lies About the Safety of the Genetically Engineered Foods You're Eating.* Fairfield, IA: Yes Books; 2003.
2. Walton RG. *Survey of Aspartame Studies: Correlation of Outcomes and Funding sources.* 1998.
3. Graff G, Cullen S, Bradford K, Zilberman D, Bennett A. The public-private structure of intellectual property ownership in agricultural biotechnology. *Nature Biotechnology.* 2003;21(9). Available at: http://are.berkeley.edu/~zilber11/papers/publicprivate.pdf.
4. Suurkula J. Dysfunctional science: Towards a "pseudoscientific world order?" *Physicians and Scientists for Responsible Application of Science and Technology.* 2000.
5. Guyenet, Stephan. "By 2606, the US Diet will be 100 Percent Sugar." Whole Health Source: Nutrition and Health Science; February 18, 2012. Available at: https://wholehealthsource.blogspot.com/2012/02/by-2606-us-diet-will-be-100-percent.html
6. University of California San Francisco. "How Much Is Too Much? The growing concern over too much added sugar in our diets." Sugar Science: The Unsweetened Truth. Available at: http://sugarscience.ucsf.edu/the-growing-concern-of-overconsumption.html#.XebenNV7mUm
7. Young, Kelly. "Artificial Sweeteners Not Tied to Lower BMI and May Even Increase It." NEJM Journal Watch. July 17, 2017. Available at: https://www.jwatch.org/fw113100/2017/07/17/artificial-sweeteners-not-tied-lower-bmi-and-may-even?query=pfwRSTOC&jwd=000020054348&jspc=
8. Jennifer A. Nettleton, et al. "Diet Soda Intake and Risk of Incident Metabolic Syndrome and Type 2 Diabetes in the Multi-Ethnic Study of Atherosclerosis (MESA)." Diabetes Care 2009 Apr; 32(4): 688-694. https://doi.org/10.2337/dc08-1799
9. Soffritti M, Padovani M, Tibaldi E, Falcioni L, Manservisi F, Belpoggi F. "The carcinogenic effects of aspartame: The urgent need for regulatory re-evaluation." *Am J Ind Med.* 2014 Apr;57(4):383-97. doi: 10.1002/ajim.22296.

Get To Know Fake Meat

1. Impossible Foods. "Impossible Foods Receives No-Questions Letter From US Food and Drug Administration." July 23, 2018. Available at: https://impossiblefoods.com/announcements/fda-no-questions-letter/
2. FDA US Food & Drug Administration: Center For Food Safety & Applied Nutrition. "Re: GRAS Notice No. GRN 000737." Available at: https://res.cloudinary.com/dlvhhibcv/image/upload/Documents/2018-07-23_GRN_737_Response_Letter.pdf
3. Impossible Foods. "Why Does the Package Have a 'Bioengineered' Symbol?" Available at: https://faq.impossiblefoods.com/hc/en-us/articles/360036138833-Why-does-the-package-have-a-bioengineered-symbol-

4. GMO Free USA. "Reports of Impossible Burger Health Reactions Lead to National Health Survey." September 30, 2019. Available at: https://www.csrwire.com/press_releases/42725-Reports-of-Impossible-Burger-Health-Reactions-Lead-to-National-Health-Survey?fbclid=IwAR3-FjsnF3Wgtg5MeFdQ0Lh2ct-djrrRORyyT4iMHnCpTFDVENPyyAhNLqc
5. Impossible Burger. "What are the ingredients?" Available at: https://faq.impossiblefoods.com/hc/en-us/articles/360018937494-What-are-the-ingredients-
6. Zinöcker, Marit K, and Inge A Lindseth. "The Western Diet-Microbiome-Host Interaction and Its Role in Metabolic Disease." *Nutrients* vol. 10,3 365. 17 Mar. 2018, doi:10.3390/nu10030365

Hydrate Your Cells

1. Cowan, Thomas. "New Biology of Water." The Body Electric Summit.
2. Gratrix, Nikki. "Resolving Trauma with Bioenergetics." The Body Electric Summit.
3. Cowan, Thomas. "Cancer and the New Biology of Water." Chelsea Green Publishing, 2019.
4. Pollack, Gerald. "The Fourth Phase of Water: Beyond Solid, Liquid and Vapor." Ebner and Sons Publishers, 2013 (http:// www.ebnerandsons.com)
5. Pollack, Gerald. "Cells, Gels and the Engines of Life." Ebner and Sons Publishers, 2001.
6. Batmanghelidj, F. "You're Not Sick, You're Thirsty: Water for Health, for Healing, for Life. Warner Books, 2003.
7. Pollack, GH: Is the cell a gel—and why does it matter? Invited review, Japanese Journal of Physiology. 51(6):649-60, 2001.
8. Loudon, Irvine. "A brief history of homeopathy." *Journal of the Royal Society of Medicine* vol. 99,12 (2006): 607-10. doi:10.1258/jrsm.99.12.607

Say Yes to rBGH-free Milk Products

1. Epstein S. Unlabeled milk from cows treated with biosynthetic growth hormones: a case of regulatory abdication. *International Journal of Health Services*. 1996;261:173–185.
2. Renehan AG, Painter JE, O'Halloran D, et al. Circulating insulin-like growth factor II and colorectal adenomas. *J Clin Endocrinol Metab.* 2000;85(9):3402–3408.
3. Rinaldi S, Cleveland R, Norat T, et al. Serum levels of IGF-I, IGFBP-3 and colorectal cancer risk: Results from the EPIC cohort, plus a meta-analysis of prospective studies. *International Journal of Cancer.* 2010;126(7):1702–1715.
4. Epstein S. Role of the insulin-like growth factors in cancer development and progression. *Journal of the National Cancer Institute.* 2001;93(3):238.
5. Yu, H; Rohan T. Role of the insulin-like growth factor family in cancer development and progression. *Journal of the National Cancer Institute.* 2000;92:1472–1484.
6. Toniolo P et al. Serum insulin-like growth factor-1 and breast cancer. *International Journal of Cancer.* 2000;88(5):828–832.
7. Agurs-Collins T et al. Insulin-like growth factor-1 and breast cancer risk in post-menopausal American women. *Proceedings of the American Association of Cancer Research 40.* 1999:152.
8. Badr M, Hassan T, Tarhony S, Metwally W. Insulin-like growth factor-1 and childhood cancer risk. *Oncol Lett.* 2010;1(6):1055–1059. Available at: http://www.ncbi.nlm.nih.gov/pmc/articles/PMC3412533/.
9. Ross J, Perentesis J, Robison L, Davies S. Big babies and infant leukemia: a role for insulin-like growth factor-1? *Cancer Causes Control.* 1996;7(5):553–559.
10. Gucciardi A. Banned in 27 Countries, Monsanto's RBGH Inhabits Many U.S. Dairy Products. *NaturalSociety.com.* 2011.
11. USDA. Dairy 2007 Part I: Reference of Dairy Cattle Health and Management Practices in the United States, 2007. *Veterinary Services, Animal and Plant Health Inspection Services, U.S. Department of Agriculture.* 2007:79.
12. GAO. *Recombinant Bovine Growth Hormone: FDA Approval Should Be Withheld Until the Mastitis Issue is Resolved.* 1992:68.
13. Chopra S et al. *rBST (Nutrilac) "GAPS Analysis" Report.* Ottawa; 1998.
14. United States Department of Agriculture NASS. Livestock Slaughter. *www.usda.gov.* 2016.
15. Provincial Health Officer's Annual Report. *Food, Health and Well-Being in British Columbia.* British Columbia Ministry of Health Office of the Provincial Health Officer; 2005.
16. Hallberg M. Historical Perspective on Adjustment in the Food and Agricultural Sector. *Penn State University.* 2003.
17. Epstein, Samuel MD. *What's In Your Milk? An Expose of Industry and Government Cover-Up on the DANGERS of the Genetically Engineered (rBGH) Milk You're Drinking.* Victoria: Trafford Publishing; 2006.
18. Dohoo IR, DesCôteaux L, Leslie K, et al. A meta-analysis review of the effects of recombinant bovine somatotropin. 2. Effects on animal health, reproductive performance, and culling. *Canadian journal of veterinary research = Revue canadienne de recherche vétérinaire.* 2003;67(4):252–64.
19. Cohen R. *Milk: The Deadly Poison.* First. Englewood Cliffs, NJ: Argus Publishing; 1998.
20. Cohen R. PUS Expose: Your State's Average Pus Count. *notmilk.com*. Available at: http://www.notmilk.com/lawbreakers.html. Accessed May 7, 2015.
21. U.S. Department of Health and Human Services, Public Health Service F and DA. Grade "A" Pasteurized Milk Ordinance. *www.fda.gov.* 2009. Available at: http://www.fda.gov/downloads/Food/GuidanceRegulation/UCM209789.pdf.
22. Hudson W. CDC: "Nightmare bacteria" spreading. *CNN.com.* 2013. Available at: http://www.cnn.com/2013/03/06/health/super-bug-bacteria-spreading/.
23. Bittman M. *A Bone to Pick: The good and bad news about food, with wisdom and advice on diets, food safety, GMOs, farming and more.* New York: Pam Krauss Books; 2015.
24. Murphy R. *GAO Report regarding alleged conflicts of interest in FDA.* Washington DC\; 1994.
25. FDA. *Consumer Report.* 1988.
26. Hardin P. Personal Communication. 2016.

27. Waters A, Contente-Cuomo T, Jordan B, et al. Multidrug-Resistant Staphylococcus aureus in US Meat and Poultry. *Clin Infect Dis.* 2011;52(10):1227–1230.
28. Kusserow RP. *Audit of Issues Related to the Food and Drug Administration Review of Bovine Somatotropin (A-15-90-00046).* 1992:23.
29. FDA. *Report on the Food and Drug Administration's Review of the Safety of Recombinant Bovine Somatotropin.* 1999.
30. Cohen R. Personal Communication. *Phone Interview*. 2016.
31. Taylor M. Interim Guidance on the Voluntary Labeling of Milk and Milk Products From Cows That Have Not Been Treated With Recombinant Bovine Somatotropin. *Federal Register.* 1994;59(28). Available at: http://www.gpo.gov/fdsys/pkg/FR-1994-02-10/html/94-3214.htm.
32. Cohen R. Robert Cohen testimony before FDA panel. Available at: http://www.ecoglobe.org/nz/news1999/d049news.htm.
33. Epstein, Samuel and Hardin P. Confidential Monsanto Research Files Dispute Many bGH Safety Claims. *The Milkweed.* 1990.
34. Epstein, Samuel and Hardin P. Epstein & Hardin Respond. *The Milkweed.* 1990.

Be Informed At Restaurants

1. Refer to References in "Eat What You Can Pronounce."
2. Centers for Disease Control and Prevention. "Fast Food Consumption Among Adults in the United States, 2013-2016." October 2018. Available at: https://www.cdc.gov/nchs/products/databriefs/db322.htm

Look For The Duo

1. Refer to References in "Harness Your Power."
2. Johal GS, Huber DM. Glyphosate effects on diseases of plants. *European Journal of Agronomy*. 2009;31(3):144–152.
3. Bøhn T, Cuhra M, Traavik T, et al. Compositional differences in soybeans on the market: Glyphosate accumulates in Roundup Ready GM soybeans. *Food Chemistry.* 2014;153:207–215.
4. Lundberg DS, Lebeis SL, Paredes SH, et al. Defining the core Arabidopsis thaliana root microbiome. *Nature*. 2012;488:86–90.
5. Kremer RJ, Means NE. Glyphosate and glyphosate-resistant crop interactions with rhizosphere microorganisms. *European Journal of Agronomy.* 2009;31(3):153–161.
6. Lappe M, Bailey B, Childress C, Setchell K. Alterations in Clinically Important Phytoestrogens in Genetically Modified, Herbicide-Tolerant Soybeans. *Journal of Medicinal Food.* 2009;1(4):241–245.
7. Lissin L, Cooke J. Phytoestrogens and cardiovascular health. *J Am Coll Cardiol.* 2000;35(6):1403–1410. Available at: http://www.ncbi.nlm.nih.gov/pubmed/10807439.
8. Benbrook CM. Impacts of genetically engineered crops on pesticide use in the U.S. -- the first sixteen years. *Environmental Sciences Europe.* 2012;24(1):1–13. Available at: http://dx.doi.org/10.1186/2190-4715-24-24.
9. Beville R. How Pervasive are GMOs in Animal Feed? *GMOinside.org.* 2013. Available at: http://gmoinside.org/gmos-in-animal-feed/. Accessed November 7, 2016.
10. United States Department of Agriculture ERS. Corn: Background. *www.ers.usda.gov*. 2016. Available at: https://www.ers.usda.gov/topics/crops/corn/background/. Accessed December 17, 2016.
11. Andhra P. *Mortality in Sheep Flocks after grazing on Bt Cotton fields Warangal District, Andhra Pradesh.* Warangal District; 2006. Available at: http://gmwatch.org/latest-listing/1-news-items/6416-mortality-in-sheep-flocks-after-grazing-on-bt-cotton-fields-warangal-district-andhra-pradesh-2942006.
12. Ho M-W. GM Ban Long Overdue. *ISIS Report.* 2006. Available at: http://www.i-sis.org.uk/GMBanLongOverdue.php. Accessed September 19, 2016.
13. Vecchio L, Cisterna B, Malatesta M, Martin T, Biggiogera M. Ultrastructural analysis of testes from mice fed on genetically modified soybean. *Eur J Histochem.* 2004;48(4):448–54.
14. Al. O et. Temporary Depression of Transcription in Mouse Pre-implantation Embryos from Mice Fed on Genetically Modified Soybeans. In: *48th Symposium of the Society for Histochemistry.* Lake Maggiore (Italy); 2006.
15. Velimirov A, Binter C. Biological effects of transgenic maize NK603 x MON810 fed in long term reproduction studies in mice. In: *Forschungsberichte der Sektion IV.*; 2008.
16. Ermakova I. Experimental Evidence of GMO Hazards. In: *Scientists for a FM Free Europe, EU Parliament.* Brussels; 2007.
17. Ermakova I. Genetically modified organisms and biological risks. In: *Proceedings of International Disaster Reduction Conferences (IDRC).* Davos, Switzerland; 2006:168–172.
18. Ermakova I. GMO: Life itself intervened into the experiments. *Letter, EcosInform.* 2006;N2:3–4.
19. Ermakova I. Influence of genetically modified soya on the birth-weight and survival of rat pups. In: *Epigenetics, Transgenic Plants & Risk Assessment.*; 2013. Available at: http://somloquesembrem.org/wp-content/uploads/2013/01/Ermakovasoja.pdf.
20. Malatesta M, Boraldi F, Annovi G, et al. A long-term study on female mice fed on a genetically modified soybean: effects on liver ageing. *Histochem Cell Biol.* 2008;130(5):967–77.
21. Pusztai A. Can science give us the tools for recognizing possible health risks of GM food? *Nutr Health.* 2002;16(2):73–84.
22. Lemen J, Hammond B, Riordan S, Jiang C, Nemeth M. *Summary of Study CV-2000-260: 13-Week Dietary Subchronic Comparison Study with MON 863 Corn in Rats Preceded by a 1-Week Baseline Food Consumption Determination with PMI Certified Rodent Diet #5002; Report No. MSL-18175.* St. Louis; 2002.
23. Tudisco R, Lombardi P, Bovera F, D'Angelo D. Genetically modified soya bean in rabbit feeding: detection of DNA fragments and evaluation of metabolic effects by enzymatic analysis. *Animal Science.* 2006;82(2):193–199.
24. Malatesta M, Caporaioni C, Gavaudan S, et al. Ultrastructural morphometrical and immunocytochemical analyses of hepatocyte nuclei from mice fed on genetically modified soybean. *Cell Struct Funct*. 2002;27(4):173–80.
25. Malatesta M, Biggiogera M, Manuali E, et al. Fine structural analyses of pancreatic acinar cell nuclei from mice fed on genetically modified soybean. *Eur J Histochem.* 2003;47(4):385–8.

26. Malatesta M, Caporaioni C, Rossi L, et al. Ultrastructural analysis of pancreatic acinar cells from mice fed on genetically modified soybean. *J Anat.* 2002;201(5):409–415.
27. Finamore A, Roselli M, Britti S, et al. Intestinal and peripheral immune response to MON810 maize ingestion in weaning and old mice. *J Agric Food Chem.* 2008;56(23):11533–9. Available at: http://www.ncbi.nlm.nih.gov/pubmed/19007233.
28. Fares N, El-Sayed A. Fine structural changes in the ileum of mice fed on delta-endotoxin-treated potatoes and transgenic potatoes. *Nat Toxins.* 1998;6(6):219–33.
29. SW E, Pusztai A. Effect of diets containing genetically modified potatoes expressing Galanthus nivalis lectin on rat small intestine. *Lancet.* 1999;354(9187):1353–4.
30. Vazquez-Padron R, Moreno-Fierros L, Neri-Bazan L, et al. Characterization of the mucosal and systemic immune response induced by Cry1Ac protein from Bacillus thuringiensis HD 73 in mice. *Braz J Med Biol Res.* 2000;33(2):147–55.
31. Vazquez-Padron R, Moreno-Fierros L, Neri-Bazan L, de-la Riva G, Lopez-Revilla R. Bacillus thuringiensis Cry1Ac protoxin is a potent systemic and mucosal adjuvant. *Scand J Immunol.* 1999;49(6):578–84.
32. Kroghsbo S, Madsen C, Poulsen M, et al. Immunotoxicological studies of genetically modified rice expressing PHA-E lectin or Bt toxin in Wistar rats. *Toxicology.* 2008;245(1-2):24–34.
33. Dean A, Armstrong J. Genetically Modified Foods. *www.aaemonline.org.* 2009. Available at: http://www.aaemonline.org/gmo.php. Accessed September 15, 2016.
34. Smith JM. *Seeds of Deception: Exposing Industry and Government Lies About the Safety of the Genetically Engineered Foods You're Eating.* Fairfield, IA: Yes Books; 2003.
35. Samsel A, Seneff S. Glyphosate's Suppression of Cytochrome P450 Enzymes and Amino Acid Biosynthesis by the Gut Microbiome: Pathways to Modern Diseases. *Entropy.* 2013;15(4):1416–1463. Available at: http://www.mdpi.com/1099-4300/15/4/1416.
36. Thongprakaisang S, Thiantanawat A, Rangkadilok N, Suriyo T, Satayavivad J. Glyphosate induces human breast cancer cells growth via estrogen receptors. *Food Chem. Toxicol.* 2013;59:129–36. Available at: http://www.ncbi.nlm.nih.gov/pubmed/23756170.
37. Benachour N, Séralini GE. Glyphosate formulations induce apoptosis and necrosis in human umbilical, embryonic, and placental cells. *Chemical Research in Toxicology.* 2009;22(1):97–105.
38. International Agency for Research on Cancer. *IARC Monographs Volume 112: evaluation of five organophosphate insecticides and herbicides.* 2015:2. Available at: http://www.iarc.fr/en/media-centre/iarcnews/pdf/MonographVolume112.pdf.
39. Yum H-Y, Lee S-Y, Lee K-E, Sohn M-H, Kim K-E. Genetically modified and wild soybeans: An immunologic comparison. *Allergy and Asthma Proceedings.* 2005;26(3):210–216(7). Available at: http://www.ingentaconnect.com/content/ocean/aap/2005/00000026/00000003/art00010.
40. Nordlee J, Taylor S, Townsend J, Thomas L, Bush R. Identification of a Brazil-Nut Allergen in Transgenic Soybeans. *The New Englad Journal of Medicine.* 1996;334:688–692. Available at: http://www.nejm.org/doi/full/10.1056/NEJM199603143341103#t=article.
41. Hardell, L and Erickson M. A Case-Controlled Study of non-Hodgkin's Lymphoma and Exposure to Pesticides. *Cancer.* 1999;86(6).
42. Fernandez-Cornejo J, Nehring R, Osteen C, et al. *Pesticide Use in U.S. Agriculture: 21 Selected Crops, 1960-2008.* Washington DC; 2014. Available at: https://www.ers.usda.gov/webdocs/publications/eib124/46734_eib124.pdf.
43. Goldburg R. FDA public hearing on genetically engineered foods.
44. Blewett TC. *Comments on behalf of Dow AgroSciences LLC on Supplemental information for petition for determination of nonregulated status for herbicide resistant DAS-40278-9 Corn. Economic and agronomic impacts of the introduction of DAS-40278-9 corn on glyphosate res.* 2011.
45. Neuman W, Pollack A. Farmers Cope With Roundup-Resistant Weeds. *The New York Times.* 2010. Available at: http://www.nytimes.com/2010/05/04/business/energy-environment/04weed.html?pagewanted=all&_r=0.
46. Rosenboro K. Why Is Glyphosate Sprayed on Crops Right Before Harvest? *Ecowatch.com.* 2016. Available at: http://www.ecowatch.com/why-is-glyphosate-sprayed-on-crops-right-before-harvest-1882187755.html.
47. Main D. Glypohsate Now the Most-Used Agricultural Chemical Ever. *www.newsweek.com.* 2016. Available at: http://www.newsweek.com/glyphosate-now-most-used-agricultural-chemical-ever-422419.
48. Deike J. Monsanto's Roundup Found in 75% of Air and Rain Samples. *www.ecowatch.com.* 2014. Available at: http://www.ecowatch.com/monsantos-roundup-found-in-75-of-air-and-rain-samples-1881869607.html. Accessed September 16, 2015.
49. Clair E, Mesnage R, Travert C, Séralini G-É. A glyphosate-based herbicide induces necrosis and apoptosis in mature rat testicular cells in vitro, and testosterone decrease at lower levels. *Toxicology in vitro : an international journal published in association with BIBRA.* 2012;26(2):269–79.
50. Vecchio L, Cisterna B, Malatesta M, Martin T, Biggiogera M. Ultrastructural analysis of testes from mice fed on genetically modified soybean. *European Journal of Histochemistry.* 2004.
51. Earth Open Source. Truth: So-called "safe" levels of Roundup may not be safe after all. *www.earthopensource.org.* 2015. Available at: http://earthopensource.org/gmomythsandtruths/sample-page/4-health-hazards-roundup-glyphosate/4-2-myth-strict-regulations-ensure-exposed-safe-levels-roundup/. Accessed September 18, 2016.
52. Bohn T, Cuhra M. How "Extreme Levels" of Roundup in Food Became the Industry Norm. *www.independentsciencenews.org.* 2014. Available at: https://www.independentsciencenews.org/news/how-extreme-levels-of-roundup-in-food-became-the-industry-norm/.
53. Leu A. Monsanto's Toxic Herbicide Glyphosate: A Review of its Health and Environmental Effects. *www.organicconsumers.org.* 2007. Available at: https://www.organicconsumers.org/news/monsantos-toxic-herbicide-glyphosate-review-its-health-and-environmental-effects.
54. The Detox Project. UCSF Presentation Reveals Glyphosate Contamination in People across America. *www.detoxproject.org.* 2016.
55. Aris A, Leblanc S. Maternal and fetal exposure to pesticides associated to genetically modified foods in Eastern Townships of Quebec, Canada. *Reproductive Toxicology.* 2011;31(4):528–33.
56. Shilhavy B. ALERT: Certified Organic Food Grown in U.S. Found Contaminated with Glyphosate Herbicide. *Health Impact News.* 2014. Available at: http://healthimpactnews.com/2014/alert-certified-organic-food-grown-in-u-s-found-contaminated-with-glyphosate-herbicide/. Accessed November 7, 2016.

57. Linda K. *Comments about the Federal Register document "Statement of Policy: Foods from Genetically Modified Plants."* 1992. Available at: www.biointegrity.org.
58. The Lancet. Health risks of genetically modified foods. *The Lancet.* 1999;353(9167):1811. Available at: http://www.thelancet.com/pdfs/journals/lancet/PIIS0140-6736(99)00093-8.pdf.
59. The Royal Society of Canada. *Elements of Precaution: Recommendations for the Regulation of Food Biotechnology in Canada.* Ottawa; 2001. Available at: http://www.rsc.ca/sites/default/files/pdf/GMreportEN.pdf.
60. Kmietowicz Z. GM foods should be submitted to further studies, says BMA. *British Medical Journal.* 2004;328(7440):602. Available at: https://www.ncbi.nlm.nih.gov/pmc/articles/PMC381159/.
61. Anon. *Public Health Association of Australia: Policy-at-a-glance - Genetically Modified Foods Policy.* Available at: http://www.phaa.net.au/documents/item/235.
62. Dona A, Arvanitoyannis I. Health risks of genetically modified foods. *Critical Reviews in Food Science and Nutrition.* 2009;49(2):164–75. Available at: https://www.ncbi.nlm.nih.gov/pubmed/18989835.
63. Hilbeck A et al. No scientific consensus of GMO safety. *Environmental Sciences Europe.* 2015;27(4).
64. Consumer Reports. Consumers Want Mandatory Labeling for GMOFoods. *www.consumerreports.org.* 2015. Available at: http://www.consumerreports.org/food-safety/consumers-want-mandatory-labeling-for-gmo-foods/. Accessed November 9, 2016.
65. Just Label It! Labeling Around The World. *www.justlabelit.org.* 2016. Available at: http://www.justlabelit.org/right-to-know-center/labeling-around-the-world/. Accessed November 9, 2016.
66. The Institute for Responsible Technology. Even though Obama just signed the DARK Act... *www.responsibletechnology.org.* 2016. Available at: http://responsibletechnology.org/even-though-obama-just-signed-the-dark-act/. Accessed September 18, 2016.
67. U.S. Food and Drug Administration. FDA Has Determined That the AquAdvantage Salmon is as Safe to Eat as Non-GE Salmon. *www.fda.gov.* 2015. Available at: http://www.fda.gov/ForConsumers/ConsumerUpdates/ucm472487.htm. Accessed September 15, 2016.
68. United States Department of Agriculture; Animal and Plant Health Inspection Service. Petitions for Determination of Nonregulated Status. *www.aphis.usda.gov.* 2016. Available at: https://www.aphis.usda.gov/aphis/ourfocus/biotechnology/permits-notifications-petitions/petitions/petition-status. Accessed December 31, 2016.
69. Malatesta M, Tiberi C, Baldelli B, et al. Reversibility of hepatocyte nuclear modifications in mice fed on genetically modified soybean. *European Journal of Histochemistry.* 2005;49(3):237–242. Available at: http://www.ncbi.nlm.nih.gov/pubmed/16216809.
70. Ross, Anne et al. "The Turkish Infiltration of the U.S. Organic Grain Market: How Failed Enforcement and Ineffective Regulations Made the U.S. Ripe for Fraud and Organized Crime" Cornucopia Institute; 2018. Available at: https://www.cornucopia.org/wp-content/uploads/2018/06/Turkish-Infiltration-Organic-Grain-Imports.pdf

Look For The Trio

1. See References in "Look For The Duo."
2. Caiati C, Pollice P, Favale S, Lepera ME. "The Herbicide Glyphosate and Its Apparently Controversial Effect on Human Health: An Updated Clinical Perspective." *Endocr Metab Immune Disord Drug Targets.* 2019 Oct 15. doi: 10.2174/1871530319666191015191614.
3. Duforestel M, Nadaradjane A, Bougras-Cartron G, Briand J, Olivier C, Frenel JS, Vallette FM, Lelièvre SA, Cartron PF. Glyphosate Primes Mammary Cells for Tumorigenesis by Reprogramming the Epigenome in a TET3-Dependent Manner. Front Genet. 2019 Sep 27;10:885. doi: 10.3389/fgene.2019.00885.
4. Parks CG, Hoppin JA, De Roos AJ, Costenbader KH, Alavanja MC, Sandler DP. Rheumatoid Arthritis in Agricultural Health Study Spouses: Associations with Pesticides and Other Farm Exposures. Environ Health Perspect. 2016 Nov;124(11):1728-1734.
5. Vainio H. Public health and evidence-informed policy-making: The case of a commonly used herbicide. Scand J Work Environ Health. 2019 Sep 5. pii: 3851. doi:10.5271/sjweh.3851.
6. Richardson JR, Fitsanakis V, Westerink RHS, Kanthasamy AG. Neurotoxicity of pesticides. Acta Neuropathol. 2019 Sep;138(3):343-362. doi:10.1007/s00401-019-02033-9. Epub 2019 Jun 13. Review.
7. Eriguchi M, Iida K, Ikeda S, Osoegawa M, Nishioka K, Hattori N, Nagayama H, Hara H. Parkinsonism Relating to Intoxication with Glyphosate. Intern Med. 2019 Jul 1;58(13):1935-1938. doi: 10.2169/internalmedicine.2028-18.
8. Samsel, Anthony & Seneff, Stephanie. (2013). "Glyphosate's Suppression of Cytochrome P450 Enzymes and Amino Acid Biosynthesis by the Gut Microbiome: Pathways to Modern Diseases." *Entropy.* 15. 1416-1463. 10.3390/e15041416.
9. Richard, Dawn M et al. "L-Tryptophan: Basic Metabolic Functions, Behavioral Research and Therapeutic Indications." *International journal of tryptophan research: IJTR* vol. 2 (2009): 45-60. doi:10.4137/ijtr.s2129
10. Hardeland, Rüdiger. "Melatonin metabolism in the central nervous system." *Current neuropharmacology* vol. 8,3 (2010): 168-81. doi:10.2174/157015910792246244
11. Triarhou, Lazaros C. "Dopamine and Parkinson's Disease." Madame Curie Bioscience Database. Available at: https://www.ncbi.nlm.nih.gov/books/NBK6271/
12. Gillam, Carey. "USDA Quietly Drops Plan to Test for Monsanto's Glyphosate Weed Killer in Food." Alter Net; March 27, 2017. Available at: https://www.alternet.org/2017/03/usda-quietly-drops-plan-test-monsantos-glyphosate-weed-killer-food/
13. Seneff, Stephanie & Swanson, Nancy & Li, Chen. (2015). "Aluminum and Glyphosate Can Synergistically Induce Pineal Gland Pathology: Connection to Gut Dysbiosis and Neurological Disease." *Agricultural Sciences.* 06. 42-70. 10.4236/as.2015.61005.
14. Garry, Vincent F et al. "Birth defects, season of conception, and sex of children born to pesticide applicators living in the Red River Valley of Minnesota, USA." *Environmental health perspectives* vol. 110 Suppl 3,Suppl 3 (2002): 441-9. doi:10.1289/ehp.02110s3441
15. Marc J, Mulner-Lorillon O, Bellé R. "Glyphosate-based pesticides affect cell cycle regulation." *Biol Cell.* 2004 Apr;96(3):245-9. PubMed PMID: 15182708.
16. Gasnier C, Dumont C, Benachour N, Clair E, Chagnon MC, Séralini GE. "Glyphosate-based herbicides are toxic and endocrine disruptors in human cell lines." *Toxicology.* 2009 Aug 21;262(3):184-91.
17. Koller VJ, Fürhacker M, Nersesyan A, Mišík M, Eisenbauer M, Knasmueller S. "Cytotoxic and DNA-damaging properties of glyphosate and Roundup in human-derived buccal epithelial cells." *Arch Toxicol.* 2012 May;86(5):805-13.

18. Richard, Sophie et al. "Differential effects of glyphosate and roundup on human placental cells and aromatase." *Environmental health perspectives* vol. 113,6 (2005): 716-20. doi:10.1289/ehp.7728
19. Mesnage, R, et al. "Ethoxylated adjuvants of glyphosate-based herbicides are active principles of human cell toxicity." *Toxicology* vol. 313, 2-3 (2013): 122-128
20. Arbuckle, T E et al. "An exploratory analysis of the effect of pesticide exposure on the risk of spontaneous abortion in an Ontario farm population." *Environmental health perspectives* vol. 109,8 (2001): 851-7. doi:10.1289/ehp.01109851
21. de Cock M, Maas YG, van de Bor M. "Does perinatal exposure to endocrine disruptors induce autism spectrum and attention deficit hyperactivity disorders? Review." *Acta Paediatr.* 2012 Aug;101(8):811-8.
22. Shelton, Janie F et al. "Tipping the balance of autism risk: potential mechanisms linking pesticides and autism." *Environmental health perspectives* vol. 120,7 (2012): 944-51. doi:10.1289/ehp.1104553
23. Ewen SW, Pusztai A. "Effect of diets containing genetically modified potatoes expressing Galanthus nivalis lectin on rat small intestine." *Lancet.* 1999 Oct 16;354(9187):1353-4.
24. Samsel, A.; Seneff, S. "Glyphosate's Suppression of Cytochrome P450 Enzymes and Amino Acid Biosynthesis by the Gut Microbiome: Pathways to Modern Diseases." *Entropy* **2013**, 15, 1416-1463.
25. Swanson, N.L. "Genetically Modified Organisms and the deterioration of health in the United States. *Examiner.com* Available at: https://sustainablepulse.com/wp-content/uploads/GMO-health-1.pdf
26. FDA. "Statement of Policy – Foods Derived from New Plant Varieties." FDA Federal Register Volume 57 – 1992 Friday, May 29, 1992. Available at: https://www.fda.gov/regulatory-information/search-fda-guidance-documents/statement-policy-foods-derived-new-plant-varieties
27. Zinöcker, Marit K, and Inge A Lindseth. "The Western Diet-Microbiome-Host Interaction and Its Role in Metabolic Disease." *Nutrients* vol. 10,3 365. 17 Mar. 2018, doi:10.3390/nu10030365
28. U.S. Food and Drug Administration. "Pesticide Residue Monitoring Program Fiscal Year 2017 Pesticide Report. Available at: https://www.fda.gov/media/130291/download
29. U.S. Government Accountability Office. "Food Safety: FDA and USDA Should Strengthen Pesticide Residue Monitoring Programs and Further Disclose Monitoring Limitations" October 7, 2014. Available at: https://www.gao.gov/products/GAO-15-38
30. Environmental Working Group. "Breakfast with a Dose of Roundup?" August 15, 2018. Available at: https://www.ewg.org/childrenshealth/glyphosateincereal/
31. Cook, Kara. "Glyphosate in Beer and Wine." CALPIRG Education Fund. February 2019. Available at: https://uspirg.org/sites/pirg/files/reports/WEB_CAP_Glyphosate-pesticide-beer-and-wine_REPORT_022619.pdf

Look For The Quartet

1. Refer to References in "Look For The 100% USDA Organic Label."

Eat Real Salt

1. Mercola, Joseph. "The 13 Amazing Health Benefits of Himalayan Crystal Salt, the Purest Salt on Earth." Available at: https://products.mercola.com/himalayan-salt/
2. Harrison, Claire. "Sea Salt vs. Table Salt – The Truth." Fooducate; August 12, 2011. Available at: https://www.fooducate.com/community/post/Sea-Salt-vs-Table-Salt-The-Truth/57A33CD8-A0A2-D80E-43BA-B11D7340BAA5
3. U.S. Food & Drug Administration. "Food Additive Status List." Available at: https://www.fda.gov/food/food-additives-petitions/food-additive-status-list#ftnS
4. Real Salt. "Real Salt® Elemental Analysis." Available at: http://realsalt.redmond.life/wp-content/uploads/sites/6/2017/05/Real-Salt-Analysis.pdf
5. Real Salt. "Read Salt FAQ." Available at: http://redmonddotlife.wpengine.com/pdfs/RealSalt_FAQ.pdf
6. Real Salt. "Is Your Salt Real?" Available at: http://redmonddotlife.wpengine.com/pdfs/IsYourSaltRealBooklet.pdf
7. U.S. Food and Drug Administration. "Lowering Salt in Your Diet." Available at: https://www.fda.gov/consumers/consumer-updates/lowering-salt-your-diet
8. U.S. Food and Drug Administration. "Code of Federal Regulations Title 21, Volume 2, Subchapter B, Part 100, Subpart G, Sec. 100.155 Salt and iodized salt." Available at: https://www.accessdata.fda.gov/scripts/cdrh/cfdocs/cfcfr/cfrsearch.cfm?fr=100.155

Say Yes To Wild-Caught Fish

1. Rodríguez-Hernández Á, et al. "Comparative study of the intake of toxic persistent and semi persistent pollutants through the consumption of fish and seafood from two modes of production (wild-caught and farmed)." *Sci Total Environ.* 2017 Jan 1;575:919-931.
2. Steckert LD, Furtado WE, Jerônimo GT, Pereira SA, Jesus GFA, Mouriño JLP, Martins ML. Trace elements and microbiological parameters in farmed Nile tilapia with emphasis on muscle, water, sediment and feed. J Environ Sci Health B. 2019;54(4):237-246.
3. Jiang H, Qin D, Mou Z, Zhao J, Tang S, Wu S, Gao L. Trace elements in farmed fish (Cyprinus carpio, Ctenopharyngodon idella and Oncorhynchus mykiss) from Beijing: implication from feed. Food Addit Contam Part B Surveill. 2016 Jun;9(2):132-41.
4. Tacon AG, Metian M. Aquaculture feed and food safety. Ann N Y Acad Sci. 2008 Oct;1140:50-9.
5. Mantovani A, Maranghi F, Purificato I, Macrì A. Assessment of feed additives and contaminants: an essential component of food safety. Ann Ist Super Sanita. 2006;42(4):427-32. Review.
6. Higuera-Llantén S, Vásquez-Ponce F, Barrientos-Espinoza B, Mardones FO, Marshall SH, Olivares-Pacheco J. Extended antibiotic treatment in salmon farms select multiresistant gut bacteria with a high prevalence of antibiotic resistance genes. PLoS One. 2018 Sep 11;13(9):e0203641.
7. Miranda CD, Godoy FA, Lee MR. Current Status of the Use of Antibiotics and the Antimicrobial Resistance in the Chilean Salmon Farms. Front Microbiol. 2018 Jun 18;9:1284.
8. Cárcamo JG, Aguilar MN, Carreño CF, Vera T, Arias-Darraz L, Figueroa JE, Romero AP, Alvarez M, Yañez AJ. Consecutive emamectin

benzoate and deltamethrin treatments affect the expressions and activities of detoxification enzymes in the rainbow trout (Oncorhynchus mykiss). Comp Biochem Physiol C Toxicol Pharmacol. 2017 Jan;191:129-137. doi: 10.1016/j.cbpc.2016.10.004.

9. Barisic J, Cannon S, Quinn B. Cumulative impact of anti-sea lice treatment (azamethiphos) on health status of Rainbow trout (Oncorhynchus mykiss, Walbaum 1792) in aquaculture. Sci Rep. 2019 Nov 7;9(1):16217.
10. Domingo JL, Bocio A. Levels of PCDD/PCDFs and PCBs in edible marine species and human intake: a literature review. Environ Int. 2007 Apr;33(3):397-405. Epub 2007 Jan 30. Review.
11. Nøstbakken OJ, et al. Contaminant levels in Norwegian farmed Atlantic salmon (Salmo salar) in the 13-year period from 1999 to 2011. Environ Int. 2015 Jan;74:274-80.
12. Montory M, et al. Polychlorinated biphenyls in farmed and wild Onchorhynchus kisutch and Onchorhynchus mykiss from the Chilean Patagonia. Environ Sci Pollut Res Int. 2011 May;18(4):629-37.
13. Environmental Working Group. "PCBS in Farmed Salmon: Test results show high levels of contamination." Available at: https://www.ewg.org/research/pcbs-farmed-salmon
14. Rodríguez-Hernández, Ángel et al. "Dietary Intake of Essential, Toxic, and Potentially Toxic Elements from Mussels *(Mytilus spp.)* in the Spanish Population: A Nutritional Assessment." *Nutrients* vol. 11,4 864. 17 Apr. 2019, doi:10.3390/nu11040864
15. Boyd, Claude et al. "Certification Issues for Some Common Aquaculture Species." *Reviews In Fisheries Science & Aquaculture;* Volume 13 (4); 2007. https://doi.org/10.1080/10641260500326867
16. Schlag, Anne. "Aquaculture: an emerging issue for public concern." *Journal of Risk Research*, Vol 13(7); 2010 https://doi.org/10.1080/13669871003660742
17. European Food Safety Authority. "Opinion of the Scientific Panel on Contaminants in the food chain on a request from the European Parliament related to the safety assessment of wild and farmed fish." The EFSA Journal Vol 236. Pages 1-118, 2005. Available at: https://doi.org/10.2903/j.efsa.2005.236
18. Jacobs MN, Covaci A, Schepens P. Investigation of selected persistent organic pollutants in farmed Atlantic salmon (Salmo salar), salmon aquaculture feed, and fish oil components of the feed. Environ Sci Technol. 2002 Jul 1;36(13):2797-805.
19. Kaw HY, Kannan N. A Review on Polychlorinated Biphenyls (PCBs) and Polybrominated Diphenyl Ethers (PBDEs) in South Asia with a Focus on Malaysia. Rev Environ Contam Toxicol. 2017;242:153-181.
20. Hites R., Foran J., Schwager S., Knuth B., Hamilton C., Carpenter D. Global assessment of polybrominated diphenyl ethers in farmed and wild salmon. Organohalogen Compounds. Vol 66 (2004).
21. Jacobs M.N., Covaci A., Schepens P. Investigation of selected persistent organic pollutants in farmed Atlantic salmon (Salmo salar), salmon aquaculture feed, and fish oil components of the feed. Environ Sci Technol. (2002) Jul 1; 36(13):2797-805.
22. Karl H., Kuhlmann H., Oetjen K. (2002). Transfer of toxaphene and chlordane into farmed rainbow trout, Oncorhynchus mykiss (Walbaum) via feed. Aquaculture Research 33: 925932.
23. Nettleton J. A. (2000). Fatty acids in cultivated and wild fish. oregonstate.edu/dept/IIFET/2000/papers/nettleton 2.pdf
24. Nichols PD, Glencross B, Petrie JR, Singh SP. Readily available sources of long-chain omega-3 oils: is farmed Australian seafood a better source of the good oil than wild-caught seafood? *Nutrients.* 2014 Mar 11;6(3):1063-79. doi:10.3390/nu6031063.
25. Hites, Ronald et al., "Global Assessment of Organic Contaminants in Farmed Salmon." *Science;* Vol 303, January 4004.
26. J. Oehlenschläger, U. Ostermeyer, "Feed Additives for Influencing the Color of Fish and Crustaceans." Handbook on Natural Pigments in Food and Beverages, 2016.
27. Amaya, E et al. "Using Feed to Enhance the Color Quality of Fish and Crustaceans." Feed and Feeding Practices in Aquaculture. Woodhead Publishing Series in Food Science, Technology and Nutrition, 2015.
28. U.S. Food and Drug Administration. "Tanning Pills." Available at: https://www.fda.gov/cosmetics/cosmetic-products/tanning-pills
29. Weiss, Kenneth. "Fish Farms Become Feedlots of the Sea." Los Angeles Times, December 9, 2002. Available at: https://www.latimes.com/nation/la-me-salmon9dec09-story.html
30. Koppang EO, et al. Vaccination-induced systemic autoimmunity in farmed Atlantic salmon. J Immunol. 2008 Oct 1;181(7):4807-14.
31. University of Waterloo. "Vaccines not protecting farmed fish from disease." ScienceDaily. ScienceDaily, 22 January 2018.
32. Carolina Figueroa, Paulina Bustos, Débora Torrealba, Brian Dixon, Carlos Soto, Pablo Conejeros, José A. Gallardo. Coinfection takes its toll: Sea lice override the protective effects of vaccination against a bacterial pathogen in Atlantic salmon. *Scientific Reports*, 2017; 7 (1)
33. Koppang, Erling et al. "Vaccination-Induced Systemic Autoimmunity in Farmed Atlantic Salmon." *The Journal of Immunology;* 181:4807-4814, 2008. doi: 10.4049/jimmunol.181.7.4807
34. https://geneticliteracyproject.org/2019/03/11/fda-lifts-2016-import-ban-on-gmo-aquadvantage-salmon-confirms-fish-safe-to-consume/
35. Reiley, Laura. "The facts about farmed salmon you wish you didn't know." Tampa Bay Times, March 21, 2018. Available at: https://www.tampabay.com/things-to-do/food/cooking/The-facts-about-farmed-salmon-you-wish-you-didn-t-know_166193900/
36. Johns Hopkins Center for A Livable Future. "Global Shift in Farmed Fish Feed May Impact Nutritional Benefits Ascribed to Consuming Seafood." March 14, 2016. Available at: https://clf.jhsph.edu/about-us/news/news-2016/global-shift-farmed-fish-feed-may-impact-nutritional-benefits-ascribed
37. Little, David et al. "Poultry and Fish Production - A Framework for Their Integration in Asia." Agricultural and Aquatic Systems Programme, School of Environment, Resources and Development, Asian Institute of Technology, P.O. Box 4, Klongluang, Pathum Thani, 12120, Thailand.
38. Hardy, Ronald. "Use of Soybean Meal in the Dietsof Salmon and Trout." Aquaculture Research Institute, Hagerman Fish Culture Experiment Station, University of Idaho.

Bring Your Lunch

1. Visa: Americans Report They Spend an Average of $2,746 on Lunch Yearly; 2015. Available at: https://investor.visa.com/news/news-details/2015/Visa-Americans-Report-They-Spend-an-Average-of-2746-on-Lunch-Yearly/default.aspx

Sprout & Grind Your Grains

1. World Health Organization. "Mycotoxins." May 9, 2018. Available at: https://www.who.int/news-room/fact-sheets/detail/mycotoxins
2. United States Department of Agriculture. "Grain, Fungal Disease, and Mycotoxin Reference." Washington, D.C., September 2006. Available at: https://www.gipsa.usda.gov/fgis/publication/ref/mycobook.pdf
3. Benincasa, Paolo et al. "Sprouted Grains: A Comprehensive Review." *Nutrients* vol. 11,2 421. 17 Feb. 2019, doi:10.3390/nu11020421

Chapter 5: Shift From High Quality Processed Foods To Whole Foods

1. Zhang, Hao et al. "Role of plant MicroRNA in cross-species regulatory networks of humans." *BMC systems biology* vol. 10,1 60. 8 Aug. 2016, doi:10.1186/s12918-016-0292-1
2. Sreenivasan S, Thirumalai K, Danda R, Krishnakumar S. Effect of curcumin on miRNA expression in human Y79 retinoblastoma cells. Curr Eye Res. 2012 May; 37(5):421-8.
3. Lin Zhang, et al. Exogenous plant MIR168a specifically targets mammalian LDLRAP1: evidence of cross-kingdom regulation by microRNA *Cell Research* (2012) 22:107–126.

Count Quality, Not Calories

1. Refer to References for "Look For The 100% USDA Organic Label."
2. Doaei S, Kalantari N, Mohammadi NK, Tabesh GA, Gholamalizadeh M. "Macronutrients and the FTO gene expression in hypothalamus; a systematic review of experimental studies." *Indian Heart J.* 2017 Mar - Apr;69(2):277-281. doi:10.1016/j.ihj.2017.01.014. Epub 2017 Jan 24. Review.
3. Martinez K.B., Leone V., Chang E.B. "Western diets, gut dysbiosis, and metabolic diseases: Are they linked?" *Gut Microbes.* 2017;6:1–13. doi: 10.1080/19490976.2016.1270811.
4. Shinohara K., Ohashi Y., Kawasumi K., Terada A., Fujisawa T. "Effect of apple intake on fecal microbiota and metabolites in humans." *Anaerobe.* 2010;16:510–515.
5. Balmer, Robert. "Chapter 15 – Chemical Thermodynamics." Modern Engineering Thermodynamics; pages 591-650; 2011
6. Painter, Jim. "How Do Food Manufacturers Calculate the Calorie Count of Packaged Foods?' *Scientific American;* July 31, 2006. Available at: https://www.scientificamerican.com/article/how-do-food-manufacturers/
7. Institute of Medicine (US) Committee on Examination of Front-of-Package Nutrition Rating Systems and Symbols; Wartella EA, Lichtenstein AH, Boon CS, editors. Front-of-Package Nutrition Rating Systems and Symbols: Phase I Report. Washington (DC): National Academies Press (US); 2010. 2, History of Nutrition Labeling. Available from: https://www.ncbi.nlm.nih.gov/books/NBK209859/
8. Hall, Kevin et al. "Ultra-Processed Diets Cause Excess Calorie Intake and Weight Gain: An Inpatient Randomized Controlled Trial of Ad Libitum Food Intake," *Cell Metabolism;* 30 (2019): 1-11.

Avoid The Dirty Dozen®; Choose The Clean Fifteen®

1. Refer to References for "Look For The 100% USDA Organic Label."
2. Environmental Working Group. "Dirty DozenTM: EWG's 2019 shopper's Guide." Available at: https://www.ewg.org/foodnews/dirty-dozen.php
3. Environmental Working Group. "Clean FifteenTM: EWG's 2019 Shopper's Guide." Available at: https://www.ewg.org/foodnews/clean-fifteen.php

Don't Trust The "Gluten-Free" Label

1. Dr. Tom O'Bryan. The Gluten Summit. *theglutensummit.com.* 2015. Available at: www.theglutensummit.com. Accessed November 9, 2016.
2. Dr. Peter Osborne. 43 Facts About Gluten You Might Not Know... *www.glutenfreesociety.org.* 2014. Available at: https://www.glutenfreesociety.org/43-facts-about-gluten-you-might-not-know/. Accessed November 9, 2016.
3. Leonard M, Vasagar B. US perspective on gluten-related diseases. *Clinical and Experimental Gastroenterology.* 2014;7:25–37. Available at: http://thedr.com/wp-content/uploads/2014/11/US-perspective-on-gluten-related-diseases-Leonard-2014.pdf.
4. va Berge-Henegouwen G, Mulder C. Pioneer in the gluten free diet: Willem-Karel Dicks 1905-1962, over 50 years of gluten free diet. *Gut.* 1993;34(11):1473–5. Available at: http://www.ncbi.nlm.nih.gov/pubmed/8244125/.
5. Lanzini A, et al.. "Complete recovery of intestinal mucosa occurs very rarely in adult coeliac patients despite adherence to gluten-free diet." *Aliment Pharmacol Ther.* 2009 Jun 15;29(12):1299-308. doi:10.1111/j.1365-2036.2009.03992.x.
6. Davidson IW, Lloyd RS, Whorwell PJ, Wright R. "Antibodies to maize in patients with Crohn's disease, ulcerative colitis and coeliac disease." *Clin Exp Immunol.* 1979 Jan;35(1):147-8.
7. Kristjánsson G, et al. "Gut mucosal granulocyte activation precedes nitric oxide production: studies in coeliac patients challenged with gluten and corn." *Gut.* 2005 Jun;54(6):769-74.
8. Skerritt JH, Devery JM, Penttila IA, LaBrooy JT. "Cellular and humoral responses in coeliac disease. 2. Protein extracts from different cereals." *Clin Chem Acta.* 1991 Dec 31;204(1-3):109-22.
9. Varjonen E, et al. "Skin-prick test and RAST responses to cereals in children with atopic dermatitis. Characterization of IgE-binding components in wheat and oats by an immunoblotting method." *Clin Exp Allergy.* 1995 Nov;25(11):1100-7.
10. Cabrera-Chávez F, Iametti S, Miriani M, de la Barca AM, Mamone G, Bonomi F. "Maize prolamins resistant to peptic-tryptic digestion maintain immune-recognition by IgA from some celiac disease patients." *Plant Foods Hum Nutr.* 2012 Mar;67(1):24, 30.
11. Cabrera-Chávez F, Rouzaud-Sández O, Sotelo-Cruz N, Calderón de la Barca AM. "Transglutaminase treatment of wheat and maize prolamins of bread increases the serum IgA reactivity of celiac disease patients." *J Agric Food Chem.* 2008 Feb 27;56(4):1387-91.
12. Caminiti, Lucia et al. "Food protein induced enterocolitis syndrome caused by rice beverage." *Italian journal of pediatrics* vol. 39 31. 14 May. 2013, doi:10.1186/1824-7288-39-31
13. Balakireva AV, Zamyatnin AA. "Properties of Gluten Intolerance: Gluten Structure, Evolution, Pathogenicity and Detoxification Capabilities." *Nutrients.* 2016 Oct 18;8(10). pii: E644. Review.

14. Junker Y, et al. "Wheat amylase trypsin inhibitors drive intestinal inflammation via activation of toll-like receptor 4." *J Exp Med.* 2012 Dec 17;209(13):2395-408.
15. Elli L, et al. "Diagnosis of gluten related disorders: Celiac disease, wheat allergy and non-celiac gluten sensitivity." *World J Gastroenterol.* 2015 Jun 21;21(23):7110-9.
16. Tovoli, Francesco et al. "Clinical and diagnostic aspects of gluten related disorders." *World journal of clinical cases* vol. 3,3 (2015): 275-84. doi:10.12998/wjcc.v3.i3.275
17. Elli L, Roncoroni L, Bardella MT. "Non-celiac gluten sensitivity: Time for sifting the grain." *World J Gastroenterol.* 2015 Jul 21;21(27):8221-6. doi: 10.3748/wjg.v21.i27.8221. Review.
18. Huebener S, et al. "Specific nongluten proteins of wheat are novel target antigens in celiac disease humoral response." *J Proteome Res.* 2015 Jan 2;14(1):503-11
19. Catherine M. Bulka, Matthew A. Davis, Margaret R. Karagas, Habibul Ahsan, Maria Argos. "The Unintended Consequences of a Gluten-Free Diet." *Epidemiology,* 2017; 1

Peel Your Apples

1. Zinöcker, Marit K, and Inge A Lindseth. "The Western Diet-Microbiome-Host Interaction and Its Role in Metabolic Disease." *Nutrients* vol. 10,3 365. 17 Mar. 2018, doi:10.3390/nu10030365
2. U.S. Food and Drug Administration. "Compliance Policy Guide Sec. 562.550 Safety and Labeling of Waxed (Coated) Fruits and Vegetables." November 2005. Available at: https://www.fda.gov/regulatory-information/search-fda-guidance-documents/cpg-sec-562550-safety-and-labeling-waxed-coated-fruits-and-vegetables
3. National Organic Standards Board Technical Advisory Panel Review. Compiled by OMRI for the USDA National Organic Program. April 2, 2002.

Cook A Whole Chicken

1. Axe, Josh. "The Collagen Diet: A 28-Day Plan for Sustained Weight Loss, Glowing Skin, Great Gut Health, and a Younger You." Little, Brown Spark; 2019.
2. Lodish, H et al. "Collagen: The Fibrous Proteins of the Matrix." Molecular Cell Biology, 4th Edition. W.H. Freemanl 2000.
3. Varani, James et al. "Decreased collagen production in chronologically aged skin: roles of age-dependent alteration in fibroblast function and defective mechanical stimulation." *The American journal of pathology* vol. 168,6 (2006): 1861-8. doi:10.2353/ajpath.2006.051302
4. Bello AE, Oesser S. "Collagen hydrolysate for the treatment of osteoarthritis and other joint disorders: a review of the literature." *Curr Med Res Opin.* 2006 Nov;22(11):2221-32. Review.
5. Ulrich P, Cerami A. "Protein glycation, diabetes, and aging." *Recent Prog Horm Res.* 2001;56:1-21.
6. Ricard-Blum, Sylvie. "The collagen family." *Cold Spring Harbor perspectives in biology* vol. 3,1 a004978. 1 Jan. 2011, doi:10.1101/cshperspect.a004978

Cook One Meal Using Whole Foods

1. Environmental Working Group. "Forever Chemicals: Teflon, Scotchgard and the PFAS Contamination Cristis." Available at: https://www.ewg.org/key-issues/toxics/nonstick-chemicals
2. United States Environmental Protection Agency. "Basic Information on PFAS." Available at: https://www.epa.gov/pfas/basic-information-pfas

Save Time & Money By Batching & Storing

1. Davis D R. (February 1, 2009). "Declining fruit and vegetable nutrient composition: What is the evidence?" *American Society of Horticultural Science.*
2. George D F, Bilek M M, and McKenzie D R. "Non-thermal effects in the microwave induced unfolding of proteins observed by chaperone binding." *Bioelectromagnetics* 2008 May;29(4). 324-330.
3. Kidmose U and Kaack K. "Changes in Texture and Nutritional Quality of Green Asparagus Spears (Asparagus officinalis L.) during Microwave Blanching and Cryogenic Freezing." *Agriculturae Scandinavica;* November 2010; B1999:49(2).110-117.
4. Quan R (et al). "Effects of microwave radiation on anti- infective factors in human milk." *Pediatrics;* 89(4 part I). 667-669.
5. Song K and Milner J A. "The influence of heating on the anticancer properties of garlic." *Journal of Nutrition* 2001;131(3S).1054S-1057S.
6. Vallejo F, Tomas-Barberan F A, and Garcia-Viguera C. "Phenolic compound contents in edible parts of broccoli inflorescences after domestic cooking." *Journal of the Science of Food and Agriculture* (15 Oct 2003)

Eat A Daily Helping Of Microbes From Ferments

1. Zinöcker, Marit K, and Inge A Lindseth. "The Western Diet-Microbiome-Host Interaction and Its Role in Metabolic Disease." *Nutrients* vol. 10,3 365. 17 Mar. 2018, doi:10.3390/nu10030365
2. Guarner F., Malagelada J.R. "Gut flora in health and disease." *Lancet.* 2003;361:512–519. doi: 10.1016/S0140-6736(03)12489-0.
3. Eckburg P.B et al. "Diversity of the human intestinal microbial flora." *Science.* 2005;308:1635–1638. doi: 10.1126/science.1110591.
4. Mondot S., de Wouters T., Dore J., Lepage P. "The human gut microbiome and its dysfunctions." *Dig. Dis.* 2013;31:278–285. doi: 10.1159/000354678.

Add One Prebiotic Each Week

1. Zinöcker, Marit K, and Inge A Lindseth. "The Western Diet-Microbiome-Host Interaction and Its Role in Metabolic Disease." *Nutrients* vol. 10,3 365. 17 Mar. 2018, doi:10.3390/nu10030365
2. Guarner F., Malagelada J.R. "Gut flora in health and disease." *Lancet.* 2003;361:512–519. doi: 10.1016/S0140-6736(03)12489-0.

3. Eckburg P.B., Bik E.M., Bernstein C.N., Purdom E., Dethlefsen L., Sargent M., Gill S.R., Nelson K.E., Relman D.A. "Diversity of the human intestinal microbial flora." *Science*. 2005;308:1635–1638. doi: 10.1126/science.1110591.
4. Mondot S., de Wouters T., Dore J., Lepage P. "The human gut microbiome and its dysfunctions." *Dig. Dis.* 2013;31:278–285. doi: 10.1159/000354678.
5. Vulevic J., Juric A., Tzortzis G., Gibson G.R. "A mixture of trans-galactooligosaccharides reduces markers of metabolic syndrome and modulates the fecal microbiota and immune function of overweight adults." *J. Nutr.* 2013;143:324–331. doi: 10.3945/jn.112.166132
6. Fava F., Gitau R., Griffin B.A., Gibson G.R., Tuohy K.M., Lovegrove J.A. "The type and quantity of dietary fat and carbohydrate alter faecal microbiome and short-chain fatty acid excretion in a metabolic syndrome "at-risk" population." Int. *J. Obes.* 2013;37:216–223. doi: 10.1038/ijo.2012.33.
7. Tuohy K.M., Conterno L., Gasperotti M., Viola R. "Up-regulating the human intestinal microbiome using whole plant foods, polyphenols, and/or fiber." *J. Agric.* Food Chem. 2012;60:8776–8782. doi: 10.1021/jf2053959.
8. Gibson G.R., Roberfroid M.B. "Dietary modulation of the human colonic microbiota:introducing the concept of prebiotics." *J. Nutr.* 1995;125:1401–1412.
9. Macfarlane S., Macfarlane G.T., Cummings J.H. "Review article: Prebiotics in the gastrointestinal tract." *Aliment. Pharmacol. Ther.* 2006;24:701–714. doi: 10.1111/j.1365-2036.2006.03042.x.
10. Roberfroid M., Gibson G.R., Hoyles L., McCartney A.L., Rastall R., Rowland I., Wolvers D., Watzl B., Szajewska H., Stahl B., et al. "Prebiotic effects: Metabolic and health benefits." *Br. J. Nutr.* 2010;104:S1–S63. doi: 10.1017/S0007114510003363.
11. Gibson G.R., Scott K.P., Rastall R.A., Tuohy K.M., Hotchkiss A., Dubert-Ferrandon A., Gareau M., Murphy E.F., Saulnier D., Loh G., et al. "Dietary prebiotics: Current status and new definition." *Food Sci. Tech. Bull.: Funct. Food.* 2010;7:1–19. doi: 10.1616/1476-2137.15880.
12. Martinez K.B., Leone V., Chang E.B. "Western diets, gut dysbiosis, and metabolic diseases: Are they linked?" *Gut Microbes.* 2017;6:1–13. doi: 10.1080/19490976.2016.1270811.
13. Singh, Rasnik K et al. "Influence of diet on the gut microbiome and implications for human health." *Journal of translational medicine* vol. 15,1 73. 8 Apr. 2017, doi:10.1186/s12967-017-1175-y

Spice It Up!

1. Tarantelli, Thomas. "Adulteration with Sudan Dye Has Triggered Several Spice Recalls." June 30, 2017. Food Safety Tech. Available at: https://foodsafetytech.com/feature_article/adulteration-sudan-dye-triggered-several-spice-recalls/
2. Ocean Optics. "Adulteration of Spices." October 21, 2015. Available at: https://oceanoptics.com/adulteration-of-spices/
3. American Spice Trade Association. "Cleanliness Specifications." Available at: https://www.astaspice.org/food-safety/cleanliness-specifications/
4. FDA. "Questions & Answers on Improving the Safety of Spices." Available at: https://www.fda.gov/food/cfsan-risk-safety-assessments/questions-answers-improving-safety-spices
5. FDA. "Draft Risk Profile: Pathogens and Filth in Spices." Available at: https://www.fda.gov/media/86724/download
6. Zinöcker, Marit K, and Inge A Lindseth. "The Western Diet-Microbiome-Host Interaction and Its Role in Metabolic Disease." *Nutrients* vol. 10,3 365. 17 Mar. 2018, doi:10.3390/nu10030365

Breathe In Microbial Diversity

1. Chevalier, Gaétan et al. "Earthing: health implications of reconnecting the human body to the Earth's surface electrons." *Journal of environmental and public health* vol. 2012 (2012): 291541. doi:10.1155/2012/291541

Say No To Arsenic In Rice

1. Consumer Reports. How Much Arsenic Is in Your Rice? *www.consumerreports.org.* 2014. Available at: http://www.consumerreports.org/cro/magazine/2015/01/how-much-arsenic-is-in-your-rice/index.htm. Accessed November 8, 2016.
2. U.S. Food and Drug Administration. Draft Guidance for Industry: Inorganic Arsenic in Rice Cereals for Infants: Action Level. *fda.gov.* 2016. Available at: http://www.fda.gov/Food/GuidanceRegulation/GuidanceDocumentsRegulatoryInformation/ucm486305.htm. Accessed July 29, 2016.
3. Hughes M, Beck B, Chen Y, Lewis A, Thomas D. Arsenic Exposure and Toxicology: A Historical Perspective. *Toxicological Sciences.* 2011;123(2):305–332.
4. The Dr. Oz Show. Breaking News: FDA Confirms Concerning Arsenic Levels in Rice. *doctoroz.com.* 2012. Available at: http://www.doctoroz.com/article/breaking-news-FDA-arsenic-rice. Accessed July 29, 2016.
5. U.S. Food and Drug Administration. Arsenic in Rice and Rice Products. *fda.gov.* 2016. Available at: http://www.fda.gov/Food/FoodborneIllnessContaminants/Metals/ucm319870.htm. Accessed July 29, 2016.
6. The Daily Meal. These American Meat Products Are Banned Abroad. *www.huffingtonpost.com.* 2014. Available at: http://www.huffingtonpost.com/the-daily-meal/these-american-meat-produ_b_5153275.html.

Cycle Your Foods

1. Cassiem W, de Kock M. The anti-proliferative effect of apricot and peach kernel extracts on human colon cancer cells in vitro. BMC Complement Altern Med. 2019 Jan 29;19(1):32.
2. Saleem M, Asif J, Asif M, Saleem U. Amygdalin from Apricot Kernels Induces Apoptosis and Causes Cell Cycle Arrest in Cancer Cells: An Updated Review. Anticancer Agents Med Chem. 2018;18(12):1650-1655.
3. Fenwick GR, Heaney RK, Mullin WJ. Glucosinolates and their breakdown products in food and food plants. Crit Rev Food Sci Nutr. 1983;18(2):123-201.
4. Felker P, Bunch R, Leung AM. Concentrations of thiocyanate and goitrin in human plasma, their precursor concentrations in brassica vegetables, and associated potential risk for hypothyroidism. Nutr Rev. 2016;74(4):248-258.
5. Cho YA, Kim J. Dietary factors affecting thyroid cancer risk: a meta-analysis. Nutr Cancer. 2015;67(5):811-817.

6. Oregon State University. "Cruciferous Vegetables." Linus Pauling Institute: Micronutrient Information Center. Available at: https://lpi.oregonstate.edu/mic/food-beverages/cruciferous-vegetables#reference57

Chapter 6: Shift From Whole Food To Locally grown Whole Food

1. Refer to References for "Look For The 100% USDA Organic Label."
2. Ross, Anne et al. "The Turkish Infiltration of the U.S. Organic Grain Market: How Failed Enforcement and Ineffective Regulations Made the U.S. Ripe for Fraud and Organized Crime" Cornucopia Institute; 2018. Available at: https://www.cornucopia.org/wp-content/uploads/2018/06/Turkish-Infiltration-Organic-Grain-Imports.pdf
3. Berni, Roberto et al. "Functional Molecules in Locally-Adapted Crops: The Case Study of Tomatoes, Onions, and Sweet Cherry Fruits From Tuscany in Italy." *Frontiers in plant science* vol. 9 1983. 15 Jan. 2019, doi:10.3389/fpls.2018.01983
4. Berni R., Cantini C., Romi M., Hausman J. F., Guerriero G., Cai G. (2018a). Agrobiotechnology goes wild: ancient local varieties as sources of bioactives. Int. J. Mol. Sci. 19:2248 10.3390/ijms19082248
5. Legay S., Guerriero G., Deleruelle A., Lateur M., Evers D., André C. M., et al. . (2015). Apple russeting as seen through the RNA-seq lens: strong alterations in the exocarp cell wall. Plant Mol. Biol. 88, 21–40. 10.1007/s11103-015-0303-4.
6. Legay S., Cocco E., André C. M., Guignard C., Hausman J. F., Guerriero G. (2017). Differential lipid composition and gene expression in the semi-russeted "Cox Orange Pippin" apple variety. Front. Plant Sci. 8:1656 10.3389/fpls.2017.01656
7. Andre C. M., Larsen L., Burgess E. J., Jensen D. J., Cooney J. M., Evers D., et al. . (2013). Unusual immuno-modulatory triterpene-caffeates in the skins of russeted varieties of apples and pears. J. Agric. Food Chem. 61, 2773–2779. 10.1021/jf305190e

Eat Ecologically Grown Produce From Your Local Farmer

1. Finster ME, Gray KA, Binns HJ. "Lead levels of edibles grown in contaminated residential soils: a field survey." *Sci Total Environ.* 2004 Mar 29;320(2-3):245-57.
2. FDA. "Use Caution with Ayurvedic Products." Available at: https://www.fda.gov/consumers/consumer-updates/use-caution-ayurvedic-products
3. The Consumer Wellness Center. "A New Standard in Consumer Food Safety." Available at: http://www.lowheavymetalsverified.org/
4. Adams, Mike. "ICP-MS analysis of toxic elements (heavy metals) in 100 municipal water samples from across the United States." *Natural Science Journal;* available at: http://www.naturalsciencejournal.org/ICP-MS-Analysis-100-Municipal-Water-Samples.html
5. McWillimas, James. "Rusted Roots: Is Organic Agriculture Polluting our Food with Heavy Metals? Slate. Available at: https://slate.com/technology/2008/09/is-organic-agriculture-polluting-our-food-with-heavy-metals.html
6. Arora M, Reichenberg A, Willfors C, Austin C, Gennings C, Berggren S, Lichtenstein P, Anckarsater H, Tammimies K, Bolte S. "Fetal and postnatal metal dysregulation in autism." *Nat Commun;* June 2017. doi: 10.1038/NCOMMS15493
7. LeVaux, Ari. "Shocking Levels of Heavy Metals in Imported Food Highlight the Danger." AlterNet. July 1, 2014. Available at: https://www.alternet.org/2014/07/why-food-labelled-organic-no-guarantee-safety-shocking-levels-heavy-metals-found/
8. Gardener, Hannah, et al. "Lead and cadmium contamination in a large sample of United States infant formulas and baby foods." *Science of The Total Environment;* Vol. 651 (1), February 15, 2019, pgs: 822-827. https://doi.org/10.1016/j.scitotenv.2018.09.026
9. World Health Organization. "Childhood Lead Poisoning." 2010. Available at: https://www.who.int/ceh/publications/leadguidance.pdf
10. Clean Label Project. "Heavy Metals and Organic Press Release." Available at: https://www.cleanlabelproject.org/heavy-metals-and-organic-press-release/
11. Kim, Hyun Soo et al. "An Overview of Carcinogenic Heavy Metal: Molecular Toxicity Mechanism and Prevention." *Journal of cancer prevention* vol. 20,4 (2015): 232-40. doi:10.15430/JCP.2015.20.4.232
12. Yuan, Wenzhen et al. "Advances in Understanding How Heavy Metal Pollution Triggers Gastric Cancer." *BioMed research international* vol. 2016 (2016): 7825432. doi:10.1155/2016/7825432
13. Vella, Veronica et al. "Recent views of heavy metals as possible risk factors and potential preventive and therapeutic agents in prostate cancer." *Molecular and Cellular Endocrinology;* Vol. 457, December 2017, pgs: 57-72. https://doi.org/10.1016/j.mce.2016.10.020
14. Irfan, Shazia et al. "Comparative Evaluation of Heavy Metals in Patients with Rheumatoid Arthritis and Healthy Control in Pakistani Population." *Iranian journal of public health* vol. 46,5 (2017): 626-633.
15. Bibi M, Hashmi MZ, Malik RN. "The level and distribution of heavy metals and changes in oxidative stress indices in humans from Lahore district, Pakistan." *Hum Exp Toxicol.* 2016 Jan;35(1):78-90. doi: 10.1177/0960327115578063.
16. Menke, Andy. "Metals in Urine and Diabetes in U.S. Adults." Diabetes 65(1): 164-171. January 2016. https://doi.org/10.2337/db15-0316
17. Chen, Ya & Yang, Ching & Huang, Chun & Hung, Dong-Zong & Leung, Yuk & Liu, Shing. (2009). "Heavy metals, islet function and diabetes development." *Islets*. 1. 169-76. 10.4161/isl.1.3.9262.
18. Lee, Min-Jing et al. "Heavy Metals' Effect on Susceptibility to Attention-Deficit/Hyperactivity Disorder: Implication of Lead, Cadmium, and Antimony." *International journal of environmental research and public health* vol. 15,6 1221. 10 Jun. 2018, doi:10.3390/ijerph15061221
19. Saghazadeh A, Rezaei N. "Systematic review and meta-analysis links autism and toxic metals and highlights the impact of country development status: Higher blood and erythrocyte levels for mercury and lead, and higher hair antimony, cadmium, lead, and mercury. *Prog Neuropsychopharmacol Biol Psychiatry.* 2017 Oct 3;79(Pt B):340-368.
20. Tabatadze T, Zhorzholiani L, Kherkheulidze M, Kandelaki E, Ivanashvili T. "HAIR HEAVY METAL AND ESSENTIAL TRACE ELEMENT CONCENTRATION IN CHILDREN WITH AUTISM SPECTRUM DISORDER." *Georgian Med News*. 2015 Nov;(248):77-82.
21. U.S. Food & Drug Administration; Determining the Regulatory Status of a Food Ingredient. Available at: https://www.fda.gov/food/food-ingredients-packaging/determining-regulatory-status-food-ingredient
22. Electronic Code of Federal Regulations. Available at: https://www.ecfr.gov/cgi-bin/text-idx?c=ecfr&sid=3f34f4c22f9aa8e6d9864cc2683cea02&tpl=/ecfrbrowse/Title07/7cfr205_main_02.tpl

Eat Ecologically Raised, Pastured Eggs From Your Local Farmer

1. Centers for Disease Control and Prevention. "Prevalence of Obesity Among Adults and Youth: United States, 2015-2016; October 2017. Available at: https://www.cdc.gov/nchs/products/databriefs/db288.htm
2. Bird, Julia K et al. "Risk of Deficiency in Multiple Concurrent Micronutrients in Children and Adults in the United States." *Nutrients* vol. 9,7 655. 24 Jun. 2017, doi:10.3390/nu9070655
3. Wallace TC, McBurney M, Fulgoni VL 3rd. "Multivitamin/mineral supplement contribution to micronutrient intakes in the United States, 2007-2010." *J Am Coll Nutr.* 2014;33(2):94-102. doi: 10.1080/07315724.2013.846806.
4. Davis DR, Epp MD, Riordan HD. "Changes in USDA food composition data for 43 garden crops, 1950 to 1999." *J Am Coll Nutr.* 2004 Dec;23(6):669-82.
5. Hunter D, Foster M, McArthur JO, Ojha R, Petocz P, Samman S. "Evaluation of the micronutrient composition of plant foods produced by organic and conventional agricultural methods." *Crit Rev Food Sci Nutr.* 2011 Jul;51(6):571-82. doi: 10.1080/10408391003721701. Review.

Say No To Subsidies

1. MacDonald JM, Korb P, Hoppe RA. *Farm Size and the Organization of U.S. Crop Farming.* 2013.
2. Merino N. *Agricultural Subsidies: Opposing Viewpoints.* (Merino N, ed.). Nasso, Christine; 2010.
3. Van Hoesen S, Secretary P. How Crop Subsidies May Make You Fat. *ewg.org.* 2016. Available at: http://www.ewg.org/agmag/2016/07/how-crop-subsidies-make-you-fat.
4. United States Department of Agriculture ERS. Crops. *www.ers.usda.gov.* 2016. Available at: https://www.ers.usda.gov/topics/crops/. Accessed December 18, 2016.
5. United States Department of Agriculture Economic Research Service. Corn Background. *ers.usda.gov.* 2016. Available at: http://www.ers.usda.gov/topics/crops/corn/background.aspx. Accessed July 28, 2016.
6. United States Department of Agriculture ERS. Corn: Background. *www.ers.usda.gov.* 2016. Available at: https://www.ers.usda.gov/topics/crops/corn/background/. Accessed December 17, 2016.
7. United States Department of Agriculture. Profiling Food Consumption in America. In: *Agriculture Fact Book.*; 2003. Available at: http://www.usda.gov/documents/usda-factbook-2001-2002.pdf.
8. United States Department of Agriculture Economic Research Service. Sugar & Sweeteners Policy. *usda.gov.* 2015. Available at: http://www.ers.usda.gov/topics/crops/sugar-sweeteners/policy.aspx. Accessed July 20, 2016.
9. United States Department of Agriculture Economic Research Service. Soybeans & Oil Crops. *ers.usda.gov.* 2016. Available at: http://www.ers.usda.gov/topics/crops/soybeans-oil-crops/background.aspx. Accessed July 28, 2016.
10. United States Department of Agriculture; Economic Research Service. Recent Trends in GE Adoption. *www.ers.usda.gov.* 2016. Available at: https://www.ers.usda.gov/data-products/adoption-of-genetically-engineered-crops-in-the-us/recent-trends-in-ge-adoption.aspx. Accessed December 17, 2016.
11. Siegel KR, McKeever-Bullard K, Imperatore G, et al. Association of Higher Consumption of Foods Derived From Subsidized Commodities With Adverse Cardiometabolic Risk Among US Adults. *JAMA Internal Medicine.* 2016;176(8):1124–1132. Available at: http://archinte.jamanetwork.com/article.aspx?articleid=2530901.
12. Centers for Disease Control and Prevention. Chronic Disease Overview. *cdc.gov.* 2016. Available at: http://www.cdc.gov/chronicdisease/overview/. Accessed August 1, 2016.
13. Severson K. Obesity "a threat" to U.S. security/Surgeon general urges cultural shift. SFGate. 2003. Available at: http://www.sfgate.com/health/article/Obesity-a-threat-to-U-S-security-Surgeon-2686994.php.
14. Pace G. Obesity Bigger Threat Than Terrorism? CBSNews. 2006. Available at: http://www.cbsnews.com/news/obesity-bigger-threat-than-terrorism/.
15. Pollan M. You Are What You Grow. *The New York Times Magazine.* 2007. Available at: http://michaelpollan.com/articles-archive/you-are-what-you-grow/.
16. Block G. Foods contributing to energy intake in the US: data from NHANES III and NHANES 1999-2000. *Journal of Food Composition and Analysis*. 2004;17(3-4).
17. United States Department of Agriculture Economic Research Service. Dairy Data Overview. *ers.usda.gov.* 2016. Available at: http://www.ers.usda.gov/data-products/dairy-data.aspx. Accessed July 29, 2016.
18. The Week Staff. Farm subsidies: A welfare program for agribusiness. *theweek.com.* 2013. Available at: http://theweek.com/articles/461227/farm-subsidies-welfare-program-agribusiness.
19. Stiglitz JE. The Insanity of Our Food Policy. *The New York Times: The Opinion Pages.* 2013. Available at: http://www.aae.wisc.edu/aae375/sustainable_ag/Readings NET/The Insanity of Our Food Policy 2- NYTimes.com.pdf.
20. Mittal A. Free Trade Doesn't Help Agriculture. *fpif.org.* 2007. Available at: http://fpif.org/free_trade_doesnt_help_agriculture/.

Eat Mindfully

1. Relationships Among the Brain, the Digestive System, and Eating Behavior: Workshop Summary. Food Forum; Food and Nutrition Board; Institute of Medicine. Washington (DC): National Academies Press (US); 2015 Feb 27.
2. Lebel JL, Lu J, Dubé L. Weakened biological signals: Highly-developed eating schemas amongst women are associated with maladaptive patterns of comfort food consumption. Physiology & Behavior. 2008;94(3):384–392.
3. Finkelstein SR, Fishbach A. When healthy food makes you hungry. Journal of Consumer Research. 2010;37(3):357–367.
4. Dubé L, Bechara A, Böckenholt U, Ansari A, Dagher A, Daniel M, DeSarbo WS, Fellows LK, Hammond RA, Huang TT. Towards a brain-to-society systems model of individual choice. Marketing Letters. 2008;19(3-4):323–336.
5. Dubé L, Pingali P, Webb P. Paths of convergence for agriculture, health, and wealth. Proceedings of the National Academy of Sciences of the United States of America. 2012;109(31):12294–12301.
6. Hammond RA, Dubé L. A systems science perspective and transdisciplinary models for food and nutrition security. Proceedings of the National Academy of Sciences of the United States of America. 2012;109(31):12356–12363.

Meditate Daily

1. Goyal M, et al. Meditation programs for psychological stress and well-being: a systematic review and meta-analysis. *JAMA Intern Med.* 2014 Mar;174(3):357-68.
2. Marchand WR. Mindfulness-based stress reduction, mindfulness-based cognitive therapy, and Zen meditation for depression, anxiety, pain, and psychological distress. *J Psychiatr Pract.* 2012 Jul;18(4):233-52.
3. Zeidan, F et al. "Mindfulness meditation-related pain relief: evidence for unique brain mechanisms in the regulation of pain." *Neuroscience letters* vol. 520,2 (2012): 165-73. doi:10.1016/j.neulet.2012.03.082
4. Sojcher R, Gould Fogerite S, Perlman A. Evidence and potential mechanisms for mindfulness practices and energy psychology for obesity and binge-eating disorder. Explore (NY). 2012 Sep-Oct;8(5):271-6.
5. O'Reilly, G.A. et al. "Mindfulness-based interventions for obesity-related eating behaviours: a literature review." *Obesity Treatment.* March 18, 2014.
6. Ott MJ, Norris RL, Bauer-Wu SM. "Mindfulness meditation for oncology patients: a discussion and critical review." *Integr Cancer Ther.* 2006 Jun;5(2):98-108.
7. Merkes M. "Mindfulness-based stress reduction for people with chronic diseases." *Aust J Prim Health.* 2010;16(3):200-10. doi: 10.1071/PY09063.
8. Kang SS, et al. "Transcendental meditation for veterans with post-traumatic stress disorder." *Psychol Trauma.* 2018 Nov;10(6):675-680. doi:10.1037/tra0000346. Epub 2018 Jul 19.

Grow One Herb In Your Kitchen

1. National Center for Complementary and Integrative Health. "Aloe Vera." Available at: https://nccih.nih.gov/health/aloevera
2. Yeh, Gloria et al. "Systemic Review of Herbs and Dietary Supplements for Glycemic Control in Diabetes." Diabetes Care 2003 Apr; 26(4): 1277-1294. https://doi.org/10.2337/diacare.26.4.1277
3. Coronado GD, Thompson B, Tejeda S, Godina R. "Attitudes and beliefs among Mexican Americans about type 2 diabetes." *J Health Care Poor Underserved.* 2004 Nov;15(4):576-88.
4. Cho, Soyun et al. "Dietary Aloe Vera Supplementation Improves Facial Wrinkles and Elasticity and It Increases the Type I Procollagen Gene Expression in Human Skin in vivo." *Annals of dermatology* vol. 21,1 (2009): 6-11.
5. Patel, D K et al. "Barbaloin: a concise report of its pharmacological and analytical aspects." *Asian Pacific journal of tropical biomedicine* vol. 2,10 (2012): 835-8.
6. Babaee, Neda et al. "Evaluation of the therapeutic effects of Aloe vera gel on minor recurrent aphthous stomatitis." *Dental research journal* vol. 9,4 (2012): 381-5.
7. Gupta, Rajendra Kumar et al. "Preliminary antiplaque efficacy of aloe vera mouthwash on 4 day plaque re-growth model: randomized control trial." *Ethiopian journal of health sciences* vol. 24,2 (2014): 139-44. doi:10.4314/ejhs.v24i2.6
8. Maenthaisong R, Chaiyakunapruk N, Niruntraporn S, Kongkaew C. "The efficacy of aloe vera used for burn wound healing: a systematic review." *Burns.* 2007 Sep;33(6):713-8. Epub 2007 May 17.
9. Nejatzadeh-Barandozi, Fatemeh. "Antibacterial activities and antioxidant capacity of Aloe vera." *Organic and medicinal chemistry letters* vol. 3,1 5. 19 Jul. 2013,

Grow One Edible Plant Indoors

1. Torsvik V, Øvreås L. "Microbial diversity and function in soil: from genes to ecosystems." *Curr Opin Microbiol.* 2002 Jun;5(3):240-5. Review.
2. Torsvik, V., L. Ovreas, et al. (2002). "Prokaryotic diversity - Magnitude, dynamics, and controlling factors." *Science;* 296(5570): 1064-1066.
3. European Commission DG ENV. Technical Report; "Soil Biodiversity: functions, threats, and tools for policy makers." February 2010 Available at: https://ec.europa.eu/environment/archives/soil/pdf/biodiversity_report.pdf
4. Kent, A.D. & Triplett, E.W. (2002). Microbial communities and their interactions in soil and rhizosphere ecosystems. Annual Review of Microbiology, 56, pp. 211-236.Khalil, S. (2001).
5. Microflora in the root environment of hydroponically grown tomato: Methods for assessment and effects of introduced bacteria and Pythium ultimum. Diss. Alnarp: Swedish University of Agricultural Sciences.Khalil, S. & Alsanius, B.W. (2001).
6. Dynamics of the indigenous microflora inhabiting the root zone and the nutrient solution of tomato in a commercial closed greenhouse system. *Gartenbauwissenschaft,* 66(4), pp. 188-198.
7. Khalil, S., Hultberg, M. & Alsanius, B.W. (2009). Effects of growing medium on the interactions between biocontrol agents and tomato root pathogens in a closed hydroponic system. *Journal of Horticultural Science & Biotechnology,* 84(5), pp. 489-494.
8. Khalil, S., Hultberg, M. & Alsanius, B.W. (2011). Interactions between growing media and biocontrol agents in closed hydroponic systems. *Acta Horticulturae,* 891, pp. 51-57.
9. Khalil, S. & Olsson, O. (2013). Influence of micronutrients on the biological control of Pythium ultimum in a closed soilless system. *Canadian Journal of Plant Protection,* 1(4), pp. 134-141.
10. Koohakan, P., Ikeda, H., Jeanaksorn, T., Tojo, M., Kusakari, S.I., Okada, K. & Sato, S. (2004). Evaluation of the indigenous microorganisms in soilless culture: occurrence and quantitative characteristics in the different growing systems. *Scientia Horticulturae,* 101(1-2), pp. 179-188.Larcher, W. (2003).
11. Stanghellini ME, Rasmussen SL. Identification and origin of plant pathogenic microorganisms in recirculating nutrient solutions. Adv Space Res. 1994 Nov;14(11):349-55.
12. Jacoby, Richard et al. "The Role of Soil Microorganisms in Plant Mineral Nutrition-Current Knowledge and Future Directions." *Frontiers in plant science* vol. 8 1617. 19 Sep. 2017, doi:10.3389/fpls.2017.01617
13. Hartman K, Tringe SG. Interactions between plants and soil shaping the root microbiome under abiotic stress. *Biochem J.* 2019 Oct 15;476(19):2705-2724.

14. Wang, Rui et al. "Microbial community composition is related to soil biological and chemical properties and bacterial wilt outbreak." **Scientific reports** vol. 7,1 343. 23 Mar. 2017, doi:10.1038/s41598-017-00472-6

Grow Your Sprouts

1. Xiao Z, Lester GE, Luo Y, Wang Q. "Assessment of vitamin and carotenoid concentrations of emerging food products: edible microgreens." *J Agric Food Chem.* 2012 Aug 8;60(31):7644-51. doi: 10.1021/jf300459b. Epub 2012 Jul 30.
2. Mir SA, Shah MA, Mir MM. "Microgreens: Production, shelf life, and bioactive components." *Crit Rev Food Sci Nutr.* 2017 Aug 13;57(12):2730-2736
3. Choe U, Yu LL, Wang TTY. "The Science behind Microgreens as an Exciting New Food for the 21st Century." *J Agric Food Chem.* 2018 Nov 7;66(44):11519-11530. doi: 10.1021/acs.jafc.8b03096. Epub 2018 Oct 29. Review.

Permissions

Index

acetaldehyde ... 103
ADHD ... 34, 55, 68
aeroponics ... 352
aloe vera ... 347-348
American Pastured Poultry Producers Association ... 317, 319
ancient grains ... 216
antibiotic resistance ... 50-52, 75, 146-147
antibiotics ... 49, 51, 53, 83, 94, 146, 163, 184, 231-232
aquaponics ... 353
arsenic poisoning ... 249, 284-287
artificial flavors ... 103-105
artificial sweeteners ... 123-126
aspartame ... 124
ATP ... 136-137
autism ... 82, 96, 268, 305
autoimmune disease ... 67, 69, 96, 276, 292,
... 299-300, 304, also see inflammatory disease

batch cooking ... 262-266
Bayer ... 165-170, also see Monsanto & glyphosate
bees ... 209
Beyond Meat® ... 127-130
BHT ... 151
biosolids ... 55, 316
bone broth ... 253-255, 290, 297
bT corn ... 155, 157

CAFOs ... 44, 50-51, 57, 66-67, 71, 75, 84, 86, 184-186
calories ... 227-230, 232, 235, 297
cancer ... 103-104, 108,
... 124, 147, 164, 166, 167, 170, 185, 189, 219, 276, 285
canning food ... 372
chelator ... 164
Chez Panise ... 106
chicken, organic
... 75-79, 80-89, 90-92, also see pastured poultry
chlorine ... 71-74, 80-81, 83-84, 86-89
cholesterol ... 289-291, 294
chronic disease ... see inflammatory disease
cold frames ... 359
compost ... 105, 107-108, 238, 361, 363-368
Consumer Union Score Cards ... 49
cortisol ... 9, 341
cycling foods ... 298-306

DDT ... 238
dehydration ... 134-144
dehydrating food ... 372-373
Dietary Guidelines ... 117, 295, also see food pyramid
Dr. Joe Dispenza ... 10
Dr. Masaru Emoto ... 138

earthing/grounding ... 281-283
eggs ... 66-70, 71-74, 105
Egg Beaters® ... 119, 213-214
egg washing ... 71-74, 213-214
EOV ... 176-177, 179
Environmental Working Group (EWG) ... 142, 172, 236-239

fake meat ... 127-130, 247
Farm to Consumer Legal Defense Fund ... 77, 173
farm-raised fish ... 184-189
fasting ... 337
FDA ... 36-40, 41, 99, 100, 103-105, 145,
... 147-149, 175, 187, 250, 294-295
fermented foods ... 107, 267-272
fight-or-flight ... 9, 293-294, 337-338
Flavor and Extract Manufactures Association (FEMA) ... 104
flour mills ... 218-222
Food Additive Amendment ... 99-100
food allergies ... 68, 153-154, 276, 299-300
food irradiation ... 105
food pyramid ... 139, 12, 120, 121, 112-114, 117, 119-121
Food Safety Inspection Service (FSIS) ... 38, 71, 73, 80, 86
free-range eggs ... 90-92, 319-320

GALT ... 67-68
GAPS diet ... 254
gardening ... 208-209, 346-359
generational toxicity ... 165, 336
gliadin-free ... 245
gluten free ... 244-249, 250
gluten sensitivity ... 68-69, 244-249, 250-252, 300-303
glyphosate ... 96, 160, 163-175, 216-217, 302, 371
Glyphosate Residue Free seal ... 163-171, 172-175, 176, 180
GM salmon ... 188
GMOs ... 36-38, 44, 101, 155-161, 162-174, 188
Government Accountabilty Office (GAO) ... 100
grain-finished ... 322-324
GRAS
... 34, 37, 38, 99, 100, 104, 108, 110, 129, 157, 182, 210, 250
grass fed ... 93-97, 321
grass finished beef ... 93-97, 321-323

heavy metals ... 314-315
herbs ... 276-280, 346-348, 358-359
hydroponics ... 57, 351-353

inflammation
... 14, 69, 219, 230, 245, also see inflammatory disease

Index

inflammatory disease
.......55, 67-69, 83, 108, 115, 122, 125, 136, 155-156, 187, 340
Impossible Burger® 127-130
isoeugenol...104-105

Keys, Ancel 113, 115, 117, 118

Label Game (for kids).. 208-209
Land to Market Ecological Outcome Verified............see EVO
leaky brain..163
leaky gut.............................. 68, 155, 163, 246, 254, 299-302
Lethal Dose (LD) Testing 40
locally grown... 200-203, 308-329
low-fat 112-115, 118-120, 122, 293

maximal health...6, 8
meditation 336, 339-342
metabolic water 141
microbiome 51-53, 67-68, 81-85, 87-89, 94,
......................108, 110, 157, 163-164, 255, 269, 272, 282, 344
micronutrient deficiencies 109-111, 115, 183, 320
microRNAs...225, 309
microwave 266
mindfulness............................. 281-283, 335-338, 339-342
Misfits Market.. 201-202
Monsanto 101, 124, 147, 148, 165-170, 295
multiple sclerosis (MS)...69
mycotoxins 219

National Bioengineered Food Disclosure Law.................159
National Toxicology Program 104
natural flavors...103-105
negativity.. 13-15, 17, 46
nocebo effect 14, 16
Non-GMO Project Verified.................. 159-161, 174, 176, 180
nutritional facts/label 121, 227, 232

organic grain 159-161, 216-217, 310

pastured beef.................................. 53-54, 93-97, 321-323
pastured eggs................................... 59, 66, 90-92, 319-320
pastured pork.. 324-326
pastured poultry............................ 91-92, 310-311, 317-318
PCBs 185
pesticides.. 226-239, 285
placebo effect 14
positivity..........................7-8, 10-11, 16-17, 46, 128, 137-139
prebiotics 273-275
preservatives...107-111
pressure cooker 240-243

probiotics 269, 273-274
processed foods..4, 34, 98, 103, 333
propyl gallate...108
PTFE/PFAS checmials 260-261

radiation 105-106
rBGH 145-150, 295
recipes, whole food 212, 217, 222, 242, 253, 256-257, 267
Roundup®.. see glysophate

salt...181-183
seasonal eating.. see cycling foods
serotonin 164-165, 341
SIBO 269-270
snacks 193, 195-196
soda 131-133, 228, 230
soil health...................... 176-180, 238-239, 286-287, 351-352
soil microbiome... 177, 351-352
solarium..369
spices 276-280
sprouting grains 217
sprouts 354-355
Staph infection 83, 231
sterlized food .... 85, 272, also see chlorine
stocking up (sales) 204-206
structured water...135-139
subsidies 332-334
sugar 116, 118-119, 121, 125-126
superbugs ......51, 83, 267-269, also see antibiotic resistance

Teflon® pans 260-261
Thrive Market®...201
toxicity 40

USDA Organic Label
...............55-59, 66, 75-78, 93159-161, 171-177, 179-180, 314

vaccines (in fish)...184
victim-hood/victim-land 2-3, 18-20, 44
Virginia Association for Biological Farming (VABF) 56

Walmart® organics 76, 200
water.. 134-144, 194, 370-371
wax, food grade 250-252
weeds... 7-8, 169, 277, 279
whole foods.......... 224-226, 233-234, 240-241, 253-260, 309